Occupational Therapy Evidence in Practice for Physical Rehabilitation

Occupational Therapy Evidence in Practice for Physical Rehabilitation

Edited by

Lois M. Addy

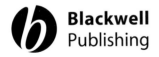
Blackwell
Publishing

© 2006 by Blackwell Publishing Ltd

Editorial offices:
Blackwell Publishing Ltd, 9600 Garsington Road, Oxford OX4 2DQ, UK
   Tel: +44 (0)1865 776868
Blackwell Publishing Inc., 350 Main Street, Malden, MA 02148-5020, USA
   Tel: +1 781 388 8250
Blackwell Publishing Asia Pty Ltd, 550 Swanston Street, Carlton, Victoria 3053, Australia
   Tel: +61 (0)3 8359 1011

First published 2006 by Blackwell Publishing Ltd

ISBN-13: 978-1-4051-4687-6
ISBN-10: 1-4051-4687-7

Library of Congress Cataloging-in-Publication Data
   Occupational therapy evidence in practice for physical rehabilitation /
      edited by Lois M Addy.
         p. ; cm.
   Includes bibliographical references and index.
   ISBN-13: 978-1-4051-4687-6 (pbk. : alk. paper)
   ISBN-10: 1-4051-4687-7 (pbk. : alk. paper)
   1. Occupational therapy.   2. Evidence-based medicine.   I. Addy, Lois M.
(Lois Margaret), 1960–. [DNLM: 1. Occupational Therapy–methods.
2. Evidence-Based Medicine.   WB 555 O1429 2006]
   RM735.O324 2006
   615.8'515–dc22
   2006010814

Set in 10/12.5 pt Palatino
by SNP Best-set Typesetter Ltd., Hong Kong
Printed and bound in India
by Replika Press Put Ltd, Kundli

For further information on Blackwell Publishing, visit our website:
www.blackwellpublishing.com

Contents

Contributors

Lois M. Addy is Senior Lecturer in the School of Professional Studies at York St. John University College, with 24 years' experience as a paediatric occupational therapist. She is author of the Speed-Up kinaesthetic handwriting programme (LDA Ltd); How to Support and Understand Children with Dyspraxia (LDA Ltd); and Get Physical inclusive PE programme (LDA Ltd); and is co-author of the Write from the Start perceptual–motor handwriting programme (LDA Ltd) and *Making Inclusion Work for Children with Dyspraxia* (Routledge Press). She has also contributed a chapter on interagency collaboration within *Developing School Provision for Children with Dyspraxia* (Sage).

Alex Clark is a Senior Lecturer in social policy, who previously taught at Exeter and Plymouth Universities. He has a general interest in the politics and structures of health and social care with a particular focus on disability studies. He is also interested in the role of the service user and anti-oppressive practice.

Janet Golledge qualified as an occupational therapist in 1980 and subsequently worked in a number of areas of physical rehabilitation. In 1988, she began working in higher education, where she currently teaches topics related to stroke rehabilitation at undergraduate and postgraduate levels. She believes strongly that occupational therapists should have a sound theoretical knowledge base to support effective practice and regularly teaches neurology-related subjects for continuing professional development short courses. Janet has also contributed a chapter to *Occupation for Occupational Therapists* (Blackwell Science) using a case study to illustrate rehabilitation post stroke.

Anne Longmore qualified in 1984 and has worked with people living with multiple sclerosis whilst being employed in a regional neurology service, social services and in a community rehabilitation team. Since 2000, Anne has been employed as a Senior Lecturer/Practitioner at York St. John University College. Her professional challenge is to encourage occupational therapists to analyse the demands of **everyday tasks** in relation to the ability of an individual.

Ruth MacDonald qualified in 1988, her clinical experience is in acute physical medicine and local authority practice. For 10 years she was Lecturer/Senior

Lecturer at York St. John University College, teaching physical rehabilitation. In 2004 she returned to clinical practice to work in rheumatology. Her publishing interests are in using evidence-based practice within rheumatology and in increasing cultural competence.

Maria Parks qualified in 1988 and went on to gain 11 years' clinical experience working for social services departments developing her expertise in housing adaptations and assistive technologies. Maria received an MSc from Brunel University in 2003 and is currently a Senior Lecturer in Occupational Therapy and Teaching Fellow at York St. John University College. Maria has taught extensively on the undergraduate programme on topics of evidence-based practice with people with physical disabilities. Her clinical interests focus on accessible environments, assistive technologies, falls prevention and older people. She has delivered in-service training to a range of older people's services on the Single Assessment Process.

Alis Racey qualified as an occupational therapist from The (former) University of Ripon and York St. John in 1998. She has worked in a range of clinical settings, and was clinical lead in orthopaedics. In 2002 she completed an MSc in advanced health care practice and joined the academic staff at York St. John University College in 2005. Her interests are in acute discharge planning and the development of care pathways and protocols to support and guide prompt treatment.

Amanda Richardson qualified as an occupational therapist in 1990 from Dorset House School of Occupational Therapy, Oxford. She was formerly employed as Regional Care Adviser for North, East and West Yorkshire by the Motor Neurone Disease Association (MNDA) from August 1999 to April 2002. This was followed by an appointment of key worker to the Mid Yorkshire Hospitals NHS Trust within a multidisciplinary and motivated motor neurone disease team, supporting an average caseload of 21 people living with motor neurone disease. She has been instrumental in developing a specialist motor neurone disease clinic, expanding the team to include specialist respiratory and gastroenterological support and palliative care link nurses, in order to fulfil current best practice guidelines. She continues her links with the MNDA and is a member of the steering group for the West Yorkshire Motor Neurone Disease Special Interest Group.

Kerry Sorby works jointly as a clinical specialist in occupational therapy (musculoskeletal team) for North Kirklees Primary Care Trust and part-time Senior Lecturer at York St. John University College. Kerry qualified in 1988 and has predominantly worked with clients with musculoskeletal dysfunction. Her main clinical interests include splinting as a therapeutic intervention and developing clinical care pathways for clients undergoing elective orthopaedic surgery. She currently teaches topics related to the rehabilitation of patients with orthopaedic and/or rheumatological conditions. In the summer of 2003, she successfully completed her MSc in allied health (hand therapy).

Acknowledgements

Thank you to Dr Christine Mayers and Janet Golledge for their support and assistance in editing this text.

Thank you to Steve Robinson for his technical support.

Thank you for my long-suffering family for their continual support, patience and encouragement.

1: Introduction

Lois M. Addy

The demand for occupational therapy to be based on sound evidence has been influential in the way we now consider practice. The ability to justify therapy based on research findings has raised the credibility of the profession considerably and for some has been seen as essential to the profession's survival. As a consequence, clinicians are now able to question practice which may have remained unchallenged for years, and have become increasingly reflective about the service occupational therapists are providing. The principle of having a therapeutic service confident in its use of justified interventions however is clouded by the reality that very few interventions have been researched thoroughly enough to appraise effectiveness (Christiansen and Lou, 2001). The challenging resolve to scour evidence and research in order to justify a technique or intervention leaves many busy clinicians feeling concerned and anxious regarding the lack of time available to prove the efficacy of their service. There may also be a concern that choosing an intervention based on the analysis of human occupation, and the resultant clinical reasoning which incorporates the client's beliefs and values, is in some way inferior to researched evidence. This concern should be confounded by the reiteration that evidence-based practice is not exclusively concerned with research findings but must combine the *best* available evidence, with clinical expertise based on occupational analysis and problem solving while maintaining a client-centred focus.

This text seeks to demonstrate the application of evidence-based practice to students and graduates of occupational therapy, utilising examples of clinical practice based on clients known to each contributor. The clients selected have a range of physical, social, psychological and cultural needs, which are addressed in various settings including home, school and hospital. The clients selected have been ordered according to their lifespan to reflect the subtle variations in practice arising from the different occupational demands of children, young adults, adults and older people. Each contributor shares his or her perception of 'best practice' based on their own clinical expertise and available evidence. All present an overview of the client's needs; the legislation and policies which have influenced his or her choice of approach; the theoretical framework underpinning the treatment, with the additional inclusion of the frame of reference, model and/or approach adopted; the rationale and justification for the choice of assessment tool and method; the clinical reasoning supporting his or her goal planning; specific aims and objectives; aspects of intervention and the supporting evidence; treatment outcomes; and personal reflection on the therapeutic process.

Each contribution is **not** intended to be prescriptive and, given altered demographics, culture, location or staffing ratio, a different approach or choice of intervention may have been adopted and the client's needs addressed very differently. However those described demonstrate the realities and complexities of occupational therapy, representing the veracity of typical occupational therapy referrals. Contributors are aware that what they perceive to be an effective approach may be disputed by others and each chapter acknowledges its limitations by concluding with a reflective discussion. At the end of each chapter a series of questions is included which intends to challenge the reader to debate how they might have addressed the client's needs, whether the reader agrees or disagrees with the therapist's clinical reasoning and suggesting what could have been done differently.

Each contribution portrays a unique situation which reflects the client's individuality, circumstantial demographics, staff resources, equipment availability, budgets, the client's support network and additional 'pressures' of work, such as waiting lists, bed demand, community resources, local authority restrictions and the client's motivation and physical health at the time of his/her involvement. We would like readers to consider how their choice of approach and intervention might have differed should one of the above variables be altered, for example in a bed shortage crisis; increase in staffing; time of year, i.e. end of the financial year.

As each of the clients selected is known to the contributor, pseudonyms have been used to maintain confidentiality. No reference has been made which would identify the location of the individuals concerned; in addition permission has been given by the clients to use any personal material included in this text, thus adhering to the Code of Ethics and Professional Conduct as defined by the College of Occupational Therapists (COT) (2005).

The concluding chapter discusses some of the moral and ethical dilemmas expressed by contributors having reflected on the therapeutic process. These are explored from a health and social care perspective. They include concerns regarding user compliance; power relationships; the tensions arising from differences between user's expectations and service restrictions; the dilemma of how to provide quality rehabilitation while accommodating a highly systematised discharge system; cognitive dissonance; the challenge of how to be client-centred while adhering to standardised care pathways; allocation of funding; and prioritisation of treatment.

What is evidence-based practice?

Before introducing each client it is important to affirm what is meant by the term evidence-based practice. It has been stated that evidence-based practice incorporates the results of both sound research and considered clinical expertise, but what is sound research? How can we be sure that the results of research are applicable to our situation? How do we obtain the evidence to justify our choice of intervention? And how can we be sure that the evidence is accurate? These questions need to be addressed before occupational therapists can substantiate their rationale for intervention.

Evidence can be defined as any empirical observation about the apparent relationship between events. Evidence is the result of systematic, planned investigations of specified problems with a predetermined outcome, which will contribute to the understanding of the phenomena in question (Cornwell, 2000). How that evidence is obtained is controversial, as in literature certain methodologies are deemed superior to others, with quantitative research often receiving higher credence than qualitative investigations. This sits uncomfortably with occupational therapists, as there is an apparent incongruence between effectiveness of research in rehabilitation and the realities and experience of clients within real contexts (Hammell and Carpenter, 2004). However, there is increasing acknowledgement that clients' experience and understanding of their disease or disability can provide a rich source of data which can support actual test results or measurable outcomes (Sackett *et al.*, 2000).

Professor David Sackett and his colleagues from the University of Oxford created a hierarchy to assist clinicians in identifying the most appropriate evidence (Sackett *et al.*, 1996). This hierarchy, although controversial, has been instrumental in initiating considerable debate by those involved in medicine and rehabilitation and has been useful in identifying the kinds of evidence most relevant to clinical practice (Fig. 1.1).

At the top of the hierarchy Sackett places systematic reviews and meta-analyses. These identify, appraise and synthesise research evidence from individual studies and therefore provide valuable sources of information. For example, the systematic review and meta-analysis of interventions which prevent falls in older adults by Chang *et al.* (2004) provides valuable justification for providing multifactorial falls risk assessments and falls management programmes, in addition to demonstrating that exercise programmes are effective in reducing the risk of falling. Systematic reviews differ from other types of review in that they follow

1.	A	Systematic reviews/meta-analyses
	B	Randomised controlled trials
	C	Experimental designs
2.	A	Cohort studies
	B	Case-control studies
3.	A	Consensus conference
	B	Expert opinion
	C	Observational study
	D	Other types of study, i.e. interviews
	E	Quasi-experimental, qualitative design
4.		Personal communication

Figure 1.1 Hierarchy of evidence, from Sackett *et al.*, 1996.

a strict protocol to ensure that as much of the relevant research base as possible has been considered and that the original studies are thoroughly synthesised and appraised. These methods minimise the risk of bias and are translucent, thus enabling replication. They are placed above randomised controlled trials in the hierarchy as they represent the amalgamated reviews of many studies.

Centres, such as the NHS Centre for Reviews and Dissemination, based at York University, and The UK Cochrane Centre and Collaboration in Oxford, were established to coordinate such reviews. The purpose of the Cochrane Centre is to *'collaborate with others to build, maintain and disseminate a database of systematic, up-to-date reviews of randomised controlled trials of health care'* (Sheldon and Chalmers, 1994) while the NHS Centre for Reviews and Dissemination undertakes a systematic review of the literature. The latter centre also has a responsibility to disseminate results of reviews through an online database and Effective Health Care Bulletins.

Randomised controlled trials are also high on Sackett's list of effective methodologies, and are often, contentiously, referred to as the 'gold standard' of research evidence. These relate to studies whereby participants are randomly assigned to either an experimental group or control group with a variable differentiating the two. Participants may know they are receiving a certain intervention or can be 'blindly' allocated to reduce prejudice. In an attempt to reduce bias the researcher may also be unaware of which group a client is assigned to; this is known as a 'double-blind' trial. If the trial is sufficiently rigorous and the results statistically significant then there is a high probability that the treatment or intervention works. Examples of these can be seen in the study by Ubhi *et al.* (2000) of the effects of botulinum toxin on the mobility of children with cerebral palsy and the study by Logan *et al.* (2003) of the effects of occupational therapy and leisure therapy on clients who have had a stroke now living in the community. For a randomised controlled trial to be universally applied it must be large enough to demonstrate sufficient power of that specific intervention (Hamer and Collinson, 1999). In reality very few of these are evident in occupational therapy research.

Randomised trials, despite their 'gold standard' label, have several limitations, for example:

- Rehabilitation is more difficult to quantify than drug treatments.
- Many rehabilitation interventions are altered to suit individual clients.
- The results of a trial may have limited applicability as a result of exclusion criteria (rules about who may not be entered into the study).
- There may be an inclusion bias, for example a selection of subjects from a group may be unrepresentative of those with that condition.
- There may be refusal of certain patient/client groups to give consent to be included in the trial.
- The analysis of only predefined objectives may exclude important qualitative aspects of the intervention (Greenhalgh, 1997).

The importance of experimental design stems from the quest for inference about causes or relationships as opposed to simply description. Researchers are rarely satisfied simply to describe the events they observe. They want to make inferences about what produced, contributed to or caused events. Experimental designs are effective in evaluating whether a certain treatment is likely to have a positive impact on the outcome of some individuals or whether it simply equates to the other treatment provided in the study (Law, 2002). For example, when Luke *et al.* (2004) considered the outcomes of using the Bobath technique to restore function in the upper limb following stroke, they found that it was not possible to demonstrate its superiority over any other approach in respect of activity or participation. They, therefore, recommended that further studies should be under-taken using more sensitive measures of upper limb function to determine the effectiveness of one approach over another. On the other hand, Vanage *et al.* (2003) used a cross-over experimental design to evaluate the benefits of an 8-week energy conservation course for persons with progressive multiple sclerosis. The results provided evidence that an energy conservation course can be an enormous benefit to these clients.

There are several drawbacks in using either randomised controlled trials or experimental designs, one of which is the need to have a clear expression of the intended outcomes of the programme or intervention. Due to the complex nature of rehabilitation, the inclusion of many variables can result in confusion and uncertainty as to the actual influences on the research group.

Another concern relates to context and complexity. Can experiments conducted in a strictly controlled environment be translated into the wider society (Shaw, 2001)? In medical research the experimental or independent variable is a single stimulus, i.e. drug, condition or treatment; in occupational therapy research, however, there is a huge range of influences which impact on the individual's performance, such as tiredness, pain threshold, motivation and the environment, to name a few. According to Shaw (2001, p. 10) *'many interventions in primary care are not 'variables' but complex social processes'* which are not easily evaluated using experimental strategies. Therefore it is important that the focus of contemporary experimental research not only considers the *outcome* but also the *process* and *context*.

Cohort studies and case-control studies take second place on Sackett's (1996) hierarchy of evidence. Cohort studies take a group of individuals and study them over a period of time. Such studies can be prospective, where specific information is identified prior to the study and collected over a period of time, or retrospective, where client's notes are used to access information over a preceding period of time. It is a very good means of evaluating the effects of an intervention over time. For example, Lincoln *et al.* (2002) sought to evaluate the benefits of providing a psychology service, including cognitive assessment and intervention, to clients with multiple sclerosis. To do so they randomly allocated clients to three cohorts from those attending a multiple sclerosis management clinic. The first group received no direct intervention. The second received a detailed cognitive assess-ment, the results of which were fed back to professionals involved in the indi-viduals' care. The third cohort received a cognitive assessment and programme designed to reduce the impact of their cognitive problems. The results failed to detect any significant effects in using either a cognitive assessment or cognitive intervention for this cohort of people. However, one of the precautions in utilising cohort studies arises from the fact that members selected may not totally share characteristics and therefore the results may be biased in respect of the client mix at a given time.

Case-control studies are similar to cohort studies but are retrospective. They select two individuals or groups of individuals with similar profiles, one with a certain condition and one without, to compare and predict possible causes of disease, disability or loss of function. For example, Polatajko et al. (2001) used two experimental case studies to explore the validity of the Cognitive Orientation to Daily Occupational Performance (CO-OP) approach with children. They used the valuable information obtained through direct observation and video footage to refine and develop their approach prior to attempting more extensive trials.

There is a range of data collection methods included in the third level of Sackett's hierarchy of evidence, providing information that is more qualitative that quantitative. Consensus conferences which draw together expert opinion, case reports, observational studies, surveys, interviews, focus groups and quasi-experimental studies all provide precious information regarding the relationships between the service and its users. These methods can provide economic evidence about the costs of interventions reflecting the value society places on these (Dowie, 1996; Maynard, 1997); evidence regarding individual's values and preferences (Benharoch and Wiseman, 2004); and contextual evidence relating to the family and social systems in which an individual's fears and goals are embedded (Hunter and Coventry, 2003).

Information arising from conferences which aim to derive a consensus opinion about a particular subject is often overlooked as an effective means of obtaining valuable evidence to support good practice. The purpose of a consensus conference is to evaluate the available scientific information on a biomedical or health-related issue and develop a statement that advances understanding of the issue under consideration which will be useful to health professionals and the public. Knowledge derived from collaboration between those with an extensive reputation for research and publication provides a rich source of information. The purpose of consensus conferences is to inform national practice through the dissemination in relevant journals and a series of conference presentations. Positive results of this approach can be seen in the National Institute of Health's Consensus Statement on Attention-Deficit/Hyperactivity Disorder (NIH, 1998) which was derived following an intense collaboration between experts over a 2-day period to inform the biomedical research and clinical practice communities of the best way to diagnose and treat children with attention deficit hyperactivity disorder (ADHD). The consensus statement provided information regarding effective treatments for ADHD and recommendations for practice. In addition, the statement identified those areas of study that deserve further investigation. More recently the BioMed Central Medical Education has issued a consensus statement regarding how to teach evidence-based practice (Dawes et al., 2005). However, this consensus conference acknowledged that the results provide a 'snapshot in time' and gave the reminder that new knowledge is continuously accumulating through healthcare research.

Cross-sectional surveys appraise or interview a sample of the population at one point in time. These are commonly used in occupational therapy to provide information relating to a specified period of time and are influential in raising key concerns and issues arising at a given time. An example is Dunford and Richards' (2003) survey, which highlighted the unacceptable number of children with developmental coordination disorder placed on waiting lists, who were waiting considerable lengths of time to be seen by an occupational therapist. This significant survey utilised questionnaires to identify the current service provision from a large random sample of child development centres from across the UK in one period. Surveys can use several data collection methods, such as interviews, questionnaires and focus groups, with results collecting either opinion or ordinal data.

Case reports provide information relating to a single person or subject. Sometimes several reports are collected together into a short series so that a comparison between subjects can be made. Case reports usually focus on individuals. However, they can also centre on institutions, facilities, education programmes, clinical sites and units (Vandenbrouke, 1999). Issues addressed in case reports may include critical incidents, ethical dilemmas, user dissonance or use of equipment or devices. References are needed to support rationales and approaches. For example, Cohen *et al.* (1995) used case reports to demonstrate the effectiveness of vestibular rehabilitation with clients suffering from coordination and balance disorders. McEwen (2001) argues that case reports are limited in that they are unable to establish cause-and-effect relationships between interventions and outcomes, and therefore their outcomes cannot be generalised to other individuals or contexts. However they can be useful in describing the therapeutic process and can highlight questions which can ultimately be used in further research. In essence, case reports are a mechanism to illustrate how clinicians integrate the best available research evidence, clinical experience and patient choice (McEwen, 2001). It is for this reason that these have been chosen as the method for presenting good practice in the subsequent chapters.

Qualitative studies, which collect data through interviews, focus groups, questionnaires, observation and surveys, have a significant part to play in evaluating individual experience in the context of everyday lives, despite being low in Sackett's (1996) hierarchy of evidence. They provide the opportunity to reflect individuals' cultural and spiritual beliefs, values and opinions, which are often neglected in quantitative research. Qualitative studies provide crucial lessons for those wanting to understand the process of implementing an intervention, what can go wrong, and what the unexpected adverse effects might be when an implementation is 'rolled out' to a larger population.

It is possible to dispute the order and importance from which 'evidence' is acquired and debate at length the arguments for and against the methods chosen by respective researchers in their endeavour to present findings which can be implemented in practice; what we cannot dispute is the fact that **all** practitioners, whatever their position, should be open to question their practice and, as such, be research active throughout their careers. This questioning reflects a dynamic service actively striving for the best for its clients. In addition all clinicians should have a forum by which best practice is shared and in which research is disseminated. Increasingly, forums, such as journal clubs, research seminars and study days, are being timetabled into the working week to ensure that clinicians have the opportunity to disseminate debate and, where appropriate, apply evidence to practice.

Clinical evidence used in Chapters 2–9

The clinical examples included in this text use a very wide range of evidence to support and justify the clinical reasoning, choice of assessment and subsequent intervention for individuals with a range of conditions across an array of ages. Examples of measures used in published research have also served to guide the choice of evaluation in the selection of appropriate outcome measures. When applying evidence to practice it is noted that there is little evidence to support particular facets of occupational therapy; this has led many occupational therapists to believe that evidence-based practice is an ideal paradigm, impossible to achieve. Students and recently qualified professionals may therefore feel at a loss to know how to justify their interventions in the absence of specific information. The following chapters will therefore demonstrate how evidence is used to support and justify a range of interventions in which occupational therapy plays a part. Emphasis may differ according to the individual and his/her condition.

Chapter 2 focuses on paediatric occupational therapy and questions whether clinical practice should be based on recent evidence, which supports the cognitive task-orientated approach to improving the motor coordination of children with developmental coordination disorder, or to continue with traditional practice, which addresses the underlying process needs of these children using sensory integration techniques, sensori-motor and perceptual–motor programmes and kinaesthetic training.

The rapid throughput experienced by those working within acute services, especially with individuals who have experienced a traumatic injury, has been a source of frustration to many occupational therapists who are aware that time is required to address both the physical and psychosocial needs of the individual. The reality of the current economic climate in the NHS necessitates individuals being discharged before all their rehabilitation needs have been addressed. This may cause professionals to feel despondent; the situation described in Chapter 3, however, concerning a young man who has experienced multiple fractures as a result of a road traffic accident, will demonstrate the significance of occupational therapy when working within the trauma case management team, and how this comprehensive team approach can lead to positive health and economic outcomes.

Individuals who have a long-term condition, such the woman with multiple sclerosis described in Chapter 4, require both long-term support and timely, and occasionally sporadic, intervention. Due to the chronic nature of this condition and timeframe involved, a different approach is required from that described in the preceding chapter. The occupational therapist in this situation does not 'don a cloak and intervene at superman speed'; rather, a collaborative problem-solving approach is the prime mode of intervention. Evidence therefore focuses on empowering the individual to self-manage symptoms in order to maintain and promote his/her quality of life for as long as is possible. Quality of life means different things to different people and therefore can be difficult to quantify, however the evidence supporting the various interventions provided in this chapter addresses the problems highlighted by the individual concerned.

The role of educator is not always acknowledged by the occupational therapy profession yet much of our practice is based on this facet. The efficacy of educational–behavioural joint protection strategies forms the evidence base when working with clients who have rheumatoid arthritis, as demonstrated in Chapter 5. One aspect of this approach is the provision of assistive devices, including orthoses. Superficially, the design and provision of 'working and resting splints' do not always seem appropriate to the domain of occupational therapy; however, when used in the context of reducing deformity and maintaining function, they demonstrate their importance in facilitating and maintaining occupational performance, particularly in relation to maintenance of vocational capacity.

Questions have arisen regarding how to evaluate and justify interventions for people who have a degenerative disorder, who are ultimately dying. Surely this is an impossible task? What sort of outcomes can be used? Chapter 6 invalidates any negativity, providing evidence to support the valuable part played by the occupational therapist as part of the palliative care team in maintaining one individual's quality of life in respect of self-care and activities for daily living. The occupational therapist provides valuable support for the carers, while addressing the individual's spiritual and emotional needs. Occupational therapists have the background experience to address both the physical and psychosocial components involved in coping with a condition such as motor neurone disease.

The systematised approach to addressing routine medical procedures may seem alien to person-centred therapy. Chapter 7 describes the effectiveness of a comprehensive integrated care pathway in addressing the needs of a gentleman who has experienced total hip replacement. The awareness of limitations to NHS expenditure supports such an approach, as has research regarding the client's experience and subsequent recovery. Creativity is demonstrated by those who wish to address such concerns. Ideas are emerging to address those aspects of rehabilitation deferred due to timely discharge, i.e. Telecare, telephone interviews.

The demographic increase in the number of older people has led to concerns regarding the number of injuries occurring each year as a consequence of falls in and around the home. The efficacy of falls prevention programmes is debated in

Chapter 8. This supports the occupational therapist as a key professional because of his/her ability to evaluate the person within the context of the home environment and the occupations undertaken therein. Evidence supports the team approach to preventing falls, but the various components analysed justify occupational therapy practice.

The complexities and individual nature of stroke challenge those seeking suitable evidence on which to base therapy. Chapter 9 includes evidence to support two specific approaches to rehabilitation: the Bobath Concept, commonly used by both physiotherapists and occupational therapists in stroke rehabilitation, and the multifactorial approach to address perceptual and cognitive concerns. Both approaches are based on sound theoretical principles, although evidence regarding efficacy is unconvincing. This chapter demonstrates how evidence which is inconclusive does not necessitate the approach or intervention being disregarded. What it does promote is the desire for clinicians to consider carefully the theoretic rationale underpinning practice, while actively questioning and evaluating practice.

At the end of each of Chapters 2–9 is a series of questions, which not only serve to challenge the reader, but which form the basis of new research questions. These, when answered, will add to the existing body of knowledge for the benefit of future practitioners. The reality of any evaluation is that from one question, new questions emerge. This demonstrates the dynamic and exciting nature of evidence-based practice.

Theoretical approaches

The previously described data collection methods have demonstrated the levels and types of evidence available to occupational therapists. However, 'pure' evidence alone is not enough to ensure good practice and is simply part of a multifaceted process whereby a client may receive the most appropriate therapy. Effective clinicians should not only base their practice on published evidence but should also draw on applicable theories, frames of reference, models and approaches to guide the clinical process. They should also draw on sound clinical reasoning skills which take into account the unique qualities, values and beliefs of the client in question. Greenhalgh (1999) states that 'the dissonance we experience when trying to apply research findings to the clinical encounter often occurs when we abandon the narrative–interpretive paradigm and try to get by on "evidence" alone'.

The College of Occupational Therapists (COT) calls for the development of explicit links between theory, research . . . and practice (Ilott and White, 2001). Despite this call, many practitioners are unclear as to the value and purpose of theory in providing a basis from which to frame their therapy (Kelly, 2004). The purpose of a theory is to provide a broad explanation of a body of facts or phenomena, in other words a system of ideas explaining something (Hagedorn, 2001). Initially many theories, such as social learning, humanistic, cognitive and psychodynamic, life-stage development and human occupation, arose from the field of medicine, social science and psychology. Many of these theories have been influential in developing practice models and/or approaches. For example, many paediatric occupational therapists use perceptual–motor training, sensory integration and/or kinaesthetic regulation, when working with children with developmental coordination disorder. These approaches were historically influenced by constructivist theorists, such as Jean Piaget (1929) and Jerome Bruner (1960), who hypothesised that children learned by actively constructing new ideas and concepts by interacting with their environment. Learning was considered to be systematic and sequential, with all children passing through a similar developmental sequence according to the maturation of the brain and engagement with their environment. Other occupational therapy practices have been influenced by theories, such as the open systems theory, which have been directly concerned with occupational performance, focusing on the person, environment, health and occupation (Reed and Sanderson, 1999).

Frames of reference arise from a theoretical position, drawing together relevant theories, in order for therapists to organise their views, values, facts and hypotheses about a given position and use this as a means of evaluating information, communicating ideas and regulating behaviour. The physiological, behavioural, cognitive, psychodynamic and humanist frames of reference are those frequently adopted by occupational therapists (Hagedorn, 2001).

These frames of reference lead to the development of distinct models of practice. Keilhofner (2002) identified eight models used by occupational therapists to guide their practice:

- The biomechanical model.
- The cognitive disabilities model.
- The model of human occupation.
- The group working model.
- The cognitive–perceptual model.
- The motor control model.
- The sensory integration model.
- The spatiotemporal adaptation model.

Models seek to provide an explanation for human behaviour in terms of occupational performance (Hagedorn, 2001). An example of this is Keilhofner's (2002) Model of Human Occupation (MOHO), which seeks to **explain** how occupation is motivated, patterned and performed. Contemporary models acknowledge the contribution of physical, social and psychological well-being, and include client satisfaction, functional capacity and measures of quality of life (Law, 2002). The Person–Environment–Occupation (PEO) model of practice (Law *et al.*, 1996) considers the person and the environment as interactive dimensions of an individual's situation. Social cognition models, such as Health Belief Model (Rosenstock, 1974) and Theory of Reasoned Action (Ajzen and Fishbein, 1980), are used to provide a theoretical framework for understanding the relationship between health beliefs and health behaviours, as demonstrated in Goodacre and Goodacre's (2003) study of the personal assistance expended by women with chronic arthritis. Currently influential is the International Classification of Functioning model (ICF) (WHO, 2001) which provides descriptions of conditions in terms of human functioning and restrictions, and serves as a framework to systematise this information. It organises this information into two sections: functioning and participation, and contextual factors. It has been influential in changing perceptions of disability from a series of medically determined criteria to highlight functionally determined requirements, which are deemed useful when quantifying financial and medical resources. For example, Rosenbaum and Stewart (2004) apply this model to guide clinical thinking in cerebral palsy, and use it as a basis for evaluating adaptive seating interventions for children with cerebral palsy (McDonald et al., 2004). Blake and Bodine (2002) used ICF criteria to assess and determine the applicability of assistive devices to clients with multiple sclerosis. However, although the ICF is radically different to previous internationally recognised categorisations of disability, it continues to base its assessment on deviations from the 'norm' and therefore its intention to be client-centred and socially inclusive could be questioned (Hammell, 2004).

An array of approaches emerges from the various models and frames of reference available to occupational therapists. These approaches determine what intervention is provided, how it is implemented and to whom. Approaches may or may not be complementary, and may cause the therapist some tension as to which to adopt given their own experience, education and belief. The increasing access to information via the internet and televisation of medical issues has led to consumers being aware of the therapeutic choices available to them. As a consequence there is an expectation that services should be able to deliver the full range of intervention methods. An example of this occurred when Andreas Pető's approach to educating children with cerebral palsy was televised in a series of two BBC documentaries. Occupational therapists and physiotherapists alike were inundated with requests for conductive education to be introduced locally (Maguire and Nanton, 2005). Previously, therapists addressed the needs of these children using Bobath techniques (Bobath, 1993). However, the principles underpinning both conductive education and the Bobath techniques are diametrically opposed to one another, in that one uses manual facilitation and inhibition of irregular movement to guide and direct motor control, the other uses verbal prompting and movement patterns which resist manual handling to achieve the same purpose.

A similar quandary is often experienced by occupational therapists working in busy orthopaedic departments. If a client has suffered a brain injury following a road traffic accident, either a biomechanical approach or a neurodevelopmental approach could be adopted. However, despite the fact that both approaches arise from the physiological frame of reference, they actually contradict one another. One uses a predominantly reductionist approach, whereby rehabilitation focuses on the musculoskeletal or the neurological injury, while the other is much more holistic and humanistic, treating the trauma from both a physical and psychological perspective. The frustration for the therapist occurs when they would ideally adopt a neurodevelopmental approach but because of bed shortages or demands for high throughput, he/she is forced into using a reductionist approach.

In spite of an increasing emphasis on theories, frames of reference, approaches and models in occupational therapy education, there remains reluctance, by many clinicians, to utilise these in practice. Forsyth *et al.* (2005) suggest there are several reasons why practitioners do not find theory and research relevant to their everyday work, one of which is the constant demand and constraints of practice settings which leave limited time for reflection and innovation. Additionally there is an academic–practice gap, whereby theoretical positions are often deemed unnecessary in clinical practice (Elliot *et al.*, 2002). It is hoped that, as evidence-based practice becomes increasingly integrated into clinical practice, this perspective will change.

Government directives

In determining that an effective, dynamic occupational therapy service needs to utilise quality available evidence, and that treatment adopted should be based on a sound theoretical basis leading to a clear frame of reference, model or/and approach, a further factor must be added to the equation, that of government directives and policy changes. The influence of government legislation has challenged, and in some situations completely changed, the focus of many areas of occupational therapy practice, as can be seen in some of the case studies presented. Especially influential have been the introduction of clinical governance in 1998, and the subsequently staggered publication of national service frameworks. Clinical governance was introduced as a framework by which NHS organisations would be accountable for continually improving the quality of their services and safeguarding high standards of care, by creating an environment in which excellence in care is paramount (Scally and Donaldson, 1998). The national service frameworks (NSFs), arising from clinical governance, are long-term recommendations, developed by a group of experts (incorporating health professionals and service users) for improving specific areas of care. They set measurable goals within set timeframes. These goals have been significant in changing therapeutic practice; for example, the move towards 'intermediate care' in 2001, although not a new concept, has significantly changed the way occupational therapists work with the older person and is the central focus of the national agenda for the development and modernisation of NHS services for older people (Department of Health, 2001, 2002).

Clinical reasoning

The implementation of good practice based on sound evidence requires each occupational therapist to use clinical reasoning to determine the applicability of the findings to each client's needs and circumstances. Clinical reasoning is the thinking, decision making and knowledge that therapists use when conducting their work. This includes the way in which they seek information, interpret the client's overall situation and how they derive the best course of action with a particular client (Higgs and Jones, 2000; Mitchell and Unsworth, 2005).

It is really important not to neglect clinical intuition, professional judgement and experience alongside hard evidence. One is not subordinate to the other (Blair and Robertson, 2005). One offers proof of the validity of an intervention, the other provides us with meaning and understanding. Both are essential to effective occupational therapy and it is the collation of these *active ingredients that interact in dynamic and unpredictable ways*' that makes occupational therapy such an exciting yet complex intervention (Creek *et al.*, 2005).

The mental strategies and high-level cognitive patterns and processes that underlie the process of naming, framing and solving problems utilise four types of reasoning: procedural, narrative, interactive and conditional (Mattingly and Fleming, 1994). The individual reports used within the text reflect these varying approaches.

Procedural reasoning originates from scientific reasoning and primarily focuses on a client's physical performance difficulties, directly addressing the disability itself. It provides the basis from which goals, aims and objectives are defined and treatment selected. It requires the occupational therapist to draw on his/her clinical knowledge of the nature of the disorder in order to address the client's needs. Many occupational therapists working in busy orthopaedic departments use such an approach as they often have less time available to them to individualise treatment regimes due to throughput and so deliver a more procedural service. These include packages of care, the provision of protocols or teaching packages.

Most clinicians use narrative reasoning with its roots in phenomenological approach towards client care to assist in their clinical decision making. According to Boden (1998, p. 664), *'we assume that we can explain or make sense of what people do by referring to their intentions, goals, aims, interests, ambitions, desires, wants, motives, needs . . . in a word, to their purposes'*. However this requires the therapist to reflect on a client's story of events arranged in a time sequence and offering some sort of meaning. The meaning can be explicit, but more frequently it is implicit. Our narratives include everything from the autobiographical snippets we gain from clients in daily conversation to their ambitions and desires. Narrative information orders, deepens and enhances both memory and meaning. It is often these key pieces of personal information which help the occupational therapist to learn about his/her client's goals, desires and concerns, and, when incorporating these with information regarding the client's clinical condition, to select the most appropriate approach and intervention.

Narrative reasoning can be extended in its use to provide qualitative evidence of the effectiveness of an intervention. Biographical research uses individuals' experience from periods of their lives to provide insight into the impact of illness or disability on their life. It can also provide objective insight into individual perceptions of health care delivery, including occupational therapy. For example, Curtin and Clarke's (2005) article relating to young people's perceptions of living with an impairment concluded by challenging therapists to focus on the individual, and listen to their unique stories, desires, needs and aspirations. They suggest that the health professional's role should not only focus on extending occupational performance, but also to be proactive in enabling individuals to accept themselves for who they are and become resilient to societal barriers. This can be extended further by emphasising the role occupational therapists have in promoting societal inclusion at all levels.

Interactive reasoning arises from narrative reasoning and involves the client in the decision-making process (Unsworth, 2004). It involves getting to know the client as an individual and relies on achieving a successful therapeutic relationship. The level of emphasis placed on procedural or interactive reasoning depends on the working context of the occupational therapist.

Evidence of conditional reasoning can also be seen in the case studies provided. Conditional reasoning is a form of clinical thinking that *'involves wider social, cultural and temporal considerations'* (Mitchell and Unsworth, 2005) The occupational therapist incorporates information relating to the client's *potential* in the context of his/her existing and predicted situations. For example, in considering a child with cerebral palsy, it is possible to consider his neurological status, observe his functional performance, evaluate the education system being adopted, appraise the child's support network and collaborate with the family to set flexible, though realistic, goals to increasing the child's occupational performance and to predict increasing functional achievement over the following year. Similar reasoning is required when working with clients who have suffered a stroke or who have multiple sclerosis.

Each type of clinical reasoning, despite their seemingly subjective, qualitative approach to information gathering, is essential to informing best practice. Greenhalgh (1999) states that *'appreciating the narrative nature of illness experience and the intuitive and subjective aspects of clinical method does not require us to reject the principles of evidence based medicine. Nor does such an approach demand an inversion of the hierarchy of evidence so that personal anecdote carries more weight in decision making than the randomised controlled trial.'* She suggests that instead of seeking to remove all elements of subjectivity in a clinical interaction, contextualised information gathered through communication with the client can, together with the results of rigorous clinical research trials and observational studies, enable a clinician reach an acceptable, *integrated* clinical judgment. Neistadt (1996) found that this multidimensional thinking not only validates the profession, but increases job satisfaction.

Clinical reasoning, therefore, allows the occupational therapist to consider relevant information regarding the client's condition, the frames of reference, models and approaches available to them, alongside personal information gained from narrative encounters, before beginning the therapeutic process.

Assessment

Information gained will be used initially to guide the choice of assessment. Once again, the chosen assessment should be meaningful and relevant to the client and, if standardised, should be justified in terms of reliability and validity. According to Alsop and Lloyd (2002), understanding the psychometric properties of standardised assessments is a fundamental skill required by occupational therapists today and critical thinking is an essential prerequisite to managing a work environment which is constantly changing. The ability to appreciate the face, content, predictive and construct validity of a test, along with its reliability and responsiveness, is crucial to substantiating practice; it is too easy to administer an assessment selected according to personal recommendation or referred to in a publication, without personally evaluating its applicability and merits to a selected population. What is very important is that the assessment is valid for the purpose and the population, while also being responsive to change. Ideally the assessment should be subject to minimal measurement error (Jerosch-Herold, 2005). Taking the time to understand the psychometric qualities of measures will provide practice and subsequent confidence in interpreting much of the current research. It is unaccepted practice to use assessments without critically appraising their effectiveness and appropriateness as a clinical utility, however given the limited time available to most clinicians such scrutiny demands an allocated time. Journal clubs and multidisciplinary team meetings provide a prime forum in which to analyse such measures (Sherratt, 2005).

Many standardised assessments have limited applicability when evaluating subjective aspects of practice such as the client's well-being and life satisfaction. There is a variety of assessments which address these areas, including those which focus on individual's perceptions of competence, social cognition and quality of life. For example, the Perceived Efficacy and Goal Setting Scale (Missiuna and Pollock, 2000) is a useful tool in determining how children perceive their abilities and difficulties. The Mayers' Lifestyle Questionnaire (Mayers, 1998) has tremendous scope in identifying areas of need from the client's perspective and is used extensively by professionals working within social services. Other assessments such as the Quality of Life in Later Life (QuiLL) (Evans et al., 2005) focuses exclusively on the needs of the older person. These assessments should become familiar to occupational therapists who wish to provide a person-centred service.

The process of agreeing on a desirable and achievable future state is generally considered a key element in the rehabilitation process. Therefore following assessment, goal planning is essential to direct the therapeutic intervention. Due to constraints and cost implications it has become increasingly important to set precise, specific goals within a given timeframe. This is encouraged as good practice and is presented within each of the case studies. Depending on the area of practice, long-term goals can be established which may cover a period up to 12 months; medium-term goals can be determined which cover a period between 1 and 2 months and short-/immediate-term goals can refer to the initial weeks of involvement. As befitting good practice, each goal should be specific, measurable, agreed upon, realistic and time limited (SMART). These 'marry' together the appropriate priorities and expectations of the client together with the realities of organisational objectives.

Outcome measurement

Following any therapeutic intervention, evaluation is paramount. According to Jerosch-Herold (2005) *'in a climate of finite resources all health care professionals face an increasing need to document outcomes as a means to demonstrating that the therapy provided is effective.'* Occupational therapists have been basing their effectiveness on *'the state or change in state that is hoped or intended for an intervention or course of action to achieve'* (Wade, 1999). The methodological tools used in assessment and research design can also prove effective in measuring change following therapeutic intervention (Wade, 1999). According to Law (2002, p. 2), *'the consistent use of measurement enables occupational therapists to identify the ambiguous outcomes of effective occupational therapy services, thus clarifying the contribution of occupational therapy to the health and well being of persons needing our services and to others on the healthcare team.'* However, before adopting any outcome measurement, it is essential to determine exactly *what* outcomes are being considered. These may be (Clark *et al.*, 2001):

- Improvements in health or quality of life.
- Improvement in function or level of independence.
- Client's determined treatment goals.
- Occupational therapy determined outcomes.
- Client satisfaction.
- Reduced length of stay in hospital.
- Reduction in readmission rates.

For example, measures such as the Canadian Occupational Performance Measure (COPM) (Law *et al.*, 1998) and the Morriston Occupational Therapy Outcome Measure (MOTOM) (James and Corr, 2004) were specifically developed to measure changes in occupational therapy performance rather than service satisfaction. The Barthel Index (Shah Version), adapted to increase its sensitivity, is widely used to determine changes in self-care activities (Shah, 1994; Patel *et al.*, 2000). Additionally, the Nottingham Extended Activities of Daily Living (NEADL) scale has proved a reliable tool for measuring changes in functional activities for those who have suffered a stroke (Parker *et al.*, 2001). In contrast, the nine-hole peg test (Mathiowetz *et al.*, 1985) was developed to measure changes in dexterity and has been used to measure the manipulation of clients who have experienced a stroke (Turner-Stokes and Turner-Stokes, 1997) and also clients who have multiple sclerosis (Stevenson *et al.*, 2000).

Reflective practice

The therapeutic process cannot conclude simply with an analysis of results. A time of reflection is paramount in order to consolidate and appraise the clinical experience. According to Blair and Robertson (2005), reflective practice involves thinking about practice from an active and conscious attempt to understand the integration of theory with experience and a personal learning experience; this can take place during or after the event. They suggest that a 'good practitioner' is not only one who is informed, rational and objective, but also is one who is able to deliberate rather than simply calculate.

Blair and Robertson (2005) acknowledge that reflective practice begins with the premise that occupational therapy is a complex intervention, in that there are *'messy, convoluted and often intractable situations to contend with in daily therapeutic interventions.'* The number of 'active ingredients' involved in the occupational therapy process make it difficult to identify or predict factors influential in achieving or hindering the outcome (Creek *et al.*, 2005; Paterson and Dieppe, 2005). Reflection, therefore, is an essential component of the whole occupational therapy process and an aspect of rehabilitation that needs to be allocated time.

Conclusion

In conclusion it has been recognised that evidence-based practice involves more than the interpretation of published research; it involves effective clinical reasoning based on clinical knowledge, and interactions with clients, taking into account their characteristics, unique situations, spiritual beliefs, culture, desires and values. The skills required by an effective practitioner include:

- A knowledge of disease mechanisms and pathophysiology.
- The ability to analyse research data and interpret psychometric tests.
- The ability to draw upon individuals' values and beliefs pertinent to their situation.
- A thorough knowledge of the theoretical philosophies underpinning occupational therapy.
- A sound understanding of the frames of reference available.
- An appreciation of a range and models and approaches.
- The ability to analyse and extract relevant information pertinent to the therapeutic context.
- The ability to be critically reflective, in order to provide the best service possible to the clients in our care.

In addition these skills must accommodate government directives and primary and social care directives.

Both qualified and student occupational therapists should be active supporters of evidence-based practice and, by being so, influential in broadening the criteria of what is considered evidence. As professionals there is a need to recognise that our learning is not complete on qualification but simply beginning, acknowledging that clinical expertise involves more than attaining a certain level of clinical competence, but a commitment to learning as well (Kamhi, 1995). In reality the process of understanding and embedding evidence-based practice is a lifelong professional learning experience rather than the simple application of a set of rules (Forsyth *et al.*, 2005). It is not simply an ideal which can be adopted or rejected at will, but a standard of practice emphasised within the professional Code of Practice which states that *'occupational therapists have a responsibility to contribute to the continuing development of the profession by utilising critical evaluation, and participating in audit and research'* (COT, 2005, section 5.6.1).

Increasing familiarity with a framework for achieving best practice will ultimately lead occupational therapists into direct involvement in research. As can be seen in the following reflection of clinical interventions, the contemplative evaluation of the therapeutic process highlights gaps in approaches, methods or processes which can then be addressed through clinically based research. Action research and participant research will increasingly become part of practice, with occupational therapists becoming actively involved in evaluating and refining the services they provide. Ultimately all occupational therapists that use evidential knowledge will be involved in generating it. This knowledge generation will emerge from cooperation and teamwork and be supported by researchers rather than directed by them, thus reducing the gulf between academics and practitioners, and providing a bridge between research, theory and practice. This, according to Boyce and Lysack (2000), will have the benefit that research will be grounded in, and designed to respond to, real life situations and shaped by local circumstances. As a consequence, any changes which are required as a result of the evaluation will be more acceptable, owing to the engagement of the clinician with the investigation process (Davies, 1999).

References

Ajzen, I. and Fishbein, M. (1980) *Understanding Attitudes and Predicting Social Behaviour.* Prentice Hall, Engelwood Cliffs

Alsop, A. and Lloyd, C. (2002) The purpose and practicalities of postgraduate education. *British Journal of Occupational Therapy*, **65**(5), 245–251

Benharoch, J. and Wiseman, T. (2004) Participation in occupations: some experiences of people with Parkinson's disease. *British Journal of Occupational Therapy*, **67**(9), 380–387

Blair, S.E. and Robertson, L.J. (2005) Hard complexities–soft complexities: an exploration of philosophical positions related to evidence in occupational therapy. *British Journal of Occupational Therapy*, **68**(6), 269–276

Blake, D.J. and Bodine, C. (2002) An overview of assistive technology for persons with multiple sclerosis. *Journal of Rehabilitation Research and Development*, **39**(2), 299–312

Bobath, K. (1993) *A Neurophysiological Basis for the Treatment of Cerebral Palsy (Clinics in Development Medicine).* MacKeith Press, London

Boden, M.A. (1998) Consciousness and human identity: An interdisciplinary perspective. In: *Consciousness and Human Identity.* Ed. Cornwell, J., pp. 1–20. Oxford University Press, Oxford

Boyce, W. and Lysack, C. (2000) Community participation uncovering its meanings. In: *Selected Readings In Community Based Rehabilitation: CBR in Transition (series 1).* Ed. Thomas, M. and Thomas M.J., pp. 39–54. Action for Disability, Newcastle upon Tyne

Bruner, J. (1960) *The Process of Education*. Harvard University, Cambridge, Mass.

Chang, J.T., Morton, S.C., Rubenstein, L.Z., Mojica, W.A., Maglione, M., Suttorp, M.J., Roth, E.A. and Shekelle, P.G. (2004) Interventions for the prevention of falls in older adults: systematic review and meta-analysis of randomised clinical trials. *British Medical Journal*, **328(7441)**, 680

Christiansen, C. and Lou, J. (2001) Ethical considerations related to evidence-based practice. *American Journal of Occupational Therapy*, **55(3)**, 345–349

Clarke, C., Sealey-Lapes, C. and Kotsch, L. (2001) *Outcome Measures. Information Pack for Occupational Therapists*. College of Occupational Therapists, London

Cohen, H., Miller, L.V., Kane-Wineland, M. and Hatfield, C.L. (1995) Case reports of vestibular rehabilitation with graded occupations. *American Journal of Occupational Therapy*, **49**, 362–367

College of Occupational Therapists (2005) *Code of Ethics and Professional Conduct*. College of Occupational Therapists, London

Cornwell, R. (2000) Essential differences between research and evidence-based practice. *Nurse Researcher*, **8(2)**, 55–68

Creek, J., Ilott, I., Cook, S. and Munday, C. (2005) Valuing occupational therapy as a complex intervention. *British Journal of Occupational Therapy*, **68(6)**, 281–284

Curtin, M. and Clarke, G. (2005) Living with impairment: learning from disabled young people's biographies. *British Journal of Occupational Therapy*, **68(9)**, 401–408

Davies, P. (1999) Introducing change. In: *Evidence-based Practice: a Primer for Health Care Professionals*. Ed. Dawes, M., Davies, P., Gray, A., Mant, J., Seers, K. and Snowball, R., pp. 241–244. Churchill Livingstone, London

Dawes, M., Summerskill, W., Glasziou, P., Cartabellotta, A., Martin, J., Hopayian, K., Porzsolt, F., Burls, A. and Osborne, J. (2005) Debate: Sicily statement on evidence-based practice. *BMC Medical*, 5.1 available from: http://www.biomedcentral.com/1472-6920/5/1

Department of Health (2001) *A Guide to Contracting for Intermediate Care Services*. HMSO, London

Department of Health (2002) *National Service Framework for Older People: Supporting Implementation – Intermediate Care: Moving Forward*. HMSO, London

Dowie, J. (1996) 'Evidence-based', 'cost-effective', and 'preference-driven' medicine: decision analysis based medical decision making is the pre-requisite. *Journal of Health Service Research Policy*, **1(2)**, 104–113

Dunford, C. and Richards, S. (2003) *Doubly Disadvantaged: Survey of Waiting Lists and Waiting Times for Occupational Therapy Services for Children with Developmental Coordination Disorder*. College of Occupational Therapists, London

Elliot, S.J., Velde, B.P. and Wittam, P.P. (2002) The use of theory in everyday practice: an exploratory study. *Occupational Therapy in Health Care*, **16(1)**, 45–62

Evans, S., Gately, C., Huxley, P., Smith, A. and Banerjee, S. (2005) Assessment of the quality of life in later life: development and validation of the QuiLL. *Quality of Life Research*, **14(5)**, 1291–1300

Forsyth, K., Summerfield Mann, L. and Keilhofner, G. (2005) Scholarship of practice: making occupation-focused, theory-driven, evidence-based practice a reality. *British Journal of Occupational Therapy*, **68(6)**, 260–268

Goodacre, L. and Goodacre, J. (2003) The negotiation and use of personal assistance by women with chronic arthritis. *British Journal of Occupational Therapy*, **66**(7), 297–301

Greenhalgh, T. (1997) How to read a paper: getting your bearings (deciding what the paper is about). *British Medical Journal*, **315**, 243–246

Greenhalgh, T. (1999) Narrative based medicine in an evidence based world. *British Medical Journal*, **318**, 323–325

Hagedorn, R. (2001) *Foundations of Practice in Occupational Therapy*. Churchill Livingstone, Edinburgh

Hamer, S. and Collinson, G. (1999) *Achieving Evidence-Based Practice: a Handbook for Practitioners*. Baillière Tindall, Edinburgh

Hammell, K.W. (2004) Deviation from the norm: a sceptical interrogation of the classification practices of the ICF. *British Journal of Occupational Therapy*, **67**(9), 408–411

Hammell, K.W. and Carpenter, C. (2004) *Qualitative Research in Evidence-Based Rehabilitation*. Churchill Livingstone, Toronto

Higgs, J. and Jones, M. (eds.) (2000) *Clinical Reasoning in the Health Professions*, 2nd edn. Butter-worth-Heinemann, Oxford

Hunter, N. and Coventry, A. (2003) A part of life's tapestry: early parenting with a spinal cord injury. *British Journal of Occupational Therapy*, **66**(10), 479–481

Ilott, I. and White, E. (2001) College of occupational therapists' research and development strategic vision and action plan. *British Journal of Occupational Therapy*, **64**(6), 270–277

James, S. and Corr, C. (2004) The Morriston Occupational Therapy Outcome Measure (MOTOM): measuring what matters. *British Journal of Occupational Therapy*, **67**(5), 210–216

Jerosch-Herold, C. (2005) An evidence-based approach to choosing outcome measures: a checklist for the critical appraisal of validity, reliability and responsiveness studies. *British Journal of Occupational Therapy*, **68**(8), 347–353

Kamhi, A.G. (1995) Research to practice: defining, developing and maintaining clinical expertise. *Language and Hearing Services in Schools*, **26**(4), 353–356

Keilhofner, G. (2002) *Model of Human Occupation*, 3rd edn. Lippincott Williams and Wilkins, Philadelphia

Kelly, G. (2004) Paediatric occupational therapy in the 21st century: a survey of UK practice. *National Association of Paediatric Occupational Therapists*, **8**(3), 17–19

Law, M. (2002) *Evidence-based Rehabilitation: a Guide to Practice*. Thorofare, Slack

Law, M., Baptiste, S., Carswell, A., McColl, M.A., Polatajko, H. and Pollock, N. (1998) *The Canadian Occupational Performance Measure*, 3rd edn. CAOT Publications ACE, Ottawa

Law, M., Cooper, B., Strong, S., Stewart, D., Rigby, P. and Letts, L. (1996) The person-environment-occupation model: a transactive approach to occupational performance. *Canadian Journal of Occupational Therapy*, **63**, 9–23

Lincoln, N.B., Dent, A., Harding, J., Weyman, N., Nicholl, C., Blumhardt, L.D. and Playford, E.D. (2002) Evaluation of cognitive assessment and cognitive intervention for people with multiple sclerosis. *Journal of Neurology, Neurosurgery, and Psychiatry*, **72**(1), 93–98

Logan, P.A., Gladman, J.R.F., Drummond, A.E.R. and Radford, K.A. (2003) A study of interventions and related outcomes in a randomised controlled trial of occupational therapy and leisure therapy for community stroke patients. Clinical Rehabilitation, **17**, 249–255

Luke, C., Dodd, K.J. and Brock, K. (2004) Outcomes of the Bobath concept on upper limb recovery following stroke. *Clinical Rehabilitation*, **18(8)**, 888–898

Maguire, G. and Nanton, R. (2005) *Looking Back and Looking Forwards; Developments in Conductive Education*. The Foundation for Conductive Education, Birmingham

Mathiowetz, V., Volland, G., Kashman, N. and Weber, K. (1985) Nine hole peg test (NHPT) In: *Measurement in Neurological Rehabilitation*. Wade, D.T. (1992), p. 171. Oxford University Press, New York

Mattingly, C. and Fleming, M.H. (1994) *Clinical Reasoning: forms of inquiry in a therapeutic practice*. FA Davis, Philadelphia

Mayers, C.A. (1998) An evaluation of the use of the Mayers' Lifestyle Questionnaire. *British Journal of Occupational Therapy*, **61**, 393–398

Maynard, A. (1997) Evidence-based medicine: an incomplete method for informing treatment choices. *Lancet*, **349**, 126–128

McDonald, R., Surtees, R. and Wirz, S. (2004) The International Classification of Functioning, Disability and Health provides a model for adaptive seating interventions for children with cerebral palsy. *British Journal of Occupational Therapy*, **67(7)**, 293–302

McEwen, I. (2001) *Writing case reports: a how-to manual for clinicians*, 2nd edn. American Physical Therapy Association, Alexandria

Missiuna, C. and Pollock, N. (2000) Perceived efficacy and goal setting in young children. *Canadian Association of Occupational Therapy*, **67**, 101–109

Mitchell, R. and Unsworth, C.A. (2005) Clinical reasoning during community health home visits: expert and novice differences. *British Journal of Occupational Therapy*, **68(5)**, 215–223

National Institute of Health Consensus Statement (1998) Diagnosis and treatment of attention deficit hyperactivity disorder. *NIH Consensus Statement*, **16(2)**, 1–37

Neistadt, M.E. (1996) Teaching strategies for the development of clinical reasoning. *American Journal of Occupational Therapy*, **50(8)**, 676–684

Parker, C.L., Gladman, J.R.F., Drummond, M.E., Lincoln, N.B., Barer, D., Logan, P.A. and Radford, K.A. (2001) A multicentre randomised controlled trial of leisure therapy and conventional occupational therapy after stroke. *Clinical Rehabilitation*, **15(1)**, 42–52

Patel, A.T., Duncan, P.W., Lai, S.-M. and Studenski, S. (2000) The relation between impairments and functional outcomes post-stroke. *Archives of Physical Medicine and Rehabilitation*, **81(10)**, 1357–1363

Paterson, C. and Dieppe, P. (2005) Characteristics and incidental (placebo) effects in complex interventions such as acupuncture. *British Medical Journal*, **330**, 1202–1205

Piaget, J. (1929) *The Child's Conception of the World*. Harcourt, Brace Jovanovich, New York

Polatajko, H., Mandich, A., Miller, L. and Macnab, J. (2001) Cognitive orientation to daily occupational performance (CO-OP): part II-the evidence. *Physical & Occupational Therapy in Paediatrics*, **20(2–3)**, 83–106

Reed, K.L. and Sanderson, S.N. (1999) *Concepts of Occupational Therapy*. Lippincott Williams and Wilkins, Baltimore

Rosenbaum, P. and Stewart, D. (2004) The World Health Organization International Classification of Functioning, Disability and Health: a model to guide clinical thinking, practice and research in cerebral palsy. *Seminars in Pediatric Neurology*, **11**(1), 5–10

Rosenstock, I. (1974) The health belief model and preventative health behaviour. *Health Education Monographs*, **2**, 354–386

Sackett, D., Richardson, W., Rosenberg, W. and Haynes, R. (1996) *Evidence-based medicine*. Churchill Livingstone, Edinburgh

Sackett, D., Strauss, S., Richardson, W., Rosenberg, W. and Haynes, R. (2000) *Evidence-based Medicine; How to Practice and Teach EBM*, 2nd edn. Churchill Livingstone, London

Scally, G. and Donaldson, L.J. (1998) Clinical governance and the drive for quality improvement in the new NHS in England. *British Medical Journal*, **317**, 61–65

Shah, S. (1994) In praise of the biometric and psychometric qualities of the Barthel Index. *Physiotherapy*, **80**, 769–771

Shaw, I. (2001) *Trent Focus for Research and Development in Primary Health Care: Introduction to Evaluating Health Services*. Trent Focus, University of Nottingham

Sheldon, T. and Chalmers, I. (1994) The UK Cochrane Centre and the NHS Centre for Reviews and Dissemination: respective roles within the information systems strategy of the NHS R&D Programme, coordination and principles underlying collaboration. *Health Economics*, **3**, 201–203

Sherratt, C. (2005) The journal club: a method for occupational therapists to ridge the theory–practice gap. *British Journal of Occupational Therapy*, **68**(7), 301–306

Stevenson, V.L., Miller, D.H., Leary, S.M., Rovaris, M., Barkhof, F., Brochet, B., Dousset, V., Dousset, V., Filippi, M., Hintzen, R., Montalban, X., Polman, C.H., Rovira, A.J., de Sa, A. and Thompson, A.J. (2000) One year follow up study of primary and transitional progressive multiple sclerosis. *Neurology and Neurosurgical Psychiatry*, **68**, 713–718

Turner-Stokes, L. and Turner-Stokes, T. (1997) The use of standardized outcome measures in rehabilitation centres in the UK. *Clinical Rehabilitation*, **11**(4), 306–313

Ubhi, T., Bhakta, B.B., Ives, H.L., Allgar, V. and Roussounis, S.H. (2000) Randomised double blind placebo controlled trial of the effect of botulinum toxin on walking in cerebral palsy. *Archives of Disease in Childhood*, **83**, 481–487

Unsworth, C.A. (2004) Clinical reasoning: How do pragmatic reasoning, worldview and client-centeredness fit? *British Journal of Occupational Therapy*, **67**(1), 11–19

Vanage, S.M., Gilbertson, K.K. and Mathiowetz, V. (2003) Effects of an energy conservation course on fatigue impact for persons with progressive multiple sclerosis. *American Journal of Occupational Therapy*, **57**(3), 315–323

Vandenbroucke, J.P. (1999) Case reports in an evidence-based world. *Journal of the Royal Society of Medicine*, **92**, 159–163

Wade, D.T. (1999) Goal planning in stroke rehabilitation: how? *Topics in Stroke Rehabilitation*, **6**, 16–36

World Health Organization (2001) *International Classification of Functioning, Disability and Health*. World Health Organization, Geneva

2: Facilitating the educational inclusion of children with developmental coordination disorder

Lois M. Addy

Introduction

The evidence base relating to children with developmental coordination disorder (DCD) has increased considerably owing to the clarification of definition and diagnostic criterion pertaining to this common childhood condition (Polatajko *et al.*, 1995; American Psychiatric Association (APA), 2000). This has led to distinctive research in areas of motor coordination which have provided occupational therapists with significant evidence on which to base their practice. The current research, utilising systematic reviews, randomised control trials and case study analysis, has challenged traditional practice which sought to identify and address the underlying process skills, i.e. visual–motor integration, kinaesthetic sensitivity, visuo-spatial awareness, deficient in the child with DCD, in favour of cognitive, task-specific approaches to therapy (Mandich *et al.*, 2001; Schoemaker and Smits-Engelsman, 2005). The evidence supporting this approach in addressing gross motor coordination is very convincing; however, its applicability to skills such as handwriting, which involves cognitive, kinaesthetic and perceptual–motor components, is more contentious (Addy, 1995; Sugden and Chambers, 1998; Rosenblum *et al.*, 2003; Jongmans *et al.*, 2003; Henderson and Markee, 2005). This chapter recommends that occupational therapists objectively critique both approaches, depending on the individual needs of the child, the child's age, current needs and present context.

The inclusion of children with special educational needs into mainstream schools has been one of the most positive changes in social and educational policy for decades. It has been influential in encouraging tolerance and the acceptance of difference, while highlighting the unique needs of **all** children. Provision for children with overt disabilities, although far from perfect, has developed extensively as the inclusion movement has gained momentum. There are, however, children whose difficulties are less transparent, who struggle with many aspects of the educational curriculum; this has a profound affect on their ability to learn and self-esteem. Children with developmental coordination disorder (DCD) form a high proportion of this group, with a population incidence of 5–8% of all children and a ratio of 5:1 boys to girls (Willoughby and Polatajko, 1995; Wilson and McKenzie, 1998; Dewey and Wilson, 2001). These children present with difficulties in motor coordination and perceptual processing which significantly impact on their academic performance. It is for this reason that DCD is often termed the 'hidden handicap' and why occupational therapists working within the field of paediatrics are so heavily involved.

The ability of the occupational therapist to analyse the motor, cognitive and perceptual components of occupational performance has been instrumental in identifying the occupational therapist as the lead professional involved with many of these children. The extent of this involvement was highlighted in a survey commissioned by the College of Occupational Therapists to determine the numbers of children involved and how this impacts on occupational therapy resources. Of the 134 paediatric occupational therapy service providers surveyed, 30.4% of the total caseload involved working with children with DCD and accounted for 61.7% of the total number waiting for assessment (Dunford and Richards, 2003).

These children are characterised by their poor motor coordination (gross and fine), planning difficulty, movement organisation and difficulties interpreting perceptual information. This affects their participation in physical education (PE) and many other aspects of the curriculum involving writing skills, practical skills, manual dexterity, organisation and effective planning. In addition, the awareness that the child's performance is different to that of his/her peers has a profound effect on the child's self-confidence, self-esteem and social interaction, and has strong implications for secondary anxiety and behavioural disorders (Smyth and Anderson, 2000; Summers and Larkin, 2002).

This chapter follows the journey of Peter (pseudonym) who was given the diagnosis of DCD at the age of 6.7 years. It will show the effect that this has had on his ability to learn and access the UK educational curriculum. Although his association with the occupational therapy service covered a period of 3 years, only a small part of his therapy will be presented. This will focus on the occupational therapy provided 2 months following diagnosis, and will cover a period of 1 year.

Initially it is important to outline the criterion that was used to define and diagnose Peter with DCD. This has a controversial history, as variation in terminology has muddied the waters as to what exactly constitutes this childhood condition. In addition, understanding the nature and presentation of DCD can be insightful in determining why a child acts or behaves as he/she does (Addy, 2004).

Developmental coordination disorder

There have been many terms used to describe children with coordination disorders. Developmental dyspraxia (Dewey, 1995) was, and still is, a familiar term commonly used by professionals, teachers and parents alike to describe a child who struggled to plan and organise his/her movements. Sensory integrative dysfunction (Ayres, 1972) was another term frequently used to explain the possible reasons why a child may be uncoordinated. Perceptual–motor dysfunction (Clark *et al.*, 1991) was used to emphasise the effect of motor dysfunction on perceptual understanding. In addition, terms such as deficit in attention motor perception (DAMP) (Gillberg, 2003), clumsy child syndrome (Cratty, 1994) and congenital maladroit are also used. Indeed, there are so many variations in terminology that questions have arisen as to whether they refer to the same disorder or distinctive disorders. The consensus term to be used in literature and research is developmental coordination disorder and is based on the American Psychiatric Association's criteria (2000) (Fig. 2.1).

Children with DCD may initially be slow to achieve their motor milestones and seem particularly 'clumsy' and disorganised in their play. However, at a preschool level this may not seem significant as variability at this age is vast. It is when the child enters full-time education that the extent of his/her difficulties is realised. The teacher and child's parents initially perceive a mismatch between the child's comprehension and/or verbal ability and motor performance. This is represented in the child's ability to provide verbal descriptions of events, yet being unable to control a pencil to write. The child may be able to describe the rules of a game yet cannot physically organise or sequence movements to action the task. In physical education (PE) the child's movement difficulties may appear more overt, with difficulties transitioning between body positions being evident and the sequencing and timing of actions appearing erratic (Parnham and Mailloux, 1996). Inappropriate timing of movements, lack of fluency in actions and abundance of effort in performing simple tasks may also be apparent (Missiuna, 1999). Problems in ideation (forming ideas and plans) and position in space will also be evident, and the child may have difficulties generating ideas of what to do in new situations (Parnham and Mailloux, 1996). In addition there may be concerns regarding dexterity and bilateral coordination which will affect ball control and subsequent participation in ball games (Geuze, 2005).

Perceptual difficulties further impact on motor actions, in particular poor kinaesthetic sensitivity affects motor responses (Jongmans *et al.*, 1998). Form and

---

A. Performance in daily activities that require motor coordination is substantially below that expected given the person's chronological age and measured intelligence.

B. The disturbance in criterion A significantly interferes with academic achievements or activities for daily living.

C. The disturbance is not due to a general medical condition (i.e. cerebral palsy, hemiplegia or muscular dystrophy) and does not meet criteria for pervasive development disorder.

D. If intellectual difficulties are present, the motor difficulties are in excess of those usually associated with it.

Figure 2.1 American Psychiatric Association diagnostic criteria (from American Psychiatric Association, 2000).

size constancy issues and visual–spatial processing are also a concern (Wilson and McKenzie, 1998).

In addition to the motor concerns, a small percentage of children with DCD have verbal developmental dyspraxia which affects their expressive language skills. This is an extremely frustrating aspect of DCD as the child may be able spontaneously to respond to an interaction, but cannot repeat this when consciously attempting to respond on cue (Hill, 1998; Rintala *et al.*, 1998).

Co-morbidity

Despite the clarity of the APA (2000) diagnostic criteria, many of the symptoms of DCD overlap with other childhood disorders. Kaplan *et al.* (1998, p. 472) state *'although there is often one feature of these children's difficulties that stands out from all others it is rarely the case that it is an entirely isolated problem.'* In addition to the characteristics previously described, DCD overlaps with attention deficit/hyperactivity disorder (ADHD) (Pitcher *et al.*, 2003). Kadesjö and Gillberg (2001) found that 47% of their children with ADHD also had DCD. There was also a co-occurrence between social, emotional and behavioural difficulties, including anxiety and depression, and DCD (Rasmussen and Gillberg, 2000; Sigurdsson and Fombonne, 2002). In addition, reading, attention and motor deficits may be evident (O'Hare and Khalid, 2002). Kaplan *et al.* (1998) found that 63% of their dyslexic children also had DCD.

Overall DCD is a condition which profoundly affects all aspects of the child's occupational performance, and research has shown that if untreated, these concerns will not resolve themselves. Therefore there are many long-term implications (Losse *et al.*, 1991; Polatajko, 1999), which suggest that early treatment will result in a better outcome (Cantell *et al.*, 1994).

As the effects of DCD become more apparent during the child's school years it would seem appropriate that this should be the prime location for any occupational therapy assessment. The need to address the child's needs within the most appropriate context has been supported not only by research (Sugden and Chambers, 1998) but also by government directives and educational reforms. It is therefore important to appreciate how recent legislation in health and education has impacted on occupational therapy service delivery.

Government directives and policies

Traditionally, occupational therapists were based in child development centres, special schools or units attached to community NHS centres. Children were withdrawn from school to attend clinics or therapy groups, which were delivered for a limited period in a specified timeframe. This had the advantage that specialised equipment could be easily accessed and disruptions to therapy time would be limited. It also allowed the therapists to involve the parents, establishing relationships with both parent and child that would span years. Appointments were based around the therapist's availability rather than the child's convenience. In addition, therapy tended to be directive and goals based on perceived functional needs, and did not necessarily address these in relation to the child's education. Therapy was provided *apart* from education and the two paths rarely crossed (Addy, 2005).

With the reforms in education initiated by the Warnock Report (Department for Education and Skills, 1978), questions were raised regarding the medical versus social model of disability, and the categorisation of disability versus curriculum-based needs. The Warnock Report was followed by the 1981 Education Act, which unfortunately retained an attention to individual deficits. The Act did, however, introduce the 'statement of special educational needs' which required therapists to consider the child's education along with therapeutic provision. Later the Code of Practice provided guidance in relation to the identification and assessment of children with special educational needs (SEN) (Department for Education, 1994), emphasising the importance of school-based intervention. This demanded that every school should publish a detailed special needs policy, appoint a special educational needs co-ordinator (SENCo) and report the school's effectiveness, in addressing children's specific educational needs, on an annual basis.

The Green Paper, *Excellence for all Children; Meeting Special Educational Needs* (Department for Education and Skills, 1997), provided initiatives for improving literacy and numeracy, introducing target setting for schools and opening up new technologies to help children with SEN to reach their full potential. Around the same time, evidence was emerging of the economic benefits of inclusive schooling versus special school provision with special school costs being consistently higher than mainstream for pupils with similar levels of need (Crowther *et al.*, 1998).

The introduction of the Special Educational Needs and Disability Act (SENDA) (Department for Education and Skills, 2001) was accompanied by two Codes of Practice produced by the Disability Rights Commission; one for schools and one for post-16 education. This made it **unlawful** to discriminate against pupils with any physical or learning disability in all aspects of school life; a 'gate keeper' was established in the form of the SEN and Disability Tribunal (SENDIT), whose remit was extended to cover cases of disability discrimination.

As inclusion gained momentum, education and therapy services, which previously tended to fit children with SEN into their own respective paradigms, developed recognition that intervention programmes should be devised in partnership with each child and his/her family, and should be focused around the child's individual needs and priorities (Mackey and McQueen, 1998). Rather than simply a location change, there was also a change in method of provision, with therapists becoming more involved in advice, consultation and teaching. The priority of the therapist became to enhance the education of the child, with the therapeutic programme assuming a complementary, supportive role to the education plan. McQueen and McLellan (1994) state, '*If routine therapy were to be cross-referenced with the National Curriculum it has the potential to reduce the pressure on pupil time, curriculum content and (ultimately) therapy resources.*'

This move was further supported by the National Service Framework for Children (Department of Health, 2004) which encouraged integrated therapy as a means of providing a smooth, timely, therapy service. This also supported research, which recommended that any intervention should be *'central to a child's daily experiences and interests and should take place in the contexts of predictable routines'* and that the *'coordination between different contexts, such as school and home, further enhances opportunities to develop skills'* (Sugden and Chambers, 1998).

The current approach of integrating therapy with education has vast advantages in ensuring that therapeutic intervention is delivered in a holistic manner and is blended with functional activities for the child, thus retreating from approaches which *'compartmentalise parts of a child's body or daily life, according to which professional discipline is involved at any one time'* (Mackey and McQueen, 1998). Shifting the power differentiation previously perceived between health and education by encouraging professionals to become *'learners as well as specialists'* (Mackey and McQueen, 1998).

It was the augmented awareness of children with SEN, and improved collaboration between health and education-based services, which led Peter's teacher to refer him to the paediatric occupational therapy service, via the school community medical officer, during his second year at school. This also influenced where and how Peter's needs were assessed and addressed.

Peter's experience

Peter was born at 30 weeks gestation and incubated for a period of 2 weeks before being stable enough to go home. His motor milestones were slow; he sat independently at 12 months and walked at 20 months. Peter's mother described him as a shy, anxious child whose movements appeared awkward and laboured. As he was a first child, however, his parents were not unduly worried until the arrival of his brother 3 years later. This provided an opportunity to compare development and differences were becoming increasingly apparent as Peter commenced the small school in his home village.

His teacher's initial concerns related to his poor handwriting, limited drawing skills, difficulties in constructive play and reluctance to participate in class PE lessons. However, she felt that he had excellent comprehension and verbal skills. Peter's teacher was confused by the mismatch between his obvious intellectual skills and his practical performance in class.

Initially Peter was seen after school at the child development centre where the occupational therapist had time to converse with both Peter and his parents. This provided an opportunity for the occupational therapist to start to form a relationship with the family without disruption from the school routine or possible stigma from his peers unsure of the purpose of occupational therapy. Peter was 6.7 years on this occasion.

Peter presented as a slight, timid little boy whose movements were slow and deliberate. The occupational therapist explained to Peter why he had been asked to attend the centre and the areas of his life with which she could possibly help. The initial assessment was supported by a visit to Peter's school with his permission, to observe him interact in the classroom, view his written work and discuss his needs from the teacher's perspective.

From these initial interviews and observations, the occupational therapist began to formulate strategies from which to gain more detailed information and from which to frame her intervention. At this point theoretical rationale and appropriate models and approaches are selected to direct and inform further assessment and subsequent therapy.

Theoretical rationale

One of the key concerns highlighted by Peter was his poor fine motor coordination in respect of his handwriting; in addition, poor gross motor coordination influenced his ability to succeed in PE lessons. It was therefore appropriate to reflect on the variation in theories relating to motor learning. These include:

- Neuromaturational theories.
- Information processing theories, which incorporate connectionism and neural selection beliefs.
- Behavioural theories, which have influenced the use of operant and classical conditioning methods.
- Motor behaviour theories, which have led to the emergence of motor learning, motor control and perceptual motor approaches being adopted.
- Dynamical systems theory.

From these, two theoretical positions were particularly influential in considering how to proceed with Peter: neuromaturational theory and dynamical systems theory.

Neuromaturational theory

Neuromaturational hierarchical theories of motor development (McGraw, 1943; Gesell and Ilg, 1946) are based on the assumption that the development of movement and motor skills results from maturation of the central nervous system (CNS) which expands progressively. Motor skills develop from primitive reflexes to advanced responses which supersede basic reactions to initiate refined control through maturation and experience (Barnhart *et al.*, 2003). These motor responses are influenced by sensory feedback which serves to help to interpret environmental information. These develop memory, attention, perception, planning and execution of motor programmes and kinaesthesis. These skills are sequential, orderly and predictable. Where difficulties arise, a 'bottom-up' or 'process-orientated' approach is adopted. This focuses on identification and remediation of **underlying dysfunctional process** skills which are impacting on the child's ability successfully to perform and acquire certain skills. The expectation is that, by improving performance in an area of difficulty, improvements can be generalised in other aspects of the child's life which have not developed adequately for his/her age (Sims *et al.*, 1996; Sugden and Chambers, 1998). For example, accurate hand–eye coordination is dependent upon effective motor planning, kinaesthetic regulation, visuospatial processing and tactile feedback. Difficulties in any of these processes will impact on the child's ability to place his/her hand accurately. The supposition is that if these areas are addressed, through various therapeutic techniques, not only would hand–eye coordination improve, but other skills requiring effective motor coordination would also show signs of increased control.

Dynamical systems theory

Dynamical systems theory acknowledges that, although neuromaturational theories provide a general model of motor development, they do not account for the variability in individual performance. Dynamical systems theory proposes that motor behaviours emerge from the interaction of a variety of neural, musculoskeletal, sensory, adaptive and anticipatory mechanisms in **task-specific contexts** (Kamm *et al.*, 1990; Washington *et al.*, 2002). All these components interact in a dynamic, non-linear fashion. This theory leads to the recommendation that the focus of therapy should be directed to a specified task, emphasising the interaction between the environment, the task and the individual in the performance of functional activities. In this sense it is an active rather than a passive view of motor learning (Ketelaar *et al.*, 2001).

Dynamical systems theory leads to the adoption of 'top-down' or 'task-orientated' approaches, which focus on enhancing occupational performance by evaluating the environments and activities in which the individual's participation is limited. This approach involves the task being *'taught directly without the emphasis on underlying processes, using a variety of practices in order that the skill is generalised'* (Sugden and Chambers, 1998). It incorporates a three-step top-down approach, which initially selects a functional outcome, then identifies an individual's movement skills and patterns, before, thirdly, identifying and addressing the internal and external constraints on movement. Many approaches influenced by this thinking use verbal guidance and cognitive strategies to change motor behaviour (Miller *et al.*, 2001). The current view is that top-down approaches are consistent with contemporary principles of best practice (Dunn, 2000) but are not successful in all occupations (Henderson and Markee, 2005).

Both the neuromaturational and dynamical systems theories influenced the occupational therapist's clinical reasoning in the type of further assessment selected, and subsequent approach to therapy.

Assessment

In an ideal world Peter's needs would have been identified before the age of 6.5 years. There is strong evidence that children born before 32 weeks' gestation have statistically significant differences on all measures of motor functioning using the Movement Assessment Battery for Children (M-ABC) (Henderson and Sugden, 1992) as an outcome measure (Foulder-Hughes and Cook, 2003). This control study compared 280 pre-term babies with 210 full-term babies and found that the rate and type of motor difficulties consistent with DCD were present in 33% of pre-term babies. This study, along with other research, supports the view that early identification of motor problems is important in preventing failure in many aspects of the child's activities for daily living with the subsequent effect on self-esteem and concomitant psychosocial problems (Skinner and Piek, 2001; Mandich and Polatajko, 2005; Schoemaker and Smits-Engelsman, 2005).

Peter was assessed after school in the child development centre, so that his typical day was not disrupted. It was important to help Peter to feel comfortable about the purpose of the assessment and to support his abilities rather than inabilities. Children with DCD have *only* known what it is like to have DCD and therefore the constant request to conform and change leads to much confusion and frustration. Understandably this continuous pressure to 'fit' very rapidly influences the child's self-perception and self-esteem and hinders his/her progress. To acknowledge the child's abilities the first question directed to Peter asked, 'What are you good at?' Initially many children fail to respond to this believing that they really have no positive attributes. Their reaction helps the therapist to ascertain the child's psychological state, and gives a positive starting point on which to build the future therapeutic relationship. Having gained some background understanding of Peter's difficulties from his parents' and teacher's perspective, through the initial referral and subsequent meetings, it was essential to understand Peter's concerns. What we as adults distinguish as important may be completely irrelevant to a child. Therefore the Perceived Efficacy and Goal Setting Scale (PEGS) (Missiuna et al., 2004) was introduced to help Peter identify how he perceived his abilities and identify areas with which he felt he needed help. PEGS is a tool for children to report their perceptions of competence in performing everyday tasks. It provides the occupational therapist with a means to identify the tasks and contexts which may be concerns for children and serve as a focus for intervention.

The PEGS is based on a pictorial self-efficacy measure that focuses on 24 occupations that children are expected to perform during any typical school day; for example keeping a tidy desk/tray, participating in ball activities, writing neatly. The child is shown a pair of contrasting cards. For example one card states 'This child is good at kicking a ball' a second card will have 'This child is not good at kicking a ball'. The assessor reads out the statements and asks, 'Which is more like you?' It uses a forced choice format (Harter, 1985) to make the child to select a response before the therapist asks the second question, 'Is it a lot like you or a little?' The child's recorded responses are placed into one of four categories (Missiuna et al., 2004a, p. 21):

▨ a lot less competent.
▨ a little less competent.

▨ a little more competent.
▨ a lot more competent.

The therapist can then use the task/s which the child believes that he/she struggles with to set therapy goals collaboratively.

PEGS is a useful introductory tool, which Missiuna and Pollock (2000) claim can be used with children as young as 5–9 years. However, there are a few disadvantages to using this tool; for example, dilemmas arise when there is a mismatch between what the child **wants** to improve and what he/she **needs** to improve. Research has shown that adults and children do not always have the same priorities for intervention (Pollock and Stewart, 1998); for example a child's desire may be to play football and to score a goal, however handwriting may be a more significant concern restricting the child's ability to record information. Should the occupational therapist focus more on improving his ball skills or address his handwriting needs? This is why collaborative goal setting is essential and may include compromises from both parties. A further concern is the influence of recent events on the child's perception of his/her abilities; for example, Peter originally stated that he was very good at ball skills. This was based on a recent game of football whereby Peter's team had won, however it transpired that during the course of the game Peter had never *touched* the ball! It is therefore important that the PEGS is not the only assessment used.

Peter was also assessed using the Movement Assessment Battery for Children (M-ABC) (Henderson and Sugden, 1992). This is a simple **task-specific** motor assessment which provides an accurate measurement of manual dexterity, ball skills and static and dynamic balance (Croce *et al.*, 2001). Impairment scores are interpreted into percentile norms with children scoring below the 5th percentile having a definite motor impairment requiring intervention.

Peter was experiencing significant difficulties in writing, a task which involves complex motor and perceptual processes, therefore the occupational therapist felt it appropriate to analyse the underlying process skills demanded by the task of handwriting (Erdhardt and Meade, 2005). The Test of Visual Motor Integration (VMI) (Beery *et al.*, 2004) was used. This **process-orientated** test provided information regarding Peter's visual perception skills. This test enabled the occupational therapist to consider the impact on other areas of Peter's life, i.e. weakness in spatial relationships not only affects Peter's ability to leave appropriate spaces between words but also influences his coordination in PE.

The VMI identifies how well the brain coordinates the visual information it has received with the need to make a motor response. It requires the child to reproduce a series of shapes which are developmentally sequenced for difficulty. The VMI has been proposed as a useful screening tool for determining handwriting difficulties (Rosenblum *et al.*, 2003). However, Marr and Cermak (2002) caution that this is not an appropriate indicator for children under the age of 6, and Goyen and Duff (2005) found that there was limited correlation between scores on the VMI and handwriting dysfunction in children aged 9–12 years.

Peter's handwriting could have been directly assessed using measurements such as the Evaluation Tool of Children's Handwriting (ETCH) (Amundson, 1995). However, despite evidence supporting its reliability and validity (Diekema *et al.*, 1998; Sudsawad *et al.*, 2000; Koziatek and Powell, 2002), the handwriting policy adopted by Peter's school was not complementary with this evaluation, which utilises the D'Nealian cursive script which incorporates loops. Instead, the non-standardised criterion-referenced assessment used to evaluate the 'Write from the Start' handwriting programme (Teodorescu and Addy, 1996) was used to gain a baseline score regarding Peter's handwriting (Fig. 2.2). This was re-used as an outcome measure following a period of intervention.

Despite the common use of these assessment tools with children with DCD, caution should be applied. There appears to be no theoretical rationale for choice of form in the VMI and no non-normative standards are provided (Seitz, 2003). The M-ABC does not determine qualitative changes in movement and may not be sufficiently detailed to identify fine motor concerns, such as handwriting (Geuze *et al.*, 2001; Dunford *et al.*, 2004). When using the PEGS, therapists should be aware that young children tend to exaggerate their abilities rather than under-estimate them (Missiuna and Pollock, 2000; Wallen and Ziviani, 2005). These concerns need to be taken into account when evaluating a child's occupational performance and highlight the importance of using multi-modal methods of assessment.

Results of Peter's assessments

Goals selected by Peter following the PEGS assessment

- Writing neatly (Peter was also concerned that his writing was slow).
- Catching a ball.
- Kicking a ball.
- Doing up buttons.

Movement ABC score at 6.7 years

- Total Motor Impairment score 27 with a percentile score well below the 5%.

Visual Motor Integration score at 6.7 years

- Standard score 79.
- Percentile rank 8%.
- Age equivalent 4.6 years.

Visual perception

- Standard score 92.
- Percentile rank 30%.
- Age equivalent 5.1 years.

Motor coordination

- Standard score 75.
- Percentile rank 5%.
- Age equivalent 3.9 years.

Sample: (use non-lined paper)

    1. **Write your name (first name)**
    2. **Copy the alphabet**
    3. **Write the alphabet (assessor can provide a verbal reminder of the alphabet)**
    4. **Copy the sentence 'the quick brown fox jumped over the lazy dog'**
    5. **Free write a sentence for a minute on the subject 'all about me'**

Legibility

Definition of term
The letter and word can be clearly recognised *apart* from its context.
(Use 1, 2 and 3)

0	Attempted letters are unrecognisable as such
1	1–5 letters are recognisable when copied
2	Name is recognisable when free written along with 1–5 copied letters
3	Name is legible, and 5 additional letters are also recognisable when free written
4	Name is legible, and 10–15 letters are also recognisable when free written
5	All letters of the alphabet are recognisable

Accurate letter formation

Definition of term
The letters are formed, commencing from the line, with correct direction of flow being demonstrated.
(Use 3 and 5)

0	All letters are incorrectly formed, despite being recognisable
1	1–5 letters are correctly formed
2	6–10 letters are correctly formed
3	11–15 letters are correctly formed
4	16–20 letters are correctly formed
5	All letters are correctly formed

Uniformity of letter size

Definition of term
Letter sizes are consistent; small letters being half the dimension of ascenders and descenders
(Use 4 and 5)

0	Attempted letters are illegible
1	Letters attempted are all the same size
2	Letters attempted are inconsistently small or large
3	5–10 letters are showing differentiation in size
4	4 out of the 7 ascenders are sized correctly (b,d,f,t,h,k,l); 3 out of the 5 descenders are sized correctly (p,q g, y j)
5	All letters show appropriate differentiation in size

Figure 2.2 Handwriting criterion-referenced assessment, age 5.0–8.0 years.

Uniformity of letter slope

Definition of term
The slant of the ascending and descending letter is consistently aligned to one another, using either a backward, upward or forward slant.
(Use 4 and 5)

0   Illegible lettering
1   Attempted letters show erratic, inappropriate directionality
2   Some ascending letters show a consistent direction but this is not evident throughout the text
3   Descending letters show a consistent direction, but the direction of ascending letters remains erratic
4   The majority of ascending and descending letters show a consistency in direction and alignment
5   All letters show a consistent alignment

Spacing between words and letters

Definition of term
Spacing between words is emerging. Letters are grouped together to form appropriate words.
(Use 4 and 5)

0   No recognisable letters and no grouping attempted
1   Few letters attempted but no grouping
2   Spacing reliant on copying skills
3   Attempts are made to group letters into words but spacing is erratic
4   Spaces between words are developing with only occasional errors in spatial planning
5   Appropriate spaces between words are evident

Alignment of writing on the page

Definition of term
Writing will start at the left hand side of the page and transfer across the page in a left to right direction
(Use 5)

0   Unrecognisable letters
1   Attempted letters are placed erratically on the page
2   Words are formatted together but do not maintain a horizontal alignment
3   Alignment across the page is attempted but writing drifts as writing progresses. Further writing does not acknowledge the original starting margin.
4   Alignment across the page is attempted but writing drifts slightly as writing progresses
5   Attempted words are consistently written from left to right in a horizontal plane

---

Figure 2.2 *Continued*

Goal planning

The results of the assessment provided both objective and subjective information from which to determine therapeutic goals. These were agreed in collaboration with Peter, his teachers and parents. They were then structured using SMART principles determining a time structure for their completion.

The long-term aim was to develop Peter's gross and fine motor skills in relation to handwriting and his participation in physical education lessons.

Objective 1: to inform and educate school staff about DCD and how this condition impacts on Peter's learning and social interaction

This will help staff to understand his unique needs, adapt the environment whenever appropriate and differentiate the curriculum to maximise learning opportunities.

The occupational therapist will coordinate and present this information at a date and time negotiated with his head teacher. This will be arranged and undertaken, with Peter's full permission, by week 3.

Objective 2: to improve perceptual and fine motor skills relating to handwriting

The 'Write from the Start' perceptual–motor handwriting programme (Teodorescu and Addy, 1996) will be incorporated into his school day on a daily basis. This will be introduced by the occupational therapist who will liaise with his class teacher, learning support assistant (LSA) and parent helper. Progress will be measured using the handwriting criterion-referenced scale (Fig. 2.2) which will be scored by Peter's parents and will be reviewed in two school terms (approximately 7 months).

Objective 3: to improve motor skills in relation to the National Curriculum Physical Education Objectives for Key Stage 1

Peter will be introduced to a therapeutic motor skills group which will be task-focused and take place each week, after school, for a period of 90 minutes. The activities taught in the session will be reinforced during playtimes and within school within PE class. He will attend the group for two school terms (approximately 7 months).

Improvement will be measured against Peter's original scores from the M-ABC and, in particular, the scores for ball skills and static and dynamic balance. The aim is to decrease Peter's total motor impairment score by 5 points.

Objective 4: to increase speed of dressing and undressing preceding and following physical education lessons

Initially, compensatory techniques will be used to enable Peter to dress and undress quickly, while simultaneously introducing a dressing programme at home to be attempted during weekends and holidays. Peter's clothing will be adapted to reduce the need to tackle numerous fastenings. A sample of this will be provided within 2 weeks and a dressing programme will be provided by week 2 to help him improve his ability and speed of dressing/undressing during the weekend. Success will be measured using a structured reward chart.

Occupational therapy

Objective 1: transfer of knowledge

The first objective was selected because the educational inclusion movement has left many teachers with the complex task of understanding the varying needs of children with a range of childhood conditions. One of the most important roles for the occupational therapist, therefore, is that of educator, i.e. to inform the relevant professionals concerned about Peter's unique needs and abilities. This educational role has positive consequences in helping those working with the children to gain an understanding about the child's learning and behaviour from the child's perspective. This educative approach is influential in helping all concerned in the child's welfare and education to adapt the environment and differentiate materials according to the child's ability. The emphasis therefore shifts to changing the environment *not* the child. Evidence shows that this approach has proved very effective (Rainforth and York-Barr, 1997; Elliott and McKenney, 1998; Cousins and Thompson, 2001).

Objective 2: handwriting remediation

Difficulty with handwriting is one of the most common reasons for referring school-aged children to an occupational therapist and is a major concern for children with DCD (Rigby and Schwellnus, 1999; Mandich *et al.*, 2003). In a study by Dunford *et al.* (2005) of children with DCD, 27 teachers (79.4%) out of the 34 involved expressed concerns regarding the handwriting abilities of children with DCD. They referred to poor handwriting presentation, erratic letter formation, poor pencil control and discrepancies between handwriting and other skills. Further studies highlighted further concerns in handwriting production:

- Words and letters were often illegible, sizes inconsistent, messy and effortful (Parush *et al.*, 1998).
- Spacing, formation and alignment on the page are affected (Wilson and McKenzie, 1998).
- Visual closure, visual figure-ground discrimination and visual motor speed all affect written output (Schoemaker *et al.*, 2001).
- Pressure through the writing instrument will also be inconsistent (Case-Smith and Weintraub, 2002).

- Poor postural control will make it hard for the child to develop/maintain the degree of stability to allow for fluent, fast writing (Wann *et al.*, 1998).
- Poor perceptual–motor integration will impact on the quality and quantity of written output (Tseng and Murray, 1994; Chu, 1997; Geuze, 2005).

It can therefore be concluded that poor handwriting performance has a **marked** effect on academic performance (Graham *et al.*, 2000; Marr *et al.*, 2004; Missiuna *et al.*, 2004b).

Peter's handwriting highlighted his visual–perceptual difficulties and fine motor difficulties (Fig. 2.3), therefore a therapeutic programme was introduced

translation: Bones can't move on their own. To be able to move you need some muscles. There are lots of them. My dad knows, he is a doctor.

Legibility	4
Accurate letter formation	1
Uniformity of letter size	2
Uniformity of letter slope	1
Spacing between words and letters	2
Alignment of writing on the page	2
Total score out of a possible 30	12

Figure 2.3 Initial handwriting sample with scores.

to take Peter through a series of motor and perceptual activities related to handwriting. The 'Write from the Start' programme (Teodorescu and Addy, 1996) was selected. This programme uses a process-orientated, 'bottom-up' approach to handwriting instruction. A carefully selected and graded series of graphic activities is used to enable the child to experience various shapes, movements and connections related to writing. Additional sensory–motor activities are also used to reinforce the perceptual and motor experience.

The 'Write from the Start' programme was developed and evaluated based on the premise that, by directing the child's perceptual and motor experiences, handwriting would improve (Teodorescu and Addy, 1996; Rosenblum et al., 2003). The control trials which followed, involving over 250 children, demonstrated statistically positive changes in many components of handwriting and, in particular, those pertaining to spatial planning (Addy, 1995). Interventions using a similar approach have claimed positive results (Oliver, 1990; Lockhart and Law, 1994; Olsen, 1998; Rutberg, 1998; Peterson, 1999; Connor, 2004).

Initially the ideology underpinning the programme was explained to Peter's teacher, parents and classroom assistant. This incorporated principles of good posture, pencil grip and how to accommodate pressure through the writing instrument (Taylor, 2001). Following this, they were encouraged to follow the programme for 15–20 minutes each day. Peter's teacher was encouraged to consider other children who may benefit from help with handwriting so that a small class-based group could be formed. She was able to do this easily after the principles of the programme had been explained. Participation in a small group helped Peter to see that he was not alone in his struggles with handwriting and was motivated through both the structure and variation of the programme in addition to the support of his peers.

The introduction of the programme to the classroom was in keeping with principles of inclusion (Dunn, 2000; Mu and Royeen, 2004), but also had the benefit that consistency and practice could be established (Wright and Sugden, 1998; Pless and Carlsson, 2000). Given the shortage of occupational therapists working in paediatrics and volume of referrals, this proved an effective means of providing an intervention. The occupational therapist visited once a fortnight to monitor progress, address any concerns and provide direction where needed.

Following two school terms, a sample of Peter's handwriting was evaluated using the original criterion referenced scale (approximately 7.6 months) with positive results (Fig. 2.4).

Peter continued to use the 'Write from the Start' programme in class, supplemented by the 'Hand for Spelling' scheme (Cripps, 1995) to support his application to general writing tasks. Legibility, production and volume of output improved considerably. However, writing at speed added increasing pressure to Peter's enjoyment of the writing task; this is a common concern for children with DCD (Addy, 2004; Bezrukikh, 2005). To accommodate this he was allowed to use a dictaphone to record his weekly diary and key stories. This gave Peter an alternative method of recording his knowledge.

We eat chips and
chicken. I got a lucky
bag. Some time Later
We Set off again.

Legibility	5
Accurate letter formation	3
Uniformity of letter size	4
Uniformity of letter slope	4
Spacing between words and letters	4
Alignment of writing on the page	4
Total score out of a possible 30	24

Figure 2.4 Final handwriting sample with scores.

Objective 3: motor skills group

Gross motor/sports activities and pencil skills are of shared concern for the child with DCD (Dunford *et al.*, 2005), therefore improving Peter's motor skills was high on his personal agenda. The motor difficulties in children with DCD do not go away and have a profound effect on their self-confidence and self-esteem (Cantell and Kooistra, 2002). The majority of children with DCD are inactive in the playground, spending more time looking than participating (Smyth and Anderson, 2000; McWilliams, 2005). The resultant social isolation seems much more pronounced with boys, who typically will be active in physical sports and games from a very early age. Systematic evidence based on 23 trials involving 1821 children correlated improved motor skills with improved self-esteem (Ekeland *et al.*, 2004), therefore this was an area in which Peter needed to see success.

The PEGS assessment highlighted Peter's difficulties attempting ball games, including catch, bat and ball games and football. As Peter attended a small village school, creating a homogenous group within the school was not feasible. Therefore Peter was invited to attend an after-school programme run by both occupational therapists and physiotherapists. The venue was located at a local gym away from the hospital setting. Approximately 36 children attended and were divided into three age groups: 4–6 years, 7–9 years and 10–12 years. The advantage of such a group was that it could be non-competitive and self-paced, which according to Poulsen and Ziviani (2004) could enhance perceptions of competence and autonomy.

A cognitive–motor, task-specific ('top-down') approach was used to address Peter's motor difficulties. This considers movement as a problem-solving exercise involving action planning, action execution and action evaluation, each interacting dynamically with each other (Larkin and Parker, 2002; Sugden and Chambers, 2003).

The Cognitive Orientation to Daily Performance (CO-OP) approach was employed, which has its roots in Meichenbaum's problem solving verbal self-instructional programme (1997). CO-OP is a *'client centred, performance-based approach that enables skill acquisition through a process of strategy use and guided discovery'* (Polatajko and Mandich, 2004). There are seven key features of this approach which are essential to its success.

Motor goals

The child, in collaboration with his/her therapist and/or parent, will identify **three motor goals** which he/she would like to address. The PEGS assessment helped Peter to determine these as:

▪ To catch a ball.
▪ To kick a football.
▪ To accurately hit a ball with a bat.

To demonstrate the application of this approach, the first goal of catching a ball will be used as an example of how his learning was directed.

Dynamic performance analysis

The therapist spent some time analysing Peter's performance in throwing and catching a ball, taking into account the demands of the skill and the environmental variables. To do this Peter was observed during school play time, on the field, in the playground and in the PE hall. This is described by Polatajko *et al.* (2000) as a **dynamic performance analysis**. Peter was noted to be unable to position himself in order to execute a precise throw; could not calculate the desired effort through his upper limb proprioceptors to propel the ball; and could not accommodate the speed and size of the ball in order to catch.

Grading the task

The task was graded according to its complexity and Peter was taught cognitive strategies in order to slow down the task using the procedure 'goal, plan, check and do' with **verbal self-guidance** being encouraged as much as possible. For example, initially Peter was expected sit on the floor and roll a ball a distance of 2 m to a partner sitting opposite. Following three successful rolls, the distance is gradually increased by 0.5 m to a distance of 3 m. The grading of the task provides 'scaffolding' whereby multi-stage learning between the individual, environment and task can take place.

Feedback

Peter was then guided through the action by the therapist who provided feedback at each stage. Peter was encouraged to verbalise 'position, hold, roll' prior to each projection. Feedback served to provide information as to position, effort, posture and grip, as well as a method of motivating Peter (Magill, 2001).

Task adaptation

The tasks involved in the programme were selected as they were fun, challenging and could be adapted. Many of the tasks used to develop Peter's motor skills have since been incorporated into a school-based therapeutic PE programme, 'Get Physical' (Addy, 2006). This incorporates graded tasks and games pertinent to those goals being addressed. In this programme **task adaptation** is used to ensure success. This involves changing the nature of the demands of the task, i.e. the equipment. Therefore in developing Peter's throw and catch skills, a variety of projectiles were used: beanbags, large foam balls, Brazilian footballs, plastic footballs, balloons, medium-sized foam balls, small sponge balls and tennis bails. Additionally the rules of games were changed according to need (Dixon and Addy, 2004; Vickerman, 2005); for example, floor football was used to encourage precise rolling skills within a competitive game (Addy, 2006).

Generalisation and transfer of skills

The sixth component of this approach aims to help with the generalisation and transfer of skills by encouraging the **participation by parents and significant others** in the learning process. In Peter's case, the school became actively involved in the programme and were instrumental in utilising the actions within the class PE lessons, with the resultant benefit being felt by not only Peter but others in the class. Schmidt and Lee's (1999) study stresses the importance of selecting the right task and context, concluding that movements with no purpose and not set in context will not be as successful as those that are, and the more practice in different situations, the better. Lesson plans from the programme were provided to be implemented in school and also by Peter's parents in order to practise at home. The importance of this is reiterated by Sallis and Owen (1997), who recommend that opportunities to practise, interest in the child's activities by significant others and the quality of instruction are among the many environmental factors shown to influence skill development.

Intervention structure

The seventh and final feature of the CO-OP approach is the **intervention structure** itself and the time allocated to this. The research which supported this approach used 10 intervention sessions as the mean to address the three motor goals. Peter's sessions were structured into four 6- or 7-week programmes according to the school's term allocation. The first block focused on throwing and catching skills; the second on bat and ball skills; the third on kicking and football skills; and the fourth consolidating tasks previously acquired.

There is substantial evidence to support the CO-OP approach including systematic reviews (Pless and Carlsson, 2000; Mandich *et al.*, 2001), randomised control trials (Miller *et al.*, 2001; Sangster *et al.*, 2005) and several clinical trials (Mandich, 1997; Pless *et al.*, 2000; Segal *et al.*, 2002; Mandich *et al.*, 2003). All provided statistically significant evidence to support this approach. Indeed, Peter's Movement ABC score exceeded the goal of decreasing his Total Motor Impairment score by 5 points, by a healthy 9 points.

Objective 4: dressing skills

The fourth objective was an organisational issue which was causing Peter some distress. He simply could not get dressed and undressed quickly enough prior to and following PE lessons. He was being teased by his peers about this slowness. The difficulty proved more of a nuisance than a major concern as out of school he could wear what he liked and had plenty of time to dress. Therefore a compensatory approach was adopted so that his clothes were subtly adapted to allow them to be removed on the occasions when Peter had PE. These adaptations included replacing button holes with Velcro tabs; reattaching the cuff button with an elastic stalk to allow it to stretch negating the need to fasten a complicated button; his trouser waistband fastening was replaced with Velcro; and a matching bootlace was attached to the zipper to allow for an easy manoeuvre. On the days Peter did PE he wore his PE T-shirt instead of a vest. These adaptations proved very successful in speeding up the dressing/undressing process.

Peter was also given a dressing/undressing chart to work on at home. This was based on principles of backward chaining and was carefully graded to ensure success (Turner *et al.*, 2001). The undressing aspect was undertaken each evening, and dressing was practised over the weekend when more time was available. Peter's dressing speed increased considerably over the period of 1 year.

Critical reflection

When reflecting on Peter's therapy it is important to ask, 'Exactly **who** has the problem?' The principles of inclusion are founded on the basis that difference and diversity should be valued. However the reality of Peter's experience was that the difficulties he faced were not necessarily intrinsic to him, but rather imposed upon him by the ecological confines of the British education system and society as a whole. His handwriting struggles were made evident by the standards and expectations demanded by a National Curriculum requiring the copious use of writing as a method by which children can record their knowledge. This does not reflect the growing use of technology and reduced need to write in adult life.

The establishment of a motor skills group could seem alien to the natural context of motor learning. Henderson and Markee (2005) demonstrated how it was possible for a child with very poor coordination to succeed in becoming an accomplished rugby player and kung-fu participant. This relied on the child being self-motivated to become engaged in occupations which were purposeful, self-directed and enjoyable, within a context which would allow flexibility of task adaptation and differentiation. Perhaps the occupational therapist's role should predominantly be that of an 'enabler', seeking out the right context and task by which the child can learn alongside his/her peers, rather than as a provider of training and instruction in an alien environment. Indeed the relationship established between the therapist and Peter allowed him to ask for guidance in helping him find a suitable hobby. The occupational therapist accommodated this request by organising trial sessions in a karate class, piano lessons and a model club before Peter eventually found his niche in a local drama class.

The difficulty with such a facilitatory approach is that, fundamentally, clinical effectiveness is defined as the extent to which specific clinical interventions when deployed in the field for a particular individual or population do what they intend to do (Donaghy, 1999), the occupational therapist's role as an enabler may be difficult to quantify and qualify to an evidenced-based employing authority, despite the brief that *'professional judgements have to be informed by, but not dictated by, the evidence'* (Alsop, 1997).

Challenges to the reader

- Sensory integration is an approach commonly used to address the needs of children with DCD. Attempt to determine the evidence to affirm or dispute this approach.
- How might therapy provision change if you were referred a child of 13+ years with a diagnosis of DCD?
- How would you address the psychosocial needs of an older child with DCD?

References

Addy, L.M. (1995) *An evaluation of a perceptuo-motor approach to handwriting.* Unpublished Masters Thesis, York University

Addy, L.M. (2004) *How to Understand and Support Children with Dyspraxia.* LDA, Cambridge

Addy, L.M. (2005) Interagency collaboration. In: *Developing School Provision for Children with Dyspraxia: a Practical Guide.* Ed. Jones, N., pp. 101–110. Sage, London

Addy, L.M. (2006) *Get Physical.* LDA, Cambridge

Alsop, A. (1997) Evidence-based practice and continued professional development. *British Journal of Occupational Therapy*, **60**(11), 503

American Psychiatric Association (2000) *Diagnostic and Statistical Manual of Mental Disorders*, 4th edn – text revision. American Psychiatric Association, Washington DC

Amundson, S.J. (1995) *Evaluation Tool of Children's Handwriting* (ETCH). OT Kids, Homer

Ayres, A.J. (1972) *Sensory Integration and Learning Disorders*. Western Psychological Services, Los Angeles

Barnhart, R.C., Davenport, M.J., Epps, S.B. and Nordquist, V.M. (2003) Developmental coordination disorder. *Physical Therapy*, **83**(8), 722–731

Beery, K.E., Buktenica, N.A. and Beery, N.A. (2004) *The Beery-Buktenica Developmental Test of Visual-Motor Integration*, 5th Edn. Western Psychological Services, Los Angeles

Bezrukikh, M. (2005) Psychophysiological mechanisms of writing difficulties in schoolchildren. *Human Physiology*, **31**(5), 539–544

Cantell, M.H., Smyth, M.M. and Ahonen, T.P. (1994) Clumsiness in adolescence: educational, motor, and social outcomes of motor delay detected at 5 years. *Adapted Physical Activity Quarterly*, **11**, 115–129

Cantell, M.J. and Kooistra, L. (2002) Long-term outcomes of developmental coordination disorder. In: *Developmental Coordination Disorder*. Ed. Cermak, S. and Larkin, D., pp. 23–38. Delmar, Albany

Case-Smith, J. and Weintraub, N. (2002) Hand function and developmental coordination disorder. In: *Developmental Coordination Disorder*. Ed. Cermak, S. and Larkin, D., pp. 157–171. Delmar, Albany

Chu, S. (1997) Occupational therapy for children with handwriting difficulties: a framework for evaluation and treatment. *British Journal of Occupational Therapy*, **60**(12), 514–520

Clark, R., Mailloux, Z., Parham, L.D. and Primeau, L.A. (1991) Occupational therapy provision of children with learning disability/or mild to moderate perceptual and motor deficits. *American Journal of Occupational Therapy*, **45**, 1069–1074

Connor, C. (2004) Professional development for the future by building on the past. *Teacher Development*, **7**(1), 91–106

Cousins, R. and Thomson, D. (2001) Integrating students with physical disabilities: part 2. *British Journal of Therapy and Rehabilitation*, **8**(5), 186–190

Cratty, B.J. (1994) *Clumsy Child Syndromes: Descriptions, Evaluation, and Remediation*. Harwood Academic Publishers, Los Angeles

Cripps, C. (1995) *A Hand for Spelling*. LDA, Cambridge

Croce, R.V., Horvat, M. and McCarthy, E. (2001) Reliability and concurrent validity of the Movement Assessment Battery for Children. *Perceptual and Motor Skills*, **93**, 275–280

Crowther, D., Dyson, A. and Millward, A. (1998) *Costs and Outcomes for Pupils with Moderate Learning Difficulties in Special and Mainstream Schools*. Research Report RR89, DfEE, London

Department for Education and Skills (1978) Special Educational Needs (The Warnock Report). HMSO, London

Department for Education (1994) Code of Practice on the Identification and Assessment of Special Educational Needs. Central Office of Information, London

Department for Education and Skills (1997) Excellence for All Children: Meeting Special Educational Needs. HMSO, London

Department for Education and Skills (2001) Special Educational Needs and Disabilities Act 2001. DfES Publications, Nottingham

Department of Health (2004) National Service Framework for Children, Young People and Maternity Services. Department of Health, London

Dewey, D. (1995) What is developmental dyspraxia? *Brain and Cognition*, **29**, 254–274

Dewey, D. and Wilson, B.N. (2001) Developmental coordination disorder: what is it? *Physical and Occupational Therapy in Pediatrics*, **20**, 5–27

Diekema, S.M., Deitz, J. and Amundson, S.J. (1998) Test-retest reliability of the evaluation tool of children's handwriting-manuscript. *American Journal of Occupational Therapy*, **52**, 248–255

Dixon, G. and Addy, L.M. (2004) *Making Inclusion Work for Children with Dyspraxia: Practical Strategies for Teachers.* Routledge-Falmer, London

Donaghy, M.E. (1999) Reflections on clinical effectiveness in therapy: a practical approach. *British Journal of Therapy and Rehabilitation*, **6(6)**, 270–274

Dunford, C. and Richards, S. (2003) *'Doubly Disadvantaged' Report of a Survey on Waiting Lists and Waiting Times for Occupational Therapy Services for Children with Developmental Coordination Disorder.* College of Occupational Therapists, London

Dunford, C., Missiuna, C., Street, E. and Sibert, J. (2005) Children's perceptions of the impact of developmental coordination disorder on activities for daily living. *British Journal of Occupational Therapy*, **68(5)**, 207–214

Dunford, C., Street, E., O'Connell, H., Kelly, J. and Sibert, J.R. (2004) Are referrals to occupational therapy for developmental coordination disorder appropriate? *Archives of Disease in Childhood*, **89**, 143–147

Dunn, W. (2000) *Best Practice Occupational Therapy: in Community Service with Children and Families.* Slack, Thorofare

Ekeland, E., Heian, F., Hagen, K.B., Abbott, J. and Nordheim, L. (2004) *Exercise to Improve Self-esteem in Children and Young People.* The Cochrane Data Base of Systematic Reviews, York

Elliott, D. and McKenney, M. (1998) Four inclusion models that work. *Teaching Exceptional Children*, **30(4)**, 54–58

Erdhardt, R.P. and Meade, V. (2005) Improving handwriting without teaching handwriting: the consultative clinical reasoning process. *Australian Occupational Therapy Journal*, **52(3)**, 199–210

Foulder-Hughes, L. and Cooke, R. (2003) Do mainstream children who were born pre-term have motor problems? *British Journal of Occupational Therapy*, **66(1)**, 9–16

Gesell, A. and Ilg, F.L. (1946) *The Child from Five to Ten.* Harper, New York

Geuze, R.H., Jongmans, M.J. and Schoemaker, M.M. (2001) Clinical and research diagnostic criteria for developmental coordination disorder: a review and discussion. *Human Movement Science*, **20**, 7–47

Geuze, R.H. (2005) Motor impairment in developmental coordination disorder and activities of daily living. In: *Children with Developmental Coordination Disorder.* Ed. Sugden, D. and Chambers, M., pp. 19–46. Whurr, London

Gillberg, C. (2003) Deficits in attention, motor control, and perception: a brief review. *Archives of Disease in Childhood*, **88**, 904–910

Goyen, T.A. and Duff, S. (2005) Discriminate validity of the test of visual motor integration in relation to children with handwriting dysfunction. *Australian Occupational Therapy Journal*, **52(2)**, 109–115

Graham, S., Harris, K.R. and Fink, B. (2000) Is handwriting causally related to learning to write? Treatment of handwriting problems in beginning writers. *Journal of Educational Psychology*, **4**, 620–633

Harter, S. (1985) *Manual for the Self-Perception Profile for Children*. University of Denver, Denver

Henderson, S.E. and Markee, A. (2005) *Daniel Can Do! The Story of a Boy with Developmental Coordination Disorder*. Institute of Education, London

Henderson, S.E. and Sugden, D.A. (1992) *Movement Assessment Battery for Children*. Psychological Corporation, London

Hill, E.L. (1998) A dyspraxic deficit in specific language impairment and developmental coordination disorder? Evidence from hand and arm movements. *Developmental Medicine and Child Neurology*, **40**, 388–395

Jones, N. (2005) *Developing School Provision for Children with Dyspraxia: a Practical Guide*. Sage, London

Jongmans, M.J., Linthorst-Bakker, E., Westenberg, Y. and Smits-Engelsman, B.C.M. (2003) Use of a task-oriented self-instruction method to support children in primary school with poor handwriting quality and speed. *Human Movement Science*, **22(4–5)**, 549–566

Jongmans, M.J., Mercuri, E., Dubowitz, L.M.S. and Henderson, S.E. (1998) Perceptual-motor difficulties and their concomitants in 6 year old children born prematurely. *Human Movement Science*, **17**, 629–653

Kadasjö, B. and Gillberg, C. (2001) The co morbidity of ADHD in the general population of Swedish school-children. *Journal of Child Psychology and Child Psychiatry*, **42**, 487–492

Kamm, K., Thelen, E. and Jensen, J.L. (1990) A dynamical systems approach to motor development. *Physical Therapy*, **70**, 763–775

Kaplan, B.J., Wilson, B.N. and Dewey, D. (1998) DCD may not be a discrete disorder. *Human Movement Science*, **17**, 471–490

Ketelaar, M., Vermeer, A., t'Hart, H., van Petegem-van Beek, E. and Helders, P.J.M. (2001) Effects of a functional therapy program on motor abilities of children with cerebral palsy. *Physical Therapy*, **81(9)**, 1534–1545

Koziatek, S.M. and Powell, N.J. (2002) A validity study of the evaluation tool of children's handwriting-cursive. *American Journal of Occupational Therapy*, **56**, 446–453

Larkin, D. and Parker, H. (2002) Task specific intervention for children with developmental co-ordination disorder: a systems view. In: *Developmental Coordination Disorder*, Ed. Cermak, S. and Larkin, D., pp. 234–247. Delmar, Albany

Lockhart, J. and Law, M. (1994) The effectiveness of a multisensory writing programme for improving cursive writing ability in children with sensorimotor difficulties. *Canadian Journal of Occupational Therapy*, **61(4)**, 206–214

Losse, A., Henderson, S.E. and Elliman, D. (1991) Clumsiness in children – do they grow out of it? A 10 year follow up study. *Developmental Medicine and Child Neurology*, **33**, 55–68

Mackey, S. and McQueen, J. (1998) Exploring the association between integrated therapy and inclusive education. *British Journal of Special Education*, **25(1)**, 22–27

Magill, R.A. (2001) *Motor Learning: Concepts and applications*, 6th edn. McGraw-Hill, Madison

Mandich, A. (1997) *Cognitive strategies and motor performance in children with Developmental Co-ordination Disorder*. Unpublished Masters Thesis, University of Western Ontario, Western Ontario, Canada

Mandich, A. and Polatajko, H.J. (2005) A cognitive perspective on intervention for children with developmental coordination disorder: the CO-OP experience. In: *Children with Developmental Coordination Disorder*, Ed. Sugden, D. and Chambers, M., pp. 228–241. Whurr, London

Mandich, A., Miller, L.T. and Polatajko, H.J. (2003) A cognitive perspective on handwriting: cognitive orientation to daily occupational performance (CO-OP). *Handwriting Review*, **2**, 41–47

Mandich, A., Polatajko, H., Macnab, J. and Miller, L. (2001) Treatment of children with developmental coordination disorder: what is the evidence? *Physical and Occupational Therapy in Paediatrics*, **20(2/3)**, 51–68

Marr, D. and Cermak, S.A. (2002) Predicting handwriting performance of early elementary students with the Developmental Test of Visual-Motor Integration. *Perceptual and Motor Skills*, **95**, 661–669

Marr, D., Cermak, S., Cohn, E.S. and Henderson, A. (2004) The relationship between fine-motor play and fine-motor skill. *National Head Start Dialogue*, **7**, 84–96

McGraw, M.B. (1943) *The Neuromuscular Maturation of the Human Infant*. Columbia University Press, New York

McQueen, J. and McLellan, L. (1994) *Access to the Curriculum: a Systematic Description and Analysis of an Integrated Approach to the Education and Management of Pupils with Physical Disabilities*. University of Southampton Rehabilitation Research Unit, Southampton

McWilliams, S. (2005) Developmental coordination disorder and self-esteem: do occupational therapy groups have a positive effect? *British Journal of Occupational Therapy*, **68(9)**, 393–400

Meichenbaum, D. (1997) *Cognitive-behaviour Modification: An integrative approach*. Plenum, New York

Miller, L.T., Polatajko, H.J., Mandich, A.D. and Macnab, J.J. (2001) A pilot trial of a cognitive treatment for children with developmental coordination disorder. *Human Movement Science*, **20(1/2)**, 183–210

Missiuna, C. (1999) *Keeping Current with Children with Fine Motor Difficulties*. CanCHild, Hamilton

Missiuna, C. and Pollock, N. (2000) Perceived efficacy and goal setting in young children. *Canadian Journal of Occupational Therapy*, **67**, 101–109

Missiuna, C., Pollock, N. and Law, M. (2004a) *Perceived Efficacy and Goal Setting System (PEGS)*. Psychological Corporation, San Antonio

Missiuna, C., Rivard, L. and Pollock, N. (2004b) They're bright but can't write: developmental coordination disorder in school aged children. *Teaching Exceptional Children Plus*, **1(1)**, article 3

Mu, K. and Royeen, C.B. (2004) Interprofessional vs interdisciplinary services in school-based occupational therapy practice. *Occupational Therapy International*, **11(4)**, 244–247

O'Hare, A. and Khalid, S. (2002) The association of abnormal cerebellar function in children with developmental coordination disorder and reading difficulties. *Dyslexia*, **8**, 234–248

Oliver, C. (1990) A sensorimotor program for improving writing readiness skills in elementary-aged children. *American Journal of Occupational Therapy*, **44(2)**, 111–116

Olsen, J.Z. (1998) *Handwriting without Tears*, 8th edn. Author, Potomac

Panham, L.D. and Mailloux, Z. (1996) Sensory integration. In: *Occupational Therapy for Children*, 3rd edn. Ed. Case-Smith, J., Allen, A.S. and Nuse Pratt, P., pp. 307–356. Mosby Year Book, St Louis

Parush, S., Pindak, V., Hahn-Markowitz, J. and Mazor-Korsenty, T. (1998) Does fatigue influence children's handwriting performance? *Work*, **11**, 307–313

Peterson, C. (1999) *Effects of a handwriting intervention in at-risk first-graders*. Presentation at the American Occupational Therapy Association Conference and Exposition, Indianapolis

Pitcher, T.M., Piek, J.P. and Hay, D.A. (2003) Fine and gross motor ability in males with ADHD. *Developmental Medicine and Child Neurology*, **45(8)**, 525–535

Pless, M. and Carlsson, M. (2000) Effects of motor skill intervention on developmental coordination disorder: a meta-analysis. *Adapted Physical Activity Quarterly*, **17(4)**, 381–401

Pless, M., Carlsson, M., Sundelin, C. and Persson, K. (2000) Effects of group motor skill intervention on five to six year-old children with developmental coordination disorder. *Paediatric Physical Therapy*, **12(4)**, 183–189

Polatajko, H.J. (1999) Developmental coordination disorder; alias the clumsy child syndrome. In: *A Neurodevelopmental Approach to Specific Learning Disorder*. Ed. Whitmore, K, Hart, H. and Willems, G., pp. 119–133. MacKeith Press, London

Polatajko, H.J. and Mandich, A.D. (2004) *Enabling Occupation in Children: the Cognitive Orientation to Daily Occupational Performance (CO-OP) Approach*. CAOT Publications ACE, Ottowa

Polatajko, H.J., Fox, A.M. and Missiuna, C. (1995) An international consensus on children with developmental coordination disorder. *Canadian Journal of Occupational Therapy*, **62(1)**, 3–6

Polatajko, H.J., Mandich, A.D. and Martini, R. (2000) Dynamic performance analysis: a framework for understanding occupational performance. *American Journal of Occupational Therapy*, **54**, 55–72

Pollock, N. and Stewart, D. (1998) Occupational performance needs of school-aged children with physical disabilities in the community. *Physical and Occupational Therapy in Pediatrics*, **18**, 55–68

Poulsen, A.A. and Ziviani, J.M. (2004) Can I play too? Physical activity engagement of children with developmental coordination disorder. *Canadian Journal of Occupational Therapy*, **2(71)**, 100–107

Rainforth, B. and York-Barr, J. (1997) *Collaborative Teams for Students with Severe Disabilities: Integrating Therapy and Educational Services*. Paul Brookes, Baltimore

Rasmussen, P. and Gillberg, C. (2000) Natural outcome of ADHD with developmental coordination disorder at age 22 years: a controlled longitudinal, community-based study. *Journal of the American Academy of Child and Adolescent Psychiatry*, **39**, 1424–1431

Rigby, P. and Schwellnuss, H. (1999) Occupational therapy decision making guidelines for problems in written productivity. *Physical and Occupational Therapy in Pediatrics*, **19**, 5–7

Rintala, P., Pienimaki, K. and Ahonen, T. (1998) The effects of a psychomotor training programme on motor skill development in children with developmental language disorders. *Human Movement Science*, **17**, 721–737

Rosenblum, S., Parush, S. and Weiss, P.L. (2003) The in air phenomenon: temporal and spatial correlates of the handwriting process. *Perceptual and Motor Skills*, **96(3)**, 933–954

Rosenblum, S., Weiss, P.L. and Parush, S. (2003) Product and process evaluation of handwriting difficulties. *Educational Psychology Review*, **15(1)**, 41–81

Rutberg, J. (1998) *A comparison of two treatments for remediating handwriting disabilities*. Unpublished Doctoral Dissertation: University of Washington

Sallis, J.F. and Owen, N. (1997) *Physical Activity and Behavioural Medicine*. Sage, Thousand Oaks, California

Sangster, C.A., Beninger, C., Polatajko, H.J. and Mandich, A. (2005) Cognitive strategy generation in children with developmental coordination disorder. *Canadian Journal of Occupational Therapy*, **72(2)**, 67–77

Schmidt, R.A. and Lee, T.D. (1999) *Motor Control and Learning: a Behavioural Emphasis*, 3rd edn. Human Kinetics, Champaign

Schoemaker, M.M. and Smits-Engelsman, B.C.M. (2005) Neuromotor task training: a new approach to treat children with DCD. In: *Children with Developmental Coordination Disorder*. Ed. Sugden, D. and Chambers, M., pp. 212–227. Whurr, London

Schoemaker, M.M., Wees, M. and Van der Flapper, B. (2001) Perceptual skills of children with developmental coordination disorder. *Human Movement Science*, **20**, 111–133

Segal, R., Mandich, A. and Polatajko, H. (2002) Stigma and its management: a pilot study of parental perceptions of the experiences of children with developmental coordination disorder. *American Journal of Occupational Therapy*, **56**, 422–428

Seitz, J. (2003) The developmental test of visual-motor integration (VMI): a critique. City University of New York, *e-Working Papers in the Brain, Behavioral, and Social Sciences*. http://www.york.cuny.edu/~seitz/bio.html

Sigurdsson, E., van Os, J. and Fombonne, E. (2002) Are impaired childhood motor skills a risk factor for adolescent anxiety? Results from the 1958 birth cohorts and the National Child Development Study. *American Journal of Psychiatry*, **159**, 1044–1046

Sims, K., Henderson, S.E. and Morton, J. (1996) The remediation of clumsiness II: is kinaesthesis the answer? *Developmental Medicine and Child Neurology*, **38**, 988–997

Skinner, R.A. and Piek, J.P. (2001) Psychological implications of poor motor coordination in children and adolescents. *Human Movement Science*, **20**, 73–94

Smyth, M.M. and Anderson, H.I. (2000) Coping with clumsiness in the school playground: social and physical play in children with coordination impairments. *British Journal of Developmental Psychology*, **18**, 389–413

Sudsawad, P., Trombly, C.A., Henderson, A. and Tickle-Degnen, L. (2000) The relationship between the evaluation tool of children's handwriting and teachers' perceptions of handwriting legibility. *American Journal of Occupational Therapy*, **55**, 518–523

Sugden, D.A. and Chambers, M.E. (1998) Intervention approaches and children with developmental coordination disorder. *Paediatric Rehabilitation*, **2(4)**, 139–147

Sugden, D.A. and Chambers, M.E. (2003) Intervention in children with developmental coordination disorder: the role of parents and teachers. *British Journal of Educational Psychology*, **73**, 545–561

Sugden, D. and Chambers, M. (2005) *Children with Developmental Coordination Disorder*. Whurr, London

Summers, J. and Larkin, D. (2002) *Social relationships of children with Developmental Coordination Disorder*. Presentation at the World Federation of Occupational Therapy Conference, Sweden

Taylor, J. (2001) *Handwriting. A Teachers Guide: Multisensory approaches to assessing and improving handwriting skills*. David Fulton, London

Teodorescu, I. and Addy, L.M. (1996) *The Write from the Start Perceptuo-Motor Handwriting Programme*. LDA Ltd, Cambridge

Tseng, M.H. and Murray, E.A. (1994) Differences in perceptual-motor measures in children with good and poor handwriting. *Occupational Therapy Journal of Research*, **14(1)**, 19–36

Turner, L., Lammi, B., Friesen, K. and Phelan, N. (2001) *Dressing Workbook*. CanChild Centre for Childhood Disability Research, Canada

Vickerman, P. (2005) Adapting the PE curriculum. In: *Developing School Provision for Children with Dyspraxia: a Practical Guide*. Ed. Jones, N., pp. 86–100. Sage, London

Wallen, M. and Ziviani, J. (2005) PEGS. The perceived efficacy and goal setting system. *Australian Occupational Therapy Journal*, **52(3)**, 266–267

Wann, J.P., Mon-Williams, M. and Rushton, K. (1998) Postural control and coordination disorders: the swinging room revisited. *Human Movement Science*, **17**, 491–513

Washington, K., Deitz, J.C., White, O.R. and Schwartz, I.S. (2002) The effects of a contoured foam seat on postural alignment and upper-extremity function in infants with neuromotor impairments. *Physical Therapy*, **82(11)**, 1064–1076

Willoughby, C. and Polatajko, H.J. (1995) Motor problems in children with developmental coordination disorder: review of the literature. *American Journal of Occupational Therapy*, **49**, 787–794

Wilson, P.H. and Mc Kenzie, B.E. (1998) Information processing deficits associated with developmental coordination disorder: a meta-analysis of research findings. *Journal of Child Psychology and Psychiatry*, **39**, 829–840

Wright, H.C. and Sugden, D.A. (1998) A school based intervention programme for children with developmental coordination disorder. *European Journal of Physical Education*, **3**, 35–50

3: Early intervention: facilitating a prompt home discharge following a road traffic accident

Alis Racey

Introduction

The vital role of the occupational therapist in facilitating prompt assessment and intervention followed by smooth and timely discharge, for individuals with a post-traumatic injury, is evaluated in the context of trauma case management (Atwal and Caldwell, 2003). This chapter focuses on one individual who experienced multiple fractures following a road traffic accident. Comprehensive research involving randomised controlled trials, meta-analysis and systematic reviews support the contribution made by the occupational therapist working within the traumatic case management team (Evans *et al.*, 1995; Curtis *et al.*, 2002; Pethybridge, 2004; Taylor, 2004) in addressing early mobility and transfer skills; psychosocial support (Gustafsson *et al.*, 2000); self-care (Griffin, 2002); and education regarding healing precautions (Johnson *et al.*, 2004) within the context of the hospital and home environment. The evidence demonstrates the positive effect that rapid discharge has on the individual and his/her carers' management of the injury (Preen *et al.*, 2005), the healing process (Crotty *et al.*, 2002) and general well-being. Additional benefits relate to reduced readmission rates (Sheppherd *et al.*, 2004) and economic benefits to the National Health Service (Cameron *et al.*, 1994; Mann *et al.*, 1999).

For the young man featured in this chapter, a road traffic accident led to a serious unexpected interruption to his busy daily life. The day before the accident, Darren had had a long day at his physically demanding job after which he met his friends in the pub for a game of pool. He, like countless other people who are involved in a road traffic accident, didn't see it coming and was understandably unprepared for the disruption which followed.

Road traffic accidents occur daily and their outcomes, for many people, lead to hospital admissions and lengthy recovery programmes. The functional implications are diverse. In addition, the unexpected nature of accidents will have a psychological impact on the way that the individual is able to accept and come to terms with the event. Socially there may be a change in roles and responsibilities as well as difficulties meeting up with friends and enjoying hobbies.

Hospital resources need to be allocated in a flexible way to respond to the unplanned nature of accidents. For the occupational therapist the challenge lies in facilitating a timely discharge while addressing, and not compromising, the numerous functional difficulties which may severely restrict an individual's ability to perform their day-to-day occupations.

This chapter details the occupational therapy process from hospital admission to discharge for one particular individual admitted with fractures to an orthopaedic trauma ward. The aim of intervention at this **initial** stage is to facilitate discharge by enabling the client to perform the necessary daily functions required, while adhering to medical advice. The importance of providing a comprehensive discharge service has been supported in research by Houghton *et al.* (1996), Bridges *et al.* (1999) and McKenna *et al.* (2000). Longer-term needs will be identified and recommendations will be suggested but these will not be addressed in detail in this chapter.

Outline of the condition

Every year alarming numbers of people are seriously injured or die as a result of accidental injury. In 2004, there were 280 840 casualties reported following road traffic accidents in Great Britain, of which 3221 proved fatal (Department for Transport, 2005). Accidents resulting in injury are common during many activities such as home improvements, sports, cooking and gardening. However the impact of a road traffic accident has a significantly greater risk of resulting in a complex injury. As a consequence, for many people who have been involved in a road traffic accident, there are serious consequences in terms of time away from school or work, ability to care for children and capacity to fulfil many other life roles. Difficulties resulting from such accidents may be temporary, but for some the implications will be long term and will need to be addressed with on-going therapy intervention.

Inevitably, given the vast numbers involved, the financial cost to the National Health Service (NHS) is immense; two billion pounds each year is spent on treating injury (Department of Health, 2001a). The Government, not surprisingly, made the prevention of injury a priority as outlined in a White Paper entitled *Saving Lives: Our Healthier Nation* (Department of Health, 1999). A government task force continues work to reduce the number of accidental injuries, therefore reducing the considerable effects for the individual, society and the economy (Department of Health, 2002).

The most common outcome of trauma is limb injury (Apley and Solomon, 2001). A fracture is one type of injury which can occur; however, effects of trauma are rarely isolated to a fractured bone. When a fracture occurs soft tissue damage is likely, the extent of which is greatly influenced by the violence and impact. Soft tissue damage can include severed nerves, torn muscles, ruptured blood vessels or torn ligaments (Dandy and Edwards, 2004).

Traumatic injuries which include bone fractures are commonly addressed within orthopaedic departments. Orthopaedics as a speciality can be divided into

The principles of fracture management are:

1. Reduction of the fracture.

2. Immobilisation of the fracture fragments long enough to allow union.

3. Rehabilitation of the soft tissue and joints.

Figure 3.1 Principles of fracture management (Dandy and Edwards, 2004).

two distinct areas: trauma and elective orthopaedics. Trauma is the result of an accident which is unexpected in nature. Trauma, by definition, does not allow the planned, scheduled approach of elective surgery; hospital admissions resulting from trauma are, therefore, also unplanned and resources to deal with such admissions are more difficult to schedule.

Recovery following a fracture is determined by the timescale of bone healing. Detailed information regarding fracture healing, fracture classification and surgical management can be found in many texts such as Dandy and Edwards (2004), Apley and Solomon (2001) and Atkinson *et al.* (2005). A brief summary of the 'usual' process of fracture healing and management to provide the context on which Darren's occupational therapy was based is shown in Fig. 3.1.

The type of fracture dictates whether surgical or non-surgical reduction is required. Immobilisation can be achieved either conservatively, using splints or casts, or surgically with an internal or external fixator (Atkinson *et al.*, 2005). Once the fractured bones are united, a haematoma forms around the bone ends. This blood clot coagulates and bone cells which invade it form a hard mass which is gradually converted to callus and then bone. In the upper limb fractures to the radius/ulna can take around 6 weeks to unite, however the bone remains mobile. It takes a further 6 weeks before bone consolidation is complete. In the lower limb the healing process is longer; a fracture site around the distal third of the femur takes approximately 12 weeks to unite, whereas a fracture of the distal third of the tibia will take between 16–20 weeks to unite and consolidate (Atkinson *et al.*, 2005).

Fracture reduction and immobilisation are the remit of the doctors/surgeons. Rehabilitation, the final stage, is likely to involve other health care professionals who work with the individual to maximise functional outcomes. Immobilised limbs and reduced weightbearing status are likely to cause limitations in functional performance. An individual's unique life roles are likely to be affected and independence compromised, the extent of which is dictated by the nature and severity of the injury.

Legislation and government directives

Advances in orthopaedics are often guided by Department of Health publications which impact on resource allocation, set clinical targets and influence decision making. The NHS Plan (Department of Health, 2000) outlined targets to reduce waiting times in accident and emergency departments. This document stated that by the year 2004, no one should wait in accident and emergency for longer than 4 hours from when they arrive to the time they are either discharged, admitted to a ward or transferred. This goal has had implications on the way that individuals arriving at accident and emergency departments are assessed and treated. Assessments must be prompt and a timely decision to admit must be made so that treatment can commence without delay. Bed capacity needs to be managed effectively to meet demand. These targets aim to improve the individual's experience by providing prompt treatment.

A further way that the individual's experience in trauma orthopaedics can be improved is by ensuring that shared goals, negotiated by the multidisciplinary team, are used to promote a coordinated, timely discharge. Discharge planning was the topic of a 2004 government publication *Achieving Timely 'Simple' Discharge: a Toolkit for the Multidisciplinary Team* (Department of Health, 2004). This document provided practical steps to assist health professionals to improve discharge from the hospital to the community. Guidance included prompt assessment of the individual's needs on admission and a subsequent discharge plan to be made within 24 hours. Discharge plans must be negotiated, discussed and agreed with members of the multidisciplinary team and the client. Joint documentation is commonly used within integrated care pathways adopted by orthopaedic services to promote this coordinated approach.

A shared language and framework to describe health and health-related states, provided by the World Health Organization, was introduced in 2002 to enhance communication between health professionals. The International Classification of Functioning (ICF) provides common definitions of functioning and a means of communicating this information within the team, ensuring appropriate rehabilitation programmes and discharge arrangements. This classification acknowledges that an individual's needs may be *associated* with their medical condition. However, there is also recognition that the person's environment, support network, beliefs and personal experience also have an influence on the recovery process. These influential factors are identified during the assessment process.

Legislation has identified the need to provide housing adaptations for disabled people. The NHS and Community Care Act (Department of Health, 1990) identified that people with a disability are eligible for an assessment of their needs which may be met with housing adaptations. However, the definition of a disability, outlined in the Disability Discrimination Act (Department of Health, 1995), limits services to people who experience substantial and long-term effects on their daily performance. People who are discharged from hospital following fractures will often have substantial difficulties but are not eligible for major adaptations as the effects are not expected to be long term. For this reason, discharge provisions depend on temporary equipment, available on a short-term basis, which enables safe functioning. This may be far from ideal.

The impact of the aforementioned directives have influenced the way occupational therapy was delivered and provided for a young man following a road traffic accident.

Darren's experience

Darren O'Sullivan was admitted to the orthopaedic trauma ward late at night following a road traffic accident. He was referred to the occupational therapist the following morning by the senior house officer during the regular morning ward round.

The senior house officer reported that Darren, a 22-year-old male, lost control and fell from his motor cycle when overtaking a car. Darren sustained a closed comminuted fracture to the shaft of his right femur and a closed spiral fracture to his left tibia and fibula. Darren also sustained a Colles fracture to his right dominant wrist which was reduced in the accident and emergency department and a back slab applied.

There was no loss of consciousness and no chest pathology was identified. Darren received analgesics overnight which had adequately controlled his pain. During the ward round the radiographs were reviewed and later that day surgery was undertaken involving an intermedullary nail to provide longditudinal stability and alignment for the femoral fracture to Darren's right leg. In addition Darren's left tibia and fibular fracture were internally fixated, using plates and screws, due to the unstable nature of the fracture. No surgical action was needed for Darren's Colles fracture. A radiograph taken after the reduction showed the Colles fracture to be in a good position. The back slab was due to be changed to a rigid cast, once the swelling had subsided.

During the ward round the house officer reported that Darren lived with his parents in a semi-detached house. They had a downstairs toilet and all the bedrooms were upstairs. Darren's parents both worked and were not at home during the day. His sister lived close by. Darren was a mechanic at a local garage. The occupational therapist confirmed with the consultant that Darren was likely to need a wheelchair as the surgical procedures undertaken meant that Darren would not be able to bear weight until the fractures had healed. With this information the occupational therapist knew promptly that the provision of a wheelchair and education regarding its use would be an immediate priority. Darren had expressed concern about how long he would need to stay in hospital and when he could feasibly return to work. This indicated his desire for prompt discharge and eagerness to return to his previous roles.

Frames of reference, models and approaches

The role of the occupational therapist, when working with Darren in the acute stage, was concerned with Darren's return to his necessary roles and occupations within his home environment. In a small-scale study conducted by Griffin (2002), 19 occupational therapists working in acute orthopaedics were asked to state their aim of intervention. They identified assessment for the purpose of referral to services on discharge, discharge planning and treatment monitoring. Their intervention was characterised by assessment and intervention strategies which fitted with the short-term stay of clients in this clinical area.

Selected frames of reference, models and approaches therefore have to guide prompt and concise assessment and intervention to allow a timely return home for the individual. Any further needs must be identified and referrals made to ensure these are addressed post-discharge. An intervention approach commonly used in acute orthopaedics is **compensatory**. This allows for alterations to the way in which tasks are performed in terms of the method and the objects used (Holm *et al.*, 2003). In addition, environmental changes, aimed to facilitate independent functioning, are often made, for example temporary ramps can be provided to allow immediate access for those who are required to use a wheelchair. The compensatory approach is consistent with the biomechanical model, which predicts that when soft tissue heals and fracture sites unite, range of movement, strength and endurance will be regained which will automatically result in improvements in function (Dutton, 1995). Restoration, an alternative approach to compensation, is therefore not appropriate, as function will return as a result of the healing process rather than restorative approaches to treatment. Compensation during this stage addresses the limitations in function which occur as a result of the consultant's instruction to protect and immobilise the reduced fracture site in order to promote healing.

The **rehabilitative** frame of reference guided the occupational therapist working with Darren. This utilises a compensatory approach to address immediate needs while promoting maximum functional performance in activities of daily living using graded activities. Collaboration between the occupational therapist and the client is central to this frame of reference in order to address and seek solutions for these, often short-term, functional limitations (Seidel, 2003). It is important that an **educative approach** is also used in conjunction with a compensatory approach to explain the purpose of selected strategies to help Darren understand the healing process, the reason why precautions should be followed and the necessary timescale involved. A systematic review of a series of randomised controlled trials found that the provision of verbal and written information significantly helped individuals understand their condition, the healing process and the necessary precautions associated with it. This also resulted in increased service satisfaction (Johnson *et al.*, 2004). The provision of information promotes compliance and impacts on the successfulness of recovery (Radomski, 2002). This frame of reference was used for the duration of Darren's hospital stay.

Darren was expected to continue to use compensatory strategies following discharge which he learnt as a result of an educative approach during his hospital stay. Compensatory strategies were also used by an occupational therapist working with Darren in intermediate care. Later therapy would aim to enable Darren to return to work and would therefore utilise a **restorative approach**, following a biomechanical model, for example to develop his grip strength and range of movement in order to manipulate tools such as a wrench.

Assessment

The occupational therapist is central to the discharge arrangements, and assessment needs to happen as soon as possible to begin to identify actions which need to be taken to initiate these plans. The initial assessment began the day after surgery. Darren was feeling tired and understandably found it difficult to concentrate and the process was, therefore, continued the following day.

Central to working collaboratively with Darren was ensuring the occupational therapist had gathered an in-depth understanding of his ability and problems performing valued occupations (Cohn *et al.*, 2003). Developing a rapport with Darren was fundamental to achieving a full understanding of these factors. This relationship enabled the occupational therapist to provide support and reassurance which was necessary at this early stage post-surgery. A qualitative study by Gustafsson *et al.* (2000) used interviews to conceptualise the psychosocial rehabilitation of sixteen participants who had sustained a range of fractures. They identified that early psychosocial support had a positive effect on health-related quality of life following orthopaedic injuries. Further studies by Ponzer *et al.* (2000) and Van der Sluis *et al.* (1998) confirm these findings. Subsequent recovery is enhanced by health professionals being reassuring and building a relationship of trust. One way this was achieved was by giving information about the extent and nature of the injury and the proposed treatment.

Prior to the initial assessment the occupational therapist gathered background information about Darren's injuries, proposed surgical treatment and timescales likely for recovery and functional outcomes, both for discharge and in the long term. The medical notes reported that the surgery had gone to plan with no complications. The surgeon had written instructions for Darren to be bilaterally non-weightbearing for a period of 6 weeks. Communication with the medical staff confirmed that Darren would not be permitted to use his wrist to support his weight until a rigid cast was applied and then only minimally or as pain allowed.

An initial interview is a commonly used assessment procedure and is an essential skill for occupational therapists (Henry, 2003). The interview took the form of a conversation during which the occupational therapist asked Darren to elaborate on certain aspects of his regular roles and performance areas.

Darren's parents were present when the occupational therapist began to gather necessary information from Darren. Darren was happy for them to stay and listen to the conversation which enabled the occupational therapist to make plans with them. This was important as a client's support network has been identified as important predictor of outcome following injury (Ottosson *et al.*, 2005). Darren explained that he had a very active life, working as a mechanic for a business which was owned and run by a friend. He had an active social life and, although he lived with his parents, spent little time at home. His parents worked full-time but were willing to assist Darren at home and make any necessary environmental changes. Darren's sister was a busy mother of two small children but they expected she would be able to call in with the children most days for assistance and company.

It was important to explain to Darren and his parents that he would need to use a wheelchair for at least the first 6 weeks and would be using this when he went home from hospital. After discussing the layout of the property, it became evident that there would be some difficulties with access at home. The occupational therapist arranged to carry out a home visit without taking Darren but taking the wheelchair to check door widths and turning circles. Knowledge regarding access to each room would allow realistic goals for discharge to be set.

The conclusions from the home visit were as follows:

▨ Access: Darren could access the house along the ramped access leading to the porch and back door. The ramp was steep and Darren would need supervision or assistance to negotiate this. His parents agreed to remove some belongings to make the area more spacious. Access to the front door would not be possible for Darren in a wheelchair due the number of steps.
▨ Downstairs living area: a wheelchair would fit through the kitchen and dining room doors and into the lounge. Darren's parents agreed that the lounge area could be cleared for a single bed.
▨ Toileting: access to the downstairs toilet from the lounge was across the hall. The doors were of adequate width but the toilet was inaccessible due to a staggered doorway. Darren would need a commode or chemical toilet in the lounge.
▨ Self care: Darren was unable to access the downstairs toilet wash basin but was able to access the kitchen sink. However, the sink was a standard height, and Darren would not be able to reach the taps. He would need a bowl of water near his bed. Darren's mum was willing to bring a bowl of water to his bed side so that Darren could wash, shave and dress in the lounge.
▨ Domestic tasks: during the home visit, Darren's mother said she would leave a sandwich and drinks for Darren during the day and cook a meal for Darren at night. He could then propel the wheel chair up to the dining table and eat with his family. His sister lived close by and they expected that she would be available most days to visit during the day. Friends were also likely to call in and may bring takeaway food in for Darren.

Further functional assessments needed to be completed. Unlike other clinical settings, clinical reasoning in trauma orthopaedics often incorporates assessment and treatment within the same intervention. This is because certain predictions can, and need to, be made at this early stage of intervention. An individual, who was functionally independent prior to admission, is likely to be able to transfer from bed to wheelchair with practice. Darren was not able to transfer out of bed until his solid cast was fitted. This allowed a post-operative period of 5 days to arrange for equipment, i.e. commode, cantilever table and sliding board, to be installed at home. If these plans were made only after transfer ability had been assessed, time would be limited. On further assessment, plans can be altered if the individual does not progress as expected.

Standardised assessments were not used by the occupational therapist working with Darren. These were not commonly used by the therapy team working on the ward as it seemed possible to collect adequate information and plan treatment by carrying out functional assessments and by talking in a structured way to the client. In Griffin's study (2002), the occupational therapists working in acute orthopaedics also used few standardised assessments. Those which were used were concerned with range of movement and grip strength in people who had suffered hand injuries. The most common assessments used by the occupational therapists in Griffin's study (2002) were functional and home visits and, therefore, similar to those used with Darren.

Darren's previously independent level of function did not implicate screening forms which require information about tasks which were previously difficult for the individual, such as the Functional Independence Measure (FIM) (Uniform Data System for Medical Rehabilitation, 1997). A tool could have been used to identify priority areas for treatment, such as the Canadian Occupational Performance Measure (COPM) (Law et al., 1994) or the Mayers Lifestyle Questionnaire (Mayers, 1998) but information was collected more informally in this instance and priority areas dictated by discharge needs. In essence the assessment process is dynamic in nature and occurs as an ongoing basis throughout the therapy process (Cohn et al., 2003). Ongoing evaluation has been included in the intervention section to reflect the dynamic nature of assessment.

Clinical reasoning

The fundamental belief of the profession emphasises the importance of assessing and treating individuals in a holistic way. This was necessary in order to address the physical, psychological and social implications of the accident. A further belief is the importance of maintaining a person-centred philosophy (College of Occupational Therapists, 1994). Demands of timely discharge in the clinical area can at times challenge this principle. Darren should be included in all decision making. However, individuals are only able to stay in acute beds until they can be discharged safely. The team must prioritise the person's needs, identifying those that are essential for discharge and those which can be met at a later date, post-discharge (Atwal and Caldwell, 2003).

Clinical reasoning in orthopaedics commonly takes a procedural track, identified by Flemming (1991). This form of reasoning follows a process of identification of problems, setting goals and selecting treatment which relates to the specific diagnosis. The structured approach of integrated care pathways (ICPs) promotes condition-specific preplanned treatment and assists with communicating these stages with other members of the team. ICPs have been defined as *'structured multidisciplinary care plans which detail essential steps in the care of patients with a specific clinical problem and describe the expected progress of the patient'* (Campbell *et al.*, 1998). A pathway may have pre-set goals which the individual needs to achieve. However, if these are not relevant to a person's individual needs, amendments can be made where necessary.

ICPs are often developed locally and based on the expert opinion of health professionals working within the team, while utilising legislation and best available evidence to support practice. These usually form the treatment guideline within a team (Clark and Sheinberg, 2004).

Goal setting

Following assessment, goals are negotiated in collaboration with the client, taking into account his/her levels of pain, attitudes towards the injury and motivation to return to usual occupational roles. Goals can be subdivided into long and short term, each having their own timeframe attached. This chapter focuses on how the occupational therapist addressed Darren's immediate needs; however his long-term goals provide an indication of the whole occupational therapy process.

Long-term goals

Darren's long-term goals were to return to independent living at his parents' home and return to his paid employment as a mechanic. In order for this to happen, short-term, hospital-based goals needed to be achieved. These short-term goals would lead to a safe discharge but would not fully address return to work and independent function, for example, mobilising unaided and transferring without equipment or assistance. It was important that these needs were identified by the occupational therapist at this acute stage so that services could be arranged to meet ongoing needs at a timely interval by the appropriate service following discharge.

Short-term goals

These represent the minimum requirements to enable Darren to live at home safely with the level of support from his family with which he and his parents were happy. The goals necessitated compensatory strategies, which included altering the home environment and providing devices which would maximise independence within the constraints of his injury. Darren's parents were also involved in order to accommodate environmental changes to their home and provide assistance to Darren to enable him to perform the necessary tasks in a way that was acceptable to him.

Therefore Darren's short-term goals were that, prior to discharge, he needed to be able to:

▪ Self-propel his wheelchair short distances safely and independently.
▪ Complete necessary transfers required once discharged.
▪ Be able to wash and shave independently using a bowl of water at his bed side.

These goals would be addressed within a period of 7 days, commencing soon after his surgical recovery period (5 days post-injury). In order for the next stage of rehabilitation to occur in a timely way to meet Darren's further needs, appropriate referrals to ongoing services also needed to be completed; these arrangements would also be completed within the 7-day period.

Intervention

Goal 1   Self-propel his wheelchair short distances safely and independently

Darren was instructed by his consultant that he must be bilaterally non-weight-bearing and therefore needed to use a wheelchair until his weightbearing status had been reviewed. It was expected that, once discharged, Darren would only transfer when absolutely necessary, at first, to avoid strain on his fracture sites and to reduce oedema by keeping his legs elevated when lying or sitting on his bed.

Many considerations needed to be made in the assessment for and selection of an appropriate wheelchair. Darren was of an average height (1.7 m) and weight (95 kg) and therefore a standard size wheelchair was suitable. The wheelchair needed to be self-propelling which was difficult for Darren due to his wrist fracture. Once a solid cast was applied, the surgeon permitted Darren to use the wrist to self-propel as long as distances were kept to a minimum. This allowed Darren to be able to get around at home without assistance. Self-propelling wheelchairs, although more convenient for the individual, are wider than standard models and often access is made more difficult as a result. Darren had no difficulty gripping the wheel rim with his left hand and was previously strong in his upper body. Although he could grip the right wheel rim, this was difficult and painful, particularly at first. Darren needed to be shown how to compensate for his weaker right hand so that he could travel in a straight line. Practice in the use of the wheelchair needed to consider movement over a variety of surfaces. Polished hospital floors require considerably less effort to propel a wheelchair on than a carpeted area with limited space as would be the case in Darren's home. Therefore practice was carried out along both the long hospital corridor, and in the carpeted day room.

Weightbearing status needs to be observed, even when a person is sitting. When an individual rests his/her feet on the foot plate, weight is transferred through the limb. Depending on the stability of the fracture site this could compromise the healing process. The surgeon in this case advised that elevated leg rests were not necessary as he was confident about the fixation achieved during surgery.

The wheelchair was ordered from the integrated equipment service. These services were formed nationally in response to a government initiative to modernise and expand equipment services in health and social care by combining services which have historically run in parallel (Department of Health, 2001b). This dedicated service aims to eradicate the difficulties in acute services of meeting specific requirements and unpredictable demand with access to an often limited stock of hospital equipment available for short-term loan.

Pressure relief was not expected to be a problem in Darren's case but needs to be considered in the selection of a wheelchair. Darren would not be in the wheelchair for long periods of time and could move from side to side to relieve pressure. He needed to be educated about the potential risks involved.

It is important that a wheelchair is available for the individual to learn to transfer to and from as soon as they are able. Delays in getting up from the bed can result in medical complications. Due to Darren's wrist fracture he had to stay in bed for 5 days post-surgery until a cast was applied and he could transfer into the wheelchair. This gave the occupational therapist adequate time to obtain a wheelchair, carry out the home visit and begin to get the necessary equipment in place at home. However, careful monitoring needed to take place to ensure that this did not have an adverse effect on his medical condition. Psychologically it is important for clients to get out of bed as soon as they are medically able to. This helps the client to remain positive about their return to function and independence. While in bed, Darren was dependent on others and unaware of his ability to be able to move around on the ward.

Goal 2 Complete the necessary transfers required once discharged

When planning interventions of this type, it is important to consider the discharge environment. Darren needed to be able to transfer in a way that would enable him to perform necessary tasks which were essential for discharge. Darren could only transfer towards his left side at first so that he could rely on his left uninjured arm during the transfer.

An activity analysis enables the identification of component tasks and their requirements. Cynkin and Robinson (1990) provide a series of prompts to guide analysis of the demands of the task. These will be used to analyse Darren's necessary transfers:

▪ Description of the activity. To transfer from his bed using a sliding board to a chemical toilet, which would be placed to the left of the bed. From the toilet Darren needed to transfer to his wheelchair placed to the left of the toilet. He then needed to propel around the bed to the other side where he could transfer back into the bed to his left side.

■ Purpose. This activity represents the minimum requirement essential for discharge. A taught sequence of transfers would enable Darren to use the chemical toilet. The same method could be used to get in and out of the wheelchair if he went outside, while supervised down the ramp, or to eat at the table with his family.

■ Essential requirements. Darren would need to:

  Have adequate upper limb strength, particularly in his left arm.

  Be able to use his right arm for stability.

  Lift and place his legs.

  Have adequate knowledge of the equipment and safety factors.

  Be able to self-propel.

  Have all necessary equipment at home before discharge provided by the occupational therapist.

  Have his bed and any other furniture moved at home (to be carried out by the family).

■ Antecedent and consequent. The wheelchair would need to be positioned by Darren's family in preparation for the task. The chemical toilet could then be moved out of sight for the rest of the day.

■ Temporal activities. This sequence would only need to be carried out once a day. Darren reported that he opened his bowels once daily, usually first thing in the morning. He would have a urine bottle for the rest of the day. As Darren progressed he may choose to transfer out of bed more regularly but at first it was important that this was kept to a minimum.

A risk assessment was important to identify potential hazards. This activity can be considered to be high risk due to the need for equipment, the wheelchair, which is unfamiliar to the individual, and a significant change in the individual's functional ability. Much of the literature regarding safe handling using a sliding board has tended to include dependent individuals (Ulin *et al.*, 1997; Zhuang *et al.*, 1999). However, although the aim was for Darren to be able to complete the task independently, he required some assistance in hospital at first. Ensuring the safety of Darren and the occupational therapist was essential. Environmental hazards needed to be identified and minimised and equipment checked to ensure it was in safe working order.

Compensatory strategies need to be introduced to provide an immediate solution to concerns which, given Darren's injuries, would demand an inordinate amount of effort and energy, and which would increase the risks of further injury. Darren needed to have a single bed in the lounge. This needed to be of a comparable height to the wheelchair. A camp bed, suggested by his father would have been more convenient to move but unsuitable in terms of height and stability. The bed needed to be positioned to allow for the chemical toilet at one side and enough room for the wheelchair at the other.

There is little guidance in the literature regarding teaching clients to transfer in this way following trauma. Clinical judgement guides the stages needed and assists the practitioner to respond to the individual's ability during continual assessment and transfer practice. Grading allows the task to be broken into component parts and then taught, beginning with a reduced task, progressing to more complex ones (Holm *et al.*, 2003). Below are the treatment sessions which were required to ensure that Darren achieved his goal. These took place each day for a period of 30–45 minutes, at various times in order to observe Darren's changing levels of fatigue.

Treatment session 1

A few days after the initial interview, the occupational therapist demonstrated the functions and safety features of the wheelchair to Darren. In this way he would be familiar with it when he practised his first transfer. This also enabled the occupational therapist to have contact with Darren to ensure that they continued to develop a trusting relationship. The necessity of providing a chemical toilet was explained to Darren, and although he expressed his discomfort and embarrassment at the thought of using this, his desire for a rapid discharge helped him to accommodate and accept this equipment. The occupational therapist kept Darren informed of the delivery of the chemical toilet and any other equipment. The occupational therapist also monitored Darren's medical status and received progress updates from the physiotherapist regarding bed mobility and exercises.

Treatment session 2

The physiotherapist reported that Darren was able to sit up on the side of the bed unaided by using both elbows and his left arm and hand. The occupational therapist conducted a joint transfer assessment with the physiotherapist. Darren transferred from his bed into the wheelchair using a sliding board to his left side. Darren managed this transfer with minimal physical prompts and maximum verbal guidance. He was then wheeled to the other side of the bed and practised the same process to get back on to the bed.

Treatment session 3

The following day the same transfer was practised, this time with less verbal guidance. During this session the occupational therapist demonstrated the functions and safety features of the wheelchair to increase Darren's familiarity. Darren was also shown how to self-propel.

Treatment session 4

The same transfers were practised, this time with Darren taking responsibility for chair positioning and brakes and placing the sliding board for each transfer. He self-propelled the wheelchair while carrying the sliding board on his lap.

Treatment session 5

Darren was now confident with the transfers that had previously been practised. The sequence of transfers he would need to do at home was practised. He was able to do this safely and confidently.

Continuing practice

Darren was encouraged to practise these transfers with the nurses when he needed to use the toilet. The transfer method was documented in his care pathway so that all members of the team would know how to guide Darren.

For Darren's safety it was important that the occupational therapist ensured that he was safe to do these transfers before being allowed to do them unsupervised. This is a fine balance because if Darren received supervision for an extended time he may have become dependent on the physical prompts and reassurance offered. The Association of Chartered Physiotherapists Interested in Neurology (ACPIN) have produced guidelines on manual handling, which includes teaching someone to transfer using a sliding board (ACPIN, 2001). Although designed for a different client group, the principles can be usefully applied. If one person assists with the transfer, the individual concerned can receive assistance to set up the wheelchair, place the sliding board and remove it after the task. With supervision only, the individual would be required to do these tasks themselves. Once the person had completed these tasks consistently and safely they could be encouraged to do them independently.

Goal 3   Be able to wash and shave independently using a bowl of water at his bed side

The occupational therapists in Griffin's study (2002) identified self-care as their second most important aim in acute orthopaedics. Darren was keen to be able to wash, shave and dress independently and this needed to be achieved prior to discharge. To enable this, considerable changes needed to be made to the task method, objects and the environment.

In terms of the method, Darren would need to wash and shave at his bed side using a bowl and portable mirror. Darren needed his mother to help with preparing for the task and tidying away after. It was important that Darren was able to practise washing while sitting over the side of the bed or lying in bed on the ward. The nurses needed to be made aware that this was an aim for discharge so that he wasn't encouraged to propel to the bathroom on the ward.

Darren needed to apply the instructions about his weightbearing status when washing. By using an educative approach, the occupational therapist had informed and advised Darren on why he must not bear weight. Education relating to his weightbearing restrictions and advice about using his wrist to support his position needed to be applied to this task. In order to wash his bottom and back he was required to roll on to his side and not bridge which would involve bearing weight through his feet.

The task needed to be performed mainly unilaterally. His right hand could, however, be used to stabilise items. Darren was encouraged to keep his fingers moving to improve circulation and increase range of movement. Darren and his mother were given advice concerning how to keep the cast dry when washing.

Using these methods Darren would still not be able to wash his hair. He decided to have his hair shaved by a hairdresser who could travel to his home once he was discharged to reduce the number of times his hair would need to be washed.

Advice about the task objects was given. Pump action soap could be dispensed using one hand. A sponge could be squeezed more easily than a flannel could be wrung out. A smaller towel could be more easily negotiated for drying. Darren practised using his electric razor with one hand in hospital and was independent. In terms of the environment, a cantilever table was ordered to help Darren to have the water and mirror in a position where he could most easily reach them. His mother was willing to prepare the task.

Darren practised the task daily on the ward. He tended to wash before the occupational therapist arrived on the ward. Direct observation seemed unnecessary as Darren was able to identify problem areas and together they could problem-solve and find solutions. In this way Darren was encouraged to take responsibility for finding solutions to difficulties he encountered. Darren seemed to find this approach preferable to being observed by the occupational therapist while washing and dressing.

Referral to other services

Only those goals essential for discharge were met during the acute phase following admission. It was important, therefore, that any residual limitations were identified and services informed of Darren's discharge so that they could continue the rehabilitation process.

On discharge Darren had a solid cast on his right wrist; he was to attend the plaster room in 6 weeks to have the cast removed. Darren had an appointment to attend fracture clinic 2 weeks after discharge. He would have regular appointments and the consultant would advise when he could begin to bear weight, which was expected to be after approximately 6–8 weeks.

Darren's daily occupations would be restricted during the first 6–8 weeks; this was not due to his ability but restrictions placed on weightbearing. He was expected to continue to transfer using the same method, gaining confidence and being more proficient as pain subsided. During this period of time his opportunity for social interaction needed to be considered. Darren could not go outside unsupervised due to the steep ramped access. Opportunities for friends to visit and eventually the possibility of being able to transfer into a car needed to be considered by the occupational therapist from the **intermediate care team**. Once discharged and away from the support of the ward staff Darren may need reassurance regarding his progress. Spending time alone may lead to Darren feeling uncomfortable about the events of the night of the accident. Read *et al.* (2004) followed 65 individuals who had received traumatic injuries over a period of a year and found that 39% suffered from depression and 18% had post-traumatic stress disorder. Therefore both functional and psychological support from the intermediate care team is vital.

When the fractures began to heal intervention needed to focus on increasing Darren's mobility and transfer ability. This could occur either in the home or at an outpatient appointment. At this stage the community physiotherapist would also be involved and Darren would be invited to return to the hospital as an outpatient to receive hydrotherapy. The physiotherapist would also be able to help Darren to develop his wrist mobility and strength.

The disabled employment advisor would provide Darren with advice on benefits and allowances which he may be entitled to due to his inability to work in the short term. In the longer term, the occupational therapist working within the intermediate care team would address his work needs, introducing a work hardening programme and promoting increased wrist mobility and strength using functional tasks.

Outcome measurement

Guidance on the selection of an outcome measure can be found in various texts and publications, such as the College of Occupational Therapists information pack (Clarke, 2001). When considering outcomes, Clarke (2001) advises that it is important to be sure about what one expects to change, decide at what stage the tool should be administered and whose outcome is intended to be measured.

When considering outcome measurement, it is important to establish the indicators of the successful outcome. For an individual who has suffered extensive injuries and had surgery, like Darren, the absence of complications could be said to be a positive outcome. Due to his extensive injuries and period of time on bed rest, Darren was susceptible to developing a deep vein thrombosis, joint contractures, chest complications, pressure areas or non-/malunion. The therapy team contributed to preventing these complications by encouraging physical activity, promoting range of movement, advising on pressure relief and ensuring the protection of the fracture and surgery site during occupations.

One way to measure outcomes would be to assess the change in function by re-administering a standardised assessment. Standardised assessments were not carried out with Darren so this would not be possible. If an assessment were going to be completed again, the timing of the second phase would have to be carefully considered. Darren went home from hospital far less able than he was prior to his accident. Darren achieved the goals which were set on admission to achieve a safe timely discharge, which could be described as a positive outcome.

To evaluate critically the effectiveness of occupational therapy at this stage would be difficult due to the incomplete nature of Darren's recovery, the number of professionals involved and the unique characteristics of the individual, such as pain threshold, motivation and extent of injury. What can be evaluated are the effects of a well planned discharge regime on the individual's recovery and re-habilitation. Several studies have supported the benefits of such an approach in reducing readmission rates, increasing client's satisfaction and quality of life, not to forget the economic benefits to the NHS (Evans *et al.*, 1995; Shepperd *et al.*, 2004). Research by Curtis *et al.* (2002) demonstrated how effective multidisciplinary ICPs produce a coordinated, smooth transition from hospital to home, increasing both individual and staff satisfaction. However a systematic review of published research regarding ICPs recommended that more detailed outcomes are required to assess the continuum of care, including specific rehabilitation outcomes and long-term quality of life (Mann *et al.*, 1999). These outcomes could include issues relating to compliance, transference of skills taught within the hospital to the home and sensitive measures of functional change post-trauma (Michaels *et al.*, 1998).

Reflective analysis

Inevitably, occupational therapists need to modify their approach to meet the needs of clients in an acute setting while being mindful of bed capacity (Griffin, 1993). Darren's treatment is an example of minimum requirements for discharge being met to enable a prompt discharge. It must be noted that areas which were identified to be addressed post-discharge could have been addressed at an earlier stage if Darren had been able to stay in hospital longer or there were less pressures on the occupational therapist's time.

Darren's safety was paramount in the intervention sessions. When discharged, Darren would need to use the skills he had learnt without prompting or guidance. There was no way for the occupational therapist to know if Darren continued to complete the tasks as he had been directed. Once pain had subsided, Darren may have been tempted to become more dependent on his right hand before it had healed adequately. In addition, weightbearing status may not have been adhered to for an adequate duration. This issue of compliance is a difficult one to address. Follow-up telephone calls and subsequent home visits are often not feasible in a busy unit and would only go some way to addressing this issue.

Darren stayed in bed for 5 days post surgery. He could have been transferred out of bed for short periods using a hoist which may have increased his stimula-tion and may have been preferable for eating his meals.

Darren was not observed completing self-care activities. There is an issue here as to whether the occupational therapist can be sure that Darren was put-ting guidance into practice during the activity if this was not observed. The importance of clients being active participants in their treatment must also be considered.

Critical review

The prevention of accidental injury, including road traffic accidents is a government priority (Department of Health, 2002). The aim is to reduce the numbers of accidental deaths and serious non-fatal casualties. Two groups of pedestrians prioritised are children and older people. The numbers of pedestrian deaths and serious injuries among these populations is high but attention must be paid to how these accidents are caused so that relevant groups can be targeted. Young drivers will be targeted in the long-term plan by focusing on speed management and improved training in hazard and perceptual skills (Department of Health, 2002).

Return to work schemes need to be supportive and responsive to individuals' needs, while opportunities for re-employment need to be flexible. Financial benefits can be claimed in this country on an ongoing basis. However, if benefits were structured to make a return to work after an accident financially rewarding, opportunities offered by work hardening programmes might be used to their full potential (Mountain, 2001; Jackson et al., 2004).

The NHS plan announced major investment in intermediate care to prevent unnecessary acute admissions and to facilitate timely discharge from hospital (Department of Health, 2000). Much of these resources are directed towards older people (Department of Health, 2001c) rather than the younger population. There is a need for resources to meet the needs of *all* groups, with flexibility in the allocation of services to accommodate those who need short-term assistance and/or long-term support.

Challenge to the reader

- Are care pathways successful in prompting necessary treatment and sharing communication while being flexible enough to address patient's individual needs?
- Are there any ways that concerns regarding compliance could have been addressed?
- What factors would a standardised assessment need to include for use with an individual following the type of injuries Darren sustained?

References

Apley, A.G. and Solomon, L. (2001) *Concise System of Orthopaedics and Fractures*. Arnold, London

Association of Charted Physiotherapists Interested in Neurology (2001) *Guidance on Handling in Treatment*. ACPIN, Barnwell's Print Ltd, Norfolk

Atkinson, K., Coutts, F. and Hassenkamp, A. (2005) *Physiotherapy in Orthopaedics: a Problem-Solving Approach*. Churchill Livingstone, London

Atwal, A. and Caldwell, K. (2003) Profiting from consensus methods in occupational therapy: using a Delphi study to achieve consensus on multiprofessional discharge planning. *British Journal of Occupational Therapy*, **66(2)**, 65–70

Bridges, J., Meyer, J., Davison, D., Harris, J. and Glynn, M. (1999) Smooth passage. *Health Services Journal*, 17 June, 24–25

Cameron, I., Lyle, D. and Quine, S. (1994) Cost effectiveness of accelerated rehabilitation after proximal femoral fracture. *Journal of Clinical Epidemiology*, **47(11)**, 1307–1313

Campbell, H., Hotchkiss, R., Bradshaw, N. and Porteous, M. (1998) Integrated care pathways. *British Medical Journal*, **316**, 133–137

Clark, K. and Sheinberg, A. (2004) A model to illustrate the process of decision making in acute care discharge planning. *Australian Occupational Therapy Journal*, **51(4)**, 213–214

Clarke, N. (2001) *Outcome Measures: Information Pack for Occupational Therapists*. College of Occupational Therapists, London

Cohn, E.S., Boyt Schell, B.A. and Neistadt, M.E. (2003) Introduction to evaluation and interviewing. In: *Willard and Spackman's Occupational Therapy*. Ed. Crepeau, E.B., Cohn, E.S. and Boyt Schell, B.A., pp. 279–285. Lippincott Williams and Wilkins, Baltimore

College of Occupational Therapists (1994) *Patient Focused Care: Guidelines for BAOT Members*. College of Occupational Therapists, London

Crotty, M., Whitehead, C.H., Gray, S. and Finucane, P.M. (2002) Early discharge and home rehabilitation after hip fracture achieves functional improvements: a randomized controlled trial. *Clinical Rehabilitation*, **16(4)**, 406–413

Curtis, K., Lien, D., Chan, A., Grove, P. and Morris, R. (2002) The impact of trauma case management on patient outcomes. *Journal of Trauma – Injury Infection and Critical Care*, **53(3)**, 477–482

Cynkin, S. and Robinson, A.M. (1990) *Occupational Therapy and Activities Health: Towards Health through Activities*. Little, Brown and Co., Boston

Dandy, D.J. and Edwards, D.J. (2004) *Essential Orthopaedics and Trauma*. Churchill Livingstone, London

Department of Health (1990) *The NHS and Community Care Act*. HMSO, London

Department of Health (1995) *Disability Discrimination Act*. HMSO, London

Department of Health (1999) *Saving Lives: Our Healthier Nation*. HMSO, London

Department of Health (2000) *The NHS Plan*. HMSO, London

Department of Health (2001a) *Reforming Emergency Care*. HMSO, London

Department of Health (2001b) *Guide to Integrated Community Equipment Services*. HMSO, London

Department of Health (2001c) *National Service Framework for Older People*. HMSO, London

Department of Health (2002) *Preventing Accidental Injury: Priorities for Action*. HMSO, London

Department of Health (2004) *Achieving Timely 'Simple' Discharge: a Toolkit for the Multidisciplinary Team*. HMSO, London

Department for Transport (2005) *Transport Statistics Bulletin: Road Casualties in Great Britain, Main Results 2004*. HMSO, London

Dutton (1995) *Clinical Reasoning in Physical Disabilities*. Lippincott Williams and Wilkins, Baltimore

Evans, R., Connis, R., Hendricks, R. and Haselkorn, J. (1995) Multidisciplinary rehabilitation versus medical care: a meta-analysis. *Social Science and Medicine*, **40(12)**, 1699–1706

Flemming, M.H. (1991) The therapist with the three track mind. *American Journal of Occupational Therapy*, **45**, 1007

Griffin, S. (2002) Occupational therapy practice in acute care neurology and orthopaedics. *Journal of Allied Health*, **32**(1), 35–42

Griffin, S.D. (1993) The effect of short bed stays on the delivery of occupational therapy services in teaching hospitals. *Archives of Physical Medicine and Rehabilitation*, **74**, 1087–1090

Gustafsson, B.A., Nordstrom, G., Ponzer, S. and Lutzen, K. (2000) The role of interactive affirmation in psychosocial rehabilitation after orthopaedic injury. *Journal of Orthopaedic Nursing*, **5**, 9–14

Henry, A.D. (2003) The interview process in occupational therapy. In: *Willard and Spackman's Occupational Therapy*. Ed. Crepeau, E.B., Cohn, E.S. and Boyt Schell, B.A., pp. 285–297. Lippincott Williams and Wilkins, Baltimore

Holm, M.B., Rogers, J.C. and James, A.B. (2003) Interventions for daily living. In: *Willard and Spackman's Occupational Therapy*. Ed. Crepeau, E.B., Cohn, E.S. and Boyt Schell, B.A., pp. 491–533. Lippincott Williams and Wilkins, Baltimore

Houghton, A., Bowling, A., Clarke, K., Hopkins, A. and Jones, I. (1996) Does a dedicated discharge coordinator improve the quality of hospital discharge? *Quality in Health Care*, **5**, 89–96

Jackson, M., Harkess, J. and Ellis, J. (2004) Reporting patient's work abilities: how the use of the standardised work assessments improved clinical practice in Fife. *British Journal of Occupational Therapy*, **67**(3), 129–132

Johnson, A., Sandford, J. and Tyndall, J. (2004) *Written and Verbal Information versus Verbal Information Only for Patients being Discharged from Acute Hospital Settings to Home*. Cochrane Database for Systematic Reviews, Issue 1

Law, M., Baptiste, S., Carswell, A., Mc Coll, M., Polatajko, H. and Pollock, N. (1994) *The Canadian Occupational Performance Measure*, 2nd edn. Canadian Association of Occupational Therapists, Toronto

Mann, N.C., Mullins, R.J., MacKenzie, E.J., Jurkovich, G.J. and Mock, C.N. (1999) Systematic review of published evidence regarding trauma system effectiveness. *Journal of Trauma – Injury Infection and Critical Care*, **47**(3), S25–S33

Mayers, C.A. (1998) An evaluation of the use of the Mayers' Lifestyle Questionnaire. *British Journal of Occupational Therapy*, **61**(9), 393–398

McKenna, H., Keeney, S., Glenn, A. and Gordon, P. (2000) Discharge planning: an exploratory study. *Journal of Clinical Nursing*, **9**, 594–601

Michaels, A.J., Michaels, C.E., Moon, C.H., Zimmerman, M.A., Peterson, C. and Rodriques, J.L. (1998) Psychosocial factors limit outcomes after trauma. *Journal of Trauma*, **44**, 644–648

Mountain, G. (2001) *Work Rehabilitation and Occupational Therapy: a Review of the Literature*. College of Occupational Therapists, London

Ottosson, C., Nyren, O., Johansson, S.E. and Ponzer, S. (2005) Outcomes after minor traffic accidents: a follow-up study of orthopaedic patients in an inner-city area emergency room. *Journal of Trauma – Injury Infection and Critical Care*, **58**(3), 553–560

Pethybridge, J. (2004) How team working influences discharge planning from hospital: a study of . four multi-disciplinary teams in an acute hospital in England. *Journal of Interprofessional Care*, **18**(1), 29–41

Ponzer, S., Molin, U., Törnkist, H., Bergman, B. and Johansson, S.E. (2000) Psychosocial support in rehabilitation after orthopaedic injuries. *Journal of Trauma*, **48**, 273–279

Preen, D.B., Bailey, B.E.S., Wright, A., Kendall, P., Phillips, M., Hung, J., Hendriks, R., Mather, A. and Williams, E. (2005) Effects of a multidisciplinary, post-discharge continuance of care intervention on quality of life, discharge satisfaction, and hospital length of stay: a randomized controlled trial. *International Journal for Quality in Health Care*, **17**(1), 43–51

Radomski, M.V. (2002) Planning, guiding and documenting therapy. In: *Occupational Therapy for Physical Dysfunction*. Ed. Trombly, C.A. and Radomski, M.V., pp. 443–461. Lippincott Williams and Wilkins, Baltimore

Read, K.M., Kufera, J.A., Dischinger, P.C., Kerns, T.J., Ho, S.M., Burgess, A.R. and Burch, C.A. (2004) Life-altering outcomes after lower extremity injury sustained in motor vehicle crashes. *Journal of Trauma – Injury Infection and Critical Care*, **57**(4), 815–823

Seidel, A.C. (2003) Rehabilitative frame of reference. In: *Willard and Spackman's Occupational Therapy*. Ed. Crepeau, E.B., Cohn, E.S. and Boyt Schell, B.A., pp. 238–240. Lippincott Williams and Wilkins, Baltimore

Shepperd, S., Parkes, J., McClaren, J. and Phillips, C. (2004) *Discharge Planning from Hospital to Home*. The Cochrane Database of Systematic Reviews, Issue 1

Taylor, C. (2004) A model to illustrate the process of decision making in acute care discharge planning. *Australian Occupational Therapy Journal*, **51**(4), 213–214

Ulin, S., Chaffin, D.B., Patellos, C. and Blitz, S. (1997) A biomechanical analysis of methods used for transferring totally dependent patients. *Scientific Nursing*, **14**(1), 19–27

Uniform Data System for Medical Rehabilitation (UDSMR) (1997) *Guide for the Uniform Data Set for Medical Rehabilitation* (including the adult FIM). State University of New York at Buffalo, Buffalo

Van der Sluis, C.K., Eisma, W.H., Groothoff, J.W. and Duis, H.J. (1998) Long term physical, psychological and social consequences of severe injuries. *Injury*, **29**, 281

World Health Organization (2002) *Towards a Common Language for Functioning, Disability and Health*. World Health Organization, Geneva

Zhuang, Z., Stobbe, T.J., Hsiao, H., Collins, J.W. and Hobbs, G.R. (1999) Biomechanical evaluation of assistive devises for transferring residents. *Applied Ergonomics*, **30**, 285–294

4: Enhancing the quality of life for a person living with multiple sclerosis

Anne Longmore

Introduction

The National Health Service and Social Care Model (Department of Health, 2005b) provides a useful framework from which to demonstrate how occupational therapists can work to empower clients with long-term conditions to self-manage their symptoms and maximise independent living (Baker and Tickle Degnen, 2001). The results of adopting such an approach have been far-reaching in improving the quality of life of individuals with multiple sclerosis (Benito-Leon *et al.*, 2003). Quality of life, although a personal and multidimensional phenomenon, includes issues relating to physical health, psychological well-being, level of independence, relationships with others and spiritual beliefs. The evidence supports intervention relating to these issues and includes energy conservation (Vanage *et al.*, 2003; Mathiowetz *et al.*, 2005); sustaining activities of daily living (Månsson and Lexell, 2004); independent self-care (O'Hara *et al.*, 2002); maintaining an appropriate living environment (Peachey-Hill and Law, 2000); and the provision of timely assistive devices (Verza *et al.*, 2006), in addition to issues relating to health promotion (Neufeld and Kniepmann, 2001), coping skills (Schwartz, 1999) and vocational support (Dyck and Jongbloed, 2000). The physical and practical appreciation of clients' needs, together with the understanding of psychological concerns, endorse the occupational therapist as a key professional in this field.

In the ministerial forward in the recent national service framework for long-term conditions (Department of Health, 2005a), reference is made to the fact that services must be developed for people who are living with long-term conditions. The focus of these services is threefold: to improve quality of life, to support people in managing symptoms and to enable independent living.

This chapter will present a small part of one woman's experience in managing her long-term condition, demonstrating how occupational therapy can contribute to improving the quality of life, symptom management and maintenance of independent living. Multiple sclerosis was chosen to discuss in this context because multiple sclerosis occurs in middle adult life and is the most common neurological condition in people under 65 (Neurological Alliance, 2003). Also, unlike a complete spinal cord injury or a stroke, having multiple sclerosis is insidious and Shirley not only has to live with a diagnosis but the unpredictable nature of the disease process and the effect this has on her and particularly her family unit (Wollin, 2002).

Occupational therapy for people who have a spinal cord injury or a stroke is usually delivered by a specialist service in secondary care (Smith, 2002). However, a person living with multiple sclerosis will only be admitted to a hospital ward at a point of crisis or during a relapse; neither of which are opportune times to address health promotion or improving quality of life. The definition of quality of life used in healthcare is rooted in the World Health Organization Quality of Life 100 (WHOQOL 100) framework, which defines quality of life as an individual's perception of their position in life in the context of the culture and value systems in which they live, and in relation to their goals, expectations, standards and concerns (Power et al., 1999; Hobart et al., 2001). The important point in this definition is that quality of life can only be determined from the individual's perspective, so a person-centred approach is required.

The occupational therapy process discussed in this chapter is a 4-week period of rehabilitation that was initiated by Shirley's GP. As the focus of the intervention is on health promotion and improving quality of life, the episode of care is during a remission rather than a relapse and takes place in Shirley's home environment.

Outline of the condition: multiple sclerosis

Multiple sclerosis is a degenerative unpredictable neuro-immunological disease of the central nervous system: brain, spinal cord and optic nerves. Random attacks of inflammation damage the myelin sheath resulting in the loss of the insulation around the axons, which in turn causes scarring, therefore the velocity of the action potentials reduces (Snell, 2001). It is the location of the scarring that determines the symptoms experienced.

Symptoms that people experience include:

- Visual disturbances, such as blurring, diplopia, optic neuritis.
- Loss of balance: tremor, ataxia, vertigo, clumsiness and lack of coordination.
- Weakness and fatigue.
- Altered sensation: tingling, numbness and burning feeling.
- Altered movement: speed, weakness, spasticity, coordination and dexterity.
- Altered speech: slowing of speech, slurring of words, rhythm of speech changing and unable to portray emotion when communicating.
- Difficulty swallowing.
- Pain.
- Fatigue.
- Bladder and bowel problems.
- Problems with cognition and memory.

The first clinical signs of multiple sclerosis generally occur when a person is in their late 20s, 30s or early 40s, which in life stages terms is a time when relationships, parenting and developing careers are pertinent issues (Polman and Uitdehaag, 2000; MS Trust, 2001; De Judicibus and McCabe, 2005). However, it is important to note that, although multiple sclerosis is degenerative in nature, life expectancy is not significantly reduced (Finlayson, 2004). In the UK, 85 000 people live with multiple sclerosis and, of these, two thirds are women (National Collaborating Centre for Chronic Conditions (NCCCC), 2004).

The cause of multiple sclerosis is unknown but research indicates that there are three predetermining factors: the autoimmune system, the environment and genetics (Snell, 2001). The pathogenesis of multiple sclerosis is associated with an autoimmune process, but evidence that people with multiple sclerosis have a unique immunological abnormality is sparse (Polman and Uitdehaag, 2000). The environment is also a determinant, as the prevalence is greater in temperate countries with numbers decreasing nearer the equator. Studies in the UK suggest that the prevalence rate in England and Wales is between 100 and 120 per 100 000 but rises to 190 per 100 000 in Scotland (MS Trust, 2001). Whether this is due to environmental or genetic factors continues to be a topic for research. Although research indicates that multiple sclerosis is not directly inherited, current research is investigating whether, with a genetic predisposition, there is a reaction to some environmental agent that, upon exposure, triggers an autoimmune response (NCCCC, 2004).

Having established that multiple sclerosis is a long-term condition it is imperative that occupational therapists understand that there are different classifications of multiple sclerosis and that the clinical presentation of multiple sclerosis will be different for each person. As well as the clinical presentation being different, how this affects the person's daily life depends on much more than the disease classification.

Classification of multiple sclerosis

There are four types of multiple sclerosis:

- Benign multiple sclerosis.
- Relapsing/remitting multiple sclerosis.
- Secondary progressive multiple sclerosis.
- Primary progressive multiple sclerosis.

Statistically the majority of people living with multiple sclerosis have relapsing and remitting multiple sclerosis.

Benign multiple sclerosis

It would be extremely unusual for an occupational therapist to work with a person who has been given the diagnosis of benign multiple sclerosis. This diagnosis is only made when a person has experienced occasional relapses over a 15-year period and makes a full recovery after each relapse (MS Trust, 2001). However, in the 15 years prior to diagnosis of benign multiple sclerosis he/she may have been seen by an occupational therapist during a relapse either in secondary care or in the person's own home.

Relapsing/remitting multiple sclerosis

The majority of people living with multiple sclerosis have relapsing and remitting multiple sclerosis. There does not appear to be a consensus on the actual percentage of people with this classification, as numbers vary from 60–85%. The reason for this may be that the higher percentage is pertaining to classification at diagnosis. When a person is living with relapsing and remitting multiple sclerosis they usually experience one or two relapses each year. Unfortunately these relapses can be very disruptive as the timeframe and presentation are very unpredictable. For example, a relapse may feel like having flu, in that the person feels fatigued for 4 or 5 days and then recovers, or it may be that the person is incontinent of urine for 6 weeks.

Whilst it may be the case that after each relapse a person has 'full recovery', in many cases the person will say that although they have improved they don't feel 'back to normal'. In the case of the person with continence problems he/she may say that they are no longer incontinent but they now go to the toilet more frequently.

At this point people may begin to alter their routines and how they do ordinary everyday tasks. Fisher (1998) states that it is the role of occupational therapists to enable people to perform the actions they need and want to perform so they can engage in and do the familiar, ordinary, goal-directed activities of each day. Somerset *et al.* (2002) state that having personal control in everyday situations has a direct effect on quality of life and that family members often take over roles in the home; but the person with MS is usually reticent in criticism of the family member. For example a spouse may have taken over the task of shopping at the supermarket while his/her partner is having a relapse and may then never relinquish the role. Compensatory strategies must be reviewed during remission, otherwise personal control diminishes, dependency increases and the person is then deprived of participating in ordinary everyday tasks.

Secondary progressive multiple sclerosis

50% of people who were initially diagnosed with relapsing and remitting MS will develop secondary progressive MS within 10 years from their initial diagnosis (NCCCC, 2004). In real terms this means that there may be an increase in both the number of relapses and the number of symptoms the person is experiencing. Additionally the number of remissions may reduce and each time the person has a relapse they may be further limited or be unable to participate in everyday activities.

This may be difficult for the person and their family to accept, as for 7 or 8 years they have accepted and grown accustomed to adjusting their life for short periods of time and now they need to make major changes to their home or their daily routines. For example, if a lady had relapsing and remitting multiple sclerosis, her spouse may previously been happy to carry her up and downstairs during a relapse, as each relapse only lasted for 3 weeks. When this becomes a long-term problem, his immediate response may be to cease employment rather than considering adaptations to the home. McKeown *et al.* (2004) found that, although carers recognise that they need support, they were unwilling to ask for help and it was only at crisis point that they agreed to have input from outside agencies. Hakim *et al.* (2000) reported that caring for a family member does effect career development and 36% of relatives reduce work commitments to provide care to their relatives rather than asking for help from outside agencies. This, in turn, causes a decline in standard of living with reduced income and this continues to be a problem as the financial impact of the disease increases with age (De Judicibus and McCabe, 2005).

Primary progressive multiple sclerosis

Primary progressive multiple sclerosis is the most aggressive form of the disease, in that once a symptom presents there is a continual deterioration with no remissions. Only 10–15% of those diagnosed have this type of multiple sclerosis, and the incidence is higher when multiple sclerosis is diagnosed after the age of 45.

Coping with continuous change is challenging for the person with primary progressive multiple sclerosis, their family and the occupational therapist. For example, one week the person may report that he/she has difficulty getting out of bed and the occupational therapist supplies a piece of equipment for the person to use to move from sitting to standing. Then the following week the person reports that he/she can no longer move from lying to sitting in bed. Regular intervention from the occupational therapist will affect whether the person is able to remain in his or her own home rather than be admitted to a nursing home (Finlayson *et al.*, 2005).

The long-term nature of multiple sclerosis

Having considered that there are different classifications of multiple sclerosis it is important to note that, apart from primary progressive multiple sclerosis, the transition from independence to dependence occurs over a number of years. An example of this is how the equipment the person requires for walking changes: for 2 or 3 years the person may use a walking stick, then for 3 years he/she uses two walking sticks, then uses a Zimmer frame for 3 years and eventually 12 years after diagnosis uses an attendant wheelchair for outdoor use. In short, the person is living with a long-term condition which is unpredictable and enduring.

Whilst a person with multiple sclerosis is indeed living with a long-term condition, it is important to remember that this is different for each person and they may perceive their multiple sclerosis as episodes of illness rather than a long-term condition. There are several personal accounts which describe multiple sclerosis as living with something or someone lurking in the shadows or a enemy lying in wait for its prey (Mackie and Brattle, 1999; Nichols, 1999).

The challenge for the occupational therapist is to enable and empower the individual living with a long-term condition to participate in, and enjoy life, providing consistency and continuity while addressing both the physical and psychosocial needs of the individual.

Government directives

Government directives have been influential in the way occupational therapy is provided.

NHS and Social Care Model

The Department of Health has responded to the demand to meet the needs of those with a long-term condition by developing the **NHS and Social Care Model** (Department of Health, 2005b) (Fig. 4.1) to support local innovation and integration of services. The primary purpose of this model of care is to reduce hospital admissions for people living with long-term conditions, as the specific target is to reduce inpatient emergency bed days by 5% (Department of Health, 2005b, p. 5). However this model does provide an opportunity to change existing health and social services that are reactive, unplanned and episodic. Interestingly this model is a model for social services *and* the National Health Service which clearly shifts the focus of services from services delivered by secondary care to primary care services.

As this hierarchical model will be implemented for people living with multiple sclerosis, it is important to reflect what the profile of occupational therapy services should be in each level of care.

Level 1: supporting self health care

The core focus of this level is to provide information to the person living with MS about their clinical condition (National Multiple Sclerosis Society, 2000). The method advocated is for all primary care trusts to have an **expert patient programme** (NHS, 2005) for people living with a long-term condition. Expert patient

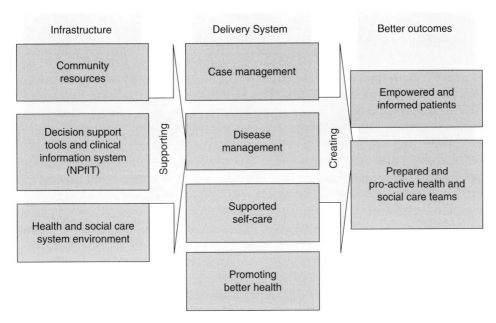

Figure 4.1 The NHS and Social Care Long-Term Conditions Model (Department of Health, 2005b).

programmes are a relatively new concept in the UK and are aimed at those living with a long-term health condition, who are able to take more control over their health by understanding and managing their conditions, leading to an improved quality of life (O'Hara *et al.*, 2000). Web resources are provided by the NHS to standardise the content of the programme. The 6-week programme (2–3 hours per week) is led by lay people and is not condition specific.

Comprehensive evidence supports such empowering programmes (Schwartz, 1999; Vanage *et al.*, 2003). However, participating in an expert patient programme is only the beginning of self-management, as the person will have to implement the strategies learnt on the programme. Occupational therapists are not involved in the organisation of expert patient programmes but may be asked to provide information or be a guest speaker at one of the sessions. Occupational therapists need to be aware of the content of these programmes and the available literature on multiple sclerosis websites, particularly the MS Society, MS Trust and MS International Federation websites. These websites have downloadable information sheets, guidance how to access services, forums for contacting other people with multiple sclerosis and research updates.

Level 2: disease/care management

In order to have effective case management or disease management a proactive approach is essential. Successful proactive approaches are dependent on partnership between the patient and the providers of health and social care to anticipate potential issues. Guidance suggests that a multidisciplinary team in the community is necessary to achieve this (Rijken and Dekker, 1998; NCCCC, 2003). The structure of these teams may vary. For example, in rural areas the team may serve the total population and use specialist services in secondary care as a resource; on the other hand, in a city there may be a specific multidisciplinary team for people with multiple sclerosis. The focus of either multidisciplinary team will be rehabilitation as defined by Wade and Bareld (2000): a reiterative, active, educational, problem-solving process focused on a person's behaviour including assessment, goal setting, intervention and evaluation. The effectiveness of any multidisciplinary team can be measured by using the MS Society measuring success toolkit, which has been in existence since 1997 (National Multiple Sclerosis Society, 2006).

Level 3: case management

If a person has multiple long-term conditions then case management is warranted. A community 'matron' manages cases but services to the person are provided by the primary care services, including the multidisciplinary team. People with primary progressive multiple sclerosis may require this form of case management due to frequent admissions and difficulties in addressing their ever-changing care packages. Older people with multiple sclerosis will also require case management due to multiple pathology, such as heart disease and chest infections, and poly pharmacy (Department of Health, 2001; Finlayson, 2004).

National Service Framework for Long-Term Conditions

In addition to the NHS and Social Care Model (2005), the National Service Framework for Long-Term Conditions (Department of Health, 2005a) will be influential in structuring services for people with MS. Introduced just 2 months after the NHS and Social Care Model, this framework aims to deliver a *'person-centred service that is efficient, supportive and appropriate from diagnosis to the end of life'* (Department of Health, 2005a, p. 5). There are eleven quality requirements recommended with an implementation date of 2015. Four of these are particular to the client in this chapter:

- Quality requirement 1: a person-centred service.
- Quality requirement 5: community rehabilitation and support.
- Quality requirement 7: providing equipment and accommodation.
- Quality requirement 10: supporting families and carers.

Guidelines

A further document, *Multiple Sclerosis: Management of Multiple Sclerosis in Primary and Secondary Care Clinical Guideline 8* (NCCCC, 2003), refers to identifying best practice from researched evidence. This uses a grading system adapted from Eccles and Mason (2001), rather than the hierarchy of evidence referred to in Chapter 1 (Sackett *et al.*, 1996).

The guidelines are a useful resource for occupational therapists and advocate a person-centred approach. Key words and phrases in the guidelines include: problem-based approach, responsive service, seamless service and active involvement of the person with multiple sclerosis. There are seven guidance statements, of which the following three are particular to the client who will be described in this chapter:

▨ 1.2 Teamwork.
▨ 1.6 Rehabilitation and maintenance of functional activities and social participation.
▨ 1.7 Managing specific impairments.

Shirley's pathway

Shirley is a 42-year-old lady who lives with her husband and two children. They live in a semi-detached house in the suburbs of a city. Shirley moved to this area when she married Richard 16 years ago. They have two daughters: Sophie who is eight and Clare who is fourteen. Richard's parents and his sister live nearby. Shirley stopped working after the birth of their second child and Richard works as a manager in a local electrical store. He recently declined promotion as he feels that his present job enables him to be available to come home quickly if Shirley needs his help during the day.

Shirley was diagnosed with multiple sclerosis 12 years ago, but hasn't used any rehabilitation services for 6 years apart from an annual appointment with a neurologist. As she was able to walk and was independent in all personal activities of daily living she had not ever thought to inform the neurologist that everyday domestic tasks were difficult.

The referral to the multidisciplinary team arose when Shirley was seen by her GP for an annual review as the practice provides an enhanced service for people with multiple sclerosis (Primary Care Contracting, 2004). At this review Shirley explained to the GP that she had stopped going out of her house on her own as she was very embarrassed that she was so uncoordinated and appeared as if she was 'drunk'. In her narrative with the GP she also described that she felt her house was chaotic and she was concerned that her children had to help her with the housework. For a person living with multiple sclerosis, having limitations in everyday occupations influences the level of personal independence and quality of life (Somerset *et al.*, 2002; Benito-Leon *et al.*, 2003; Månsson and Lexell, 2004);

this was certainly true for Shirley. Shirley felt frustrated that her role as home maintainer was being eroded and blamed her physical/neurological symptoms for the change in her status. These symptoms are frequently highlighted as the biggest source of frustration for those with multiple sclerosis (Smith and Arnett, 2005).

Shirley discussed these issues with the GP and they both decided that Shirley may benefit from input from the community rehabilitation team. The community rehabilitation team was a new service, which had been established as a response to the National Service Framework for Long-Term Conditions (Department of Health, 2005a) and as a means to provide level 2 care of the NHS and Social Care Model (Department of Health, 2005b). The community rehabilitation team considered the reasons for referral and, together with the guidance identified through the various government directives, selected specific frames of reference, models and approaches from which to base their clinical reasoning.

Models and approaches

In order for Shirley to participate in meaningful everyday occupations she needs to develop an understanding of why she has changed, how she completes tasks and how the symptoms she is experiencing effect function. Therefore a **rehabilitative frame of reference** is required (Wade and Bareld, 2000). This would enable Shirley to achieve maximum function in the performance of her daily activities (Seidel, 2003). This would involve the use both a **restorative approach** and an **educational approach**. The application of these approaches will be evident later in the chapter when discussing intervention to enable Shirley successfully to iron her clothes.

To frame the rehabilitation programme the NHS and Social Care Model (Department of Health, 2005b) was used to guide practice in the selection of appropriate assessment tools and modes of intervention. This generic model serves as an organising technique to assist in categorising ideas and structuring approaches in order to think about complex problems. In 1996, Christiansen highlighted the fact that health care was rapidly changing and that *anticipation and management* of illness would be a focus of health care in the future. Christiansen (1996) further states that 'consumers' would not only want to be involved in decision making in relation to their health, but they would also have a role in influencing and managing their own health.

The 'self management' and 'disease management' level of the NHS and Social Care Model is particularly appropriate, as Shirley is both motivated and has the cognitive ability to succeed. Enabling Shirley to have personal control through self-management and providing appropriate intervention without Shirley losing personal locus of control can only be achieved through collaborative practice.

This self-managing, person-centred philosophy is very important, as people with multiple sclerosis do not form a homogenous group. Individuality, beliefs, personal circumstances and the course of the disease result in a complex and changing range of needs and preferences (Somerset *et al.*, 2002). Vaughan *et al.* (2003) reiterated the importance of understanding that people with multiple sclerosis have *different* illness identities that will influence participation in rehabilitation and so will subsequently affect outcomes.

The Person–Environment–Occupation Model (Law *et al.*, 1996) was also used to analyse the various interactions involved in the occupations which Shirley had identified as causing her some concern (see Fig. 8.4). This model is concerned with the interaction and fit between the person, their environment and the occupation. It enables the therapist to be sensitive to the subtle changes that may occur when one part of the triad is altered. For example, a slight change to Shirley's environment may influence pacing, energy conservation and, ultimately, occupational success (Peachey-Hill and Law, 2000).

Assessment

After receiving a referral the multidisciplinary team completed a **screening assessment** within 7 working days from receipt of referral. This screening assessment parallels the single assessment process for older people (Department of Health, 2001), where basic information and overview information is gathered in order to identify need for particular services. A person-centred approach is embedded in this approach, which asks Shirley to describe 'a day in her life'; this should include any changes to her 'usual' routine rather than identifying a list of impairments and problems.

This approach is aligned to the International Classification of Function (World Health Organization, 2002) as it helps to identify participation restrictions and, to some extent, activity limitations. The severity of problem was also recorded using the language of the ICF:

1 = mild 5–24%.
2 = moderate 25–49%.
3 = severe 50–95%.
4 = complete 96–100%.

For example one participation restriction for Shirley was going out to the pub with her husband. This restriction could have been caused by any of the following factors:

- Environmental restriction: the pub that they like to go to is always crowded; the toilet is upstairs and Shirley is apprehensive that she will bump into people when she is going upstairs. The environmental restrictions are the stairs and people. Shirley rated this restriction as a 1 as she could use the toilet at home before and after she went to the pub.
- Activity limitation: Shirley feels she is no longer able to write the answers to the pub quiz. The activity limitation is being unable to write legibly. Shirley

rated this as a 3 as she felt that each week her writing was getting worse and if she couldn't write she didn't want to continue going to the pub quiz.

This screening assessment takes the form of an ethnographic interview where the interviewer is the learner and the interviewee is the information expert. During such an interview, both Shirley and the professional involved reflect on the present situation in order to derive a consensus regarding treatment goals (Bhasin and Goodman, 1992).

The following example is an extract from the interview narrative:

Shirley: 'Preparing meals is more difficult for me but I can manage. I can do everything like this morning I got up 20 minutes earlier and I made the breakfast for everyone and I'll clear the table and do the washing up before the children come home from school.'

The identified facts from this include:

- The length of time taken to complete tasks has doubled.
- Shirley feels frustrated and wants to prove to her family that she is able to maintain her roles as wife and mother.
- Shirley is frightened that other people will take over her roles.
- Shirley is motivated to continue doing normal every day tasks.

Shirley identified that to participate in everyday occupations consistently was her priority, therefore the multidisciplinary team decided that the first professional assessment should be completed by the occupational therapist (Månsson and Lexell, 1998). Had Shirley's speech been difficult to understand, or had she complained of having difficulty eating her breakfast after she prepared the meal, the speech and language therapist would have completed the first professional assessment.

The occupational therapist arranged an appointment with Shirley. Rowles (2003) described home as territory, a place of ownership that may be fiercely defended. Shirley described the kitchen as her territory and that she spent most of her day in the kitchen. The kitchen was a large modern U-shaped kitchen with floor- and wall-mounted cupboards and there was a round table with four chairs in the middle of the room. However, every worktop was cluttered with papers, a wash basket, shopping, clothes and clutter. Shirley had to move numerous magazines from the table and chairs on to the floor to create a space for the occupational therapist and her to sit down.

Working in Shirley's home enabled the occupational therapist to establish a therapeutic relationship and observe Shirley participating in everyday occupations. During the visit Shirley was introduced to the **Multiple Sclerosis Impact Scale** (MSIS-29) (Hobart et al., 2004) (Fig. 4.2). This is designed as a short, simple assessment with a summative rating scale. It is a reliable and valid measure of both the physical and psychological impact of multiple sclerosis (Riazi et al., 2002; Hobart et al., 2001).

Shirley was given the assessment in paper format and asked to read each of the 29 statements and then decide which of the five point responses best described

Multiple Sclerosis Impact Scale (MSIS-29)[a]

- The following questions ask for your views about the impact of MS on your day-to-day life **during the past two weeks**
- For each statement, please **circle** the **one** number that **best** describes your situation
- Please answer **all** questions

In the <u>past two weeks</u>, how much has your MS limited your ability to …	Not at all	A little	Moderately	Quite a bit	Extremely
1. Do physically demanding tasks?	1	2	3	4	5
2. Grip things tightly (e.g. turning on taps)?	1	2	3	4	5
3. Carry things?	1	2	3	4	5

In the <u>past two weeks</u>, how much have you been bothered by …	Not at all	A little	Moderately	Quite a bit	Extremely
4. Problems with your balance?	1	2	3	4	5
5. Difficulties moving about indoors?	1	2	3	4	5
6. Being clumsy?	1	2	3	4	5
7. Stiffness?	1	2	3	4	5
8. Heavy arms and/or legs?	1	2	3	4	5
9. Tremor of your arms or legs?	1	2	3	4	5
10. Spasms in your limbs?	1	2	3	4	5
11. Your body not doing what you want it to do?	1	2	3	4	5
12. Having to depend on others to do things for you?	1	2	3	4	5
13. Limitations in your social and leisure activities at home?	1	2	3	4	5
14. Being stuck at home more than you would like to be?	1	2	3	4	5
15. Difficulties using your hands in everyday tasks?	1	2	3	4	5
16. Having to cut down the amount of time you spent on work or other daily activities?	1	2	3	4	5
17. Problems using transport (e.g. car, bus, train, taxi, etc.)?	1	2	3	4	5
18. Taking longer to do things?	1	2	3	4	5
19. Difficulty doing things spontaneously (e.g. going out on the spur of the moment)?	1	2	3	4	5
20. Needing to go to the toilet urgently?	1	2	3	4	5
21. Feeling unwell?	1	2	3	4	5
22. Problems sleeping?	1	2	3	4	5
23. Feeling mentally fatigued?	1	2	3	4	5
24. Worries related to your MS?	1	2	3	4	5
25. Feeling anxious or tense?	1	2	3	4	5
26. Feeling irritable, impatient, or short tempered?	1	2	3	4	5
27. Problems concentrating?	1	2	3	4	5
28. Lack of confidence?	1	2	3	4	5
29. Feeling depressed?	1	2	3	4	5

[a] © Neurological Outcome Measures Unit, Institute of Neurology, University College London, WCIN 3BG, 2001.

Figure 4.2 Multiple Sclerosis Impact Scale (MSIS) (with permission of HMSO).

her situation. It took Shirley less than 5 minutes to complete the assessment and the results of her assessment were 65 in the physical scale and 22 in the psychological scale. Whilst these results demonstrate that Shirley was generally attributing 'limiting ability' to physical problems, the next stage of the assessment was to discuss the extent to which her MS affected participating in certain occupations. The following were highlighted as Shirley's concerns:

- Difficulties carrying and placing objects.
- Being clumsy.
- Tremor of arms and legs.
- Being stuck at home more than she would like to be.
- Having to cut down the amount of time spent on work or other daily activities.
- Needing to go to the toilet urgently.
- Feeling irritable, impatient or short tempered.
- Lack of confidence.

The occupational therapist then asked Shirley to describe and discuss reasoning why these activity/participation limitations were impacting her lifestyle.

- Carry things:

   Shirley: I can't do my shopping any more because I can't lift the bags out of the trolley into my car without dropping things out of the bags. This means that I have to take one of the children with me or my husband has to do the shopping on Sunday and he never gets it right.
   The most irritating thing is that I can't carry things up and down stairs. Take clothes as an example. I've spent ages ironing and folding them downstairs and then by the time I've carried them upstairs they're wrinkled.

- Being clumsy:

   Shirley: It seems as if I haven't any problems if I'm sitting down but if I'm standing up I can only use one hand at a time. The most irritating thing is that I have to sit down, for example I can't open my purse and get money out if I'm standing up. These little things are really irritating me now.

- Tremor:

   Shirley: This is weird, it seems to happen when I'm reaching upwards such as washing my hair or putting the dishes away in the high wall cupboards. I hate that other people have to help me now.

In discussion Shirley identified that these three limitations contributed to why she had highlighted the other statements. From Shirley's narrative the occupational therapist was aware that the underlying cause of all three limitations was ataxia. **Ataxia** is the collective term for motor control deficits caused by damage to the cerebellum or motor and sensory pathways providing information relating to movement (Gillen, 2000; Edwards, 2003). However, Shirley is experiencing different movement problems associated with cerebellar ataxia in particular situations.

The principal reason that Shirley is having difficulty putting her shopping in the car is that she has **dysmetria**. Dysmetria is lack of coordination of movement typified by under- or over shooting the intended position with the hand, arm, leg or eye. Dysmetria of a hand can make writing and picking things up difficult or even impossible. Dysmetria that involves undershooting is called hypometria and overshooting is called hypermetria (MS Trust, 2001). This is evident when Shirley attempts to place grocery shopping in the car boot; when she reaches to place of groceries into the car, she undershoots the movement to lift the bag over the boot ledge and, because the bags are very full and made of light plastic, items fall out either into the boot or on to the ground.

Shirley explained that she also had difficulty carrying the ironing upstairs. This task demands **multi-joint movements** at the trunk and legs to walk up the stairs, plus her upper limbs are in a flexed pattern holding the ironing. **Dys-synergy** affects her coordination in this task. Dyssynergy is the term used to describe the jerky movements, which occur as a consequence of reduced synergy in the agonist and antagonist muscles (Edwards, 2003).

Shirley's poor coordination was also apparent during bilateral tasks, such as ironing, which requires bilateral upper limb coordination while maintaining a standing position. When Shirley stands for more than 1 minute it is difficult for her to maintain postural control *and* use her arms simultaneously, therefore she adopts a compensatory position which triggers a lumbar lordosis, an anterior tilted pelvis, flexion at the hips, hyperextension of the knees, weightbearing on her heels and clawing to her toes to increase her stability (Stokes, 2002).

Shirley also experiences an **intention tremor** when reaching upwards. Tremor is a rhythmical involuntary oscillatory movement that can occur at rest or during movement (Shumway-Cook and Woollacott, 2001). An intention tremor is not present at the beginning of a movement but develops and increases towards the end of a movement. Shirley described in more detail that when washing her hair as the tremor increased her hands moved involuntarily to her face and shampoo got in her eyes. Therefore her husband or eldest daughter now washed her hair.

Further assessment could have included an assessment of Shirley's cognition using tools such the as Everyday Memory Questionnaire (Tariot, 1985). The fact that Shirley described her home as 'chaotic' may have indicated struggles with home organisation, which could be caused by short-term memory loss (Langdon and Thompson, 1999). However, concerns regarding her memory were not evident on initial assessment; also, the evidence regarding programmes to improve cognitive skills in people with multiple sclerosis is not conclusive (Lincoln *et al.*, 2002).

In addition the Nottingham Extended Activities of Daily Living Scale (SF-36) (Nicholl *et al.*, 2002), the Multiple Sclerosis Quality of Life Inventory (MSQLI) (Ritvo *et al.*, 1997), Functional Assessment of Multiple Sclerosis (FAMS) (Cella *et al.*, 1996) and Fatigue Description Scale (FDS) (Iriarte *et al.*, 1999) could have helped to inform the community rehabilitation team of Shirley's needs. These tests have been evaluated in reviews by Fischer *et al.* (1999) and Higginson *et al.* (2000).

The purpose of this current period of intervention therefore is to improve Shirley's ability to regulate and control posture and movement within the context of her everyday occupations (Giuffrida, 2003) and in doing so improve energy conservation (Hemmett *et al.*, 2004; Mallik 2005). Shumway-Cook and Woollacott

(2001) propose that learning in relation to motor control is most likely to occur in tasks and environments that are meaningful for the person. Shirley had already received printed literature about ataxia from the MS society site but the occupational therapist explained that associative learning would be used in intervention, as movement is easier to understand through observation and sensory feedback. The use of person-focused, professionally guided programmes in the management of multiple sclerosis has been found to be very effective in maintaining the individual's independence. O'Hara et al. (2002), using a randomised controlled trial involving 189 people with multiple sclerosis, found that a guided self-care programme involving both written and context-related verbal advice maintained levels of independence 6 months later in contrast to the control group which showed a significant decrease in independence.

Goal setting

The first quality requirement highlighted by the National Service Framework for Long-Term Conditions (Department of Health, 2005a) emphasises the importance of supporting people in managing their own condition, maintaining independence and achieving the best possible quality of life. Goals were set in collaboration with Shirley and would be achieved within 1 month. Shirley was particularly concerned that she was beginning to lose her role as home maintainer therefore all of the goals relate to her role as home maintainer.

Long-term goal

The long-term goal is to improve Shirley's ability to regulate and control posture and movement within the context of her everyday occupations, in order to maintain her locus of control as home maintainer.

Short-term goals

- To explain static and dynamic postural responses in relation to a variety of routine occupations.
- To apply postural adjustment and movement principles in order to successfully iron the family's clothes.
- To apply postural adjustment and movement principles to enable Shirley to issue her children's dinner money without dropping the coins.

Intervention

Intervention focused on changing skills, knowledge and attitude. Initially Shirley needed to understand how her body moved when participating in everyday occupations and appreciate her posture when in a standing position. This involved direct education by the occupational therapist. This was subsequently applied to specific practical occupations which had been identified as a particular source of frustration for Shirley. The Person–Environment–Occupation Model (Law *et al.*, 1996) was used to structure intervention; this focuses on the complex dynamic relationships between people, occupations and environments (Strong, 1999). The occupational therapist or the rehabilitation assistant visited three times each week for a period of 1 month to ensure that skills taught were fully understood and generalised within other occupations.

Goal 1: explain static and dynamic postural responses and movement in relation to a variety of routine occupations

Initially it was important to describe to Shirley 'usual' patterns of movement and how she was unconsciously compensating for her ataxia which resulted in her appearing clumsy, developing poor patterns of movement, which in turn affected her energy conservation. Information regarding movement was given both verbally and in written form, with direct examples of how this would affect function. Certain principles were then taught to correct these patterns of movement. These involved altering the centre of mass/gravity, improving postural stability, dynamic weight transference, grading movements, encouraging slow reversals of movement and the use of rhythmical movement (Stokes, 2002). These principles were then applied to specific occupations which were of particular concern to Shirley. Education regarding posture, movement, environmental adaptations and energy conservation has proved to be an effective way to increase self-efficacy and improve quality of life (Mathiowetz *et al.*, 2005).

Goal 2: application to occupation – ironing

Person

The occupation of ironing was a particular source of frustration for Shirley. Shirley did all the ironing in the home but recently had changed her routine from ironing twice a week to ironing for short periods each day. This necessitated her having her ironing board set-up permanently in the kitchen, which affected the appearance and space available in the environment.

Maintaining her stability in standing whilst ironing was a challenge for Shirley, as her centre of mass was too far forward resulting in vertical malalignment. Shirley had adopted a compensatory postural strategy by engaging more muscular effort: increased hip flexion, hyperextension of the knees and dorsiflexion of the ankles. Additionally when using her right arm to iron she did not protract and retract her shoulder girdle but used abduction and adduction at the shoulder joint. Shirley understood that by doing this she was overusing certain muscle groups and was keen to alter how she moved rather than using adaptive or compensatory strategies.

Environment

The ironing board was adjacent length wise to the worktop on the left of the fridge and there was only a 15 cm gap, therefore Shirley was unable to open the cupboards above or below the ironing board due to reduced arc of reach (Jacobs, 1999). There was a round washing basket overflowing with clothes placed on the worktop in front of the ironing board.

Occupation

Tools

The tools used included a 30 cm plastic jug for water and a lightweight steam iron, which was plugged in to the right of the ironing board above the worktop, therefore the first 30 cm of lead was on the worktop. As Shirley did all of the ironing there was a variety in shape and weight of garments varying from king-size sheets to her daughter's T-shirts.

Routines

Shirley described that as she spent most of her time in the kitchen at some point in the day she ironed the top four items in the ironing basket and if the basket was overflowing she ironed a few extra that day.

Sequence of tasks

Switch on the radio, walk to the sink and fill a jug of water, walk back to the ironing board and pour water into the iron, plug in the iron, reach forward to wash basket for one item, iron the item, place iron on worktop, fold the item on the ironing board, lift iron and iron the folded garment, place iron on the worktop, turn 180° and put item on the table.

Addressing concerns

To address these concerns Shirley needed to alter her centre of gravity at the ironing board to improve stability and arc of reach. Shirley's normal stance position involved standing with feet 15 cm apart. When ironing Shirley has to have **mediolateral stability** rather than anterior–posterior stability (required when, for example leaning forward over the sink to fill the iron's jug with water), as the motion of ironing involves a right-to-left action involving midline crossing. Mediolateral postural control is generated at the hip and trunk rather than the ankle so Shirley had to be taught to stand with her feet directly in alignment with her hips and feel the position of her hips and trunk during ironing; for example, when the iron crossed her midline from the right to the left she had to consciously transfer her body weight from her right to left leg without engaging movement at the ankles, and that when moving to the right her head should move slightly to the left. Then when ironing from the left to the right she needed to move exactly the same amount but in the opposite direction (Shumway-Cook and Woollacott, 2001). The occupational therapist identified that moving from a lateral to midline to an anterior position and then to a mid position increased the motor demands of the task, so it was decided to alter the task to exclude this sequence of movement. The task of ironing was to be adapted so that Shirley only had to move the iron from a lateral to medial to lateral position. This required a change in the environment and the occupation. The environment was adapted by placing the ironing board at right angles to the plug socket, the ironing basket to the right of the ironing board on a chair with the top of the basket in alignment with the top of the ironing board and the table to the left of the ironing board.

Equipment, such as a perching stool, could have been provided to help compensate for Shirley's postural and functional difficulties, however Shirley was reluctant to resort to this at present. There is evidence that a person's engagement with, and professionals' approach to, the provision of such devices has implications for compliance in their use (Verza et al., 2006).

With the support and guidance of the occupational therapist Shirley was able to continue to undertake the family's ironing using a better posture which enabled her to stand for longer periods. The application of postural and movement principles were also applied to other occupations involving prolonged standing, i.e. cooking.

Goal 3: application to occupation – issuing dinner money to children

Shirley's children both had school dinners and each had to take £1.40 to school each day. Shirley was becoming incredibly frustrated that it took her at least two minutes to remove her purse from her handbag and then open the purse. On two occasions her eldest daughter has got angry with Shirley and grabbed the purse and taken the money out herself. As discussed earlier Shirley wants to retain the locus of control in her own home.

Person

There were several difficulties identified by the occupational therapist when observing Shirley perform this task. Shirley used a lateral key grip rather than using a pinch grip to pick up the coins; poor postural control affected her trunk stability; Shirley held the purse at breast level rather than waist level which reduced her ability to see into the purse and when she looked down she was tilting her hips in an anterior direction by positioning the purse so high that the only way she could pick up the coins was by pronating her forearm which subsequently restricted her view, because of the position of her hand.

Environment

Shirley kept her handbag in the hall and each morning her eldest daughter carried the bag into the kitchen and placed the bag on the table. The table was cluttered with papers, and the handbag was often placed with the opening at the side rather than the top. The occupation became increasingly stressful as Shirley's eldest daughter would stand very close to Shirley and impatiently wait for the money. This is not an unusual response from a child with a parent who has multiple sclerosis; Yahav *et al.* (2005) found that children often expressed frustration and anger at the extra sense of burden and obligation, in having a parent with a deteriorating condition.

Occupation

Tools

The handbag was a soft leather shoulder bag 30 cm × 15 cm with a zip fastening and the purse was 12 cm × 9 cm with a paper money section and a zipped section for coins.

Routines

Money was removed from the purse after the children had breakfast and approximately 1 minute before they went to school.

Sequence

Walk to the table, stand at the table, open the zip of the handbag, using her right hand remove the purse, hold purse with left hand, open zipped section, pick out £1 coin and 40p change and hand money to her daughter.

Addressing concerns

To address this issue Shirley was asked if she could identify possible problem areas. She correctly identified that this was a posterior–anterior movement and that she should try moving her left leg back, a principle taught as she stood at the sink. This did improve the postural control.

The occupational therapist was then able to show Shirley that by lowering the purse to waist height and extending her right wrist into 25° extension she could use a pinch grip and see into her purse. Although this addressed the problem of dexterity the demands of the task were exacerbated by the context of the task. A coping strategy of removing the money the night before and leaving it on the hall table for the girls was a preferred option, as Shirley remained in control of the task and a stressful situation avoided. However, Shirley wanted to practise using her purse when standing so again it was arranged that the rehabilitation assistant would do this regularly for 1 month.

Outcome measures

Through her excellent level of participation and application of knowledge Shirley became an active participant in her rehabilitation and continued to identify tasks and occupations that she thought she may be able to do *better*. In this first episode of care the impairments were primarily motor but if Shirley developed fatigue or cognitive problems the same approach may not be productive. The community rehabilitation team continued to visit Shirley and work with her to achieve goals identified. The most striking change was that within the period of 1 month, Shirley had de-cluttered the kitchen as she felt that her environment contributed so much to whether she was able to participate in occupations.

A meta-analysis of the current best evidence for the use of occupational therapy with clients with multiple sclerosis suggests that occupational therapy is effective in improving capacity and ability, postural control and range of movement, and occupations relating to self-care, although more detailed analysis is recommended at a life role level (Baker and Tickle-Degnen, 2001).This is reiterated by the systematic review by Steultjens *et al.*, (2003) of occupational therapy for multiple sclerosis.

However, there is evidence that a comprehensive rehabilitation programme, such as that provided for Shirley, has a significant impact on the person's quality of life (Somerset *et al.*, 2001). A randomised controlled trial demonstrated significant improvements in all health-related quality of life domains including physical and social functioning (Patti *et al.*, 2002); this was reiterated in a follow-up study (Patti *et al.*, 2003).

Shirley achieved all her goals within the specified timeframe; in addition the MSIS 29 was repeated at the end of intervention, with the caution to the client that scores may rise rather than fall. Shirley's physical score had decreased, but only by 5 points; in addition the psychological score also decreased by 5.

This was not the conclusion of occupational therapy for Shirley as the benefits she had gained from such intensive involvement led Shirley to ask for further guidance regarding her other aspects of her occupational performance with which she was struggling. These included:

- Accessing the w.c. at her local pub.
- Writing her answers during the local pub quiz.
- Transferring her groceries into the car from the supermarket trolley.
- Reaching to take objects from a high cupboard.

Reflective analysis

The experience of Shirley leads us to ask the question: 'When is the optimal time for intervention?' Shirley was seen by the community rehabilitation team at a time when she was willing to participate in rehabilitation and not at a time of crisis. Too often occupational therapists meet the person living with multiple sclerosis at a time of crisis, i.e. during a hospital admission during a relapse or the community occupational therapist assessing for equipment or adaptations. Should a professional be introduced to the person as a potential contact shortly after diagnosis, so that any small concerns or issues can be resolved as they arise? This obviously has resource issues but is a model advocated in both the National Service Framework for Long-Term Conditions (Department of Health, 2005a) and the guidelines for multiple sclerosis (NCCCC, 2003). However the timing of contact and the provision of information should be directed by the person with multiple sclerosis, not the professional, as Ward *et al.*, (2004) have identified that too much information at the wrong time can have negative effects in that clients can begin to 'expect' and 'anticipate' alterations in function.

The current legalisation and guidelines provide the framework for a change in provision of services to people with multiple sclerosis. It is hoped, with the expert-patient programmes, individuals will become aware of how they can analyse their own occupations in order to enhance and empower themselves in participating in the normal everyday things.

Challenges to the reader

- In this chapter a rehabilitative approach was used to address the first goal. What could the occupational therapist have recommended if using an adaptive or compensatory approach?
- Which type of multiple sclerosis may not benefit from a rehabilitative approach and why?

References

Baker, N.A. and Tickle-Degnen, L. (2001) The effectiveness of physical, psychological, and functional interventions in treating clients with multiple sclerosis: a meta-analysis. *American Journal of Occupational Therapy*, **55**(3), 324–331

Benito-Leon, J., Morales, J.M., Riveera-Navarros, J. and Mitchell, A.J. (2003) A review about the impact of multiple sclerosis on health-related quality of life. *Disability and Rehabilitation*, **22**, 288–293

Bhasin, C.A. and Goodman, G.D. (1992) The use of OT FACT categories to analyse activity configurations of individuals with multiple sclerosis. *The Occupational Therapy Journal of Research*, **12**(2), 67–80

Cella, D.F., Dineen, K., Arnason, B., Reder, A., Webster, K.A. and Karabatsos, G. (1996) Value of the Multiple Sclerosis Quality of Life Instrument. *Neurology*, **4**, 187–206

Christiansen, C. (1996) Nationally speaking. Managed care: opportunities and challenges for occupational therapy in the emerging systems of the 21st century. *American Journal of Occupational Therapy*, **50**(6), 409–412

De Judicibus, M.A. and McCabe, M.P. (2005) Economic deprivation and its effects on subjective wellbeing in families of people with multiple sclerosis. *Journal of Mental Health*, **14**(1), 49–59

Department of Health (2001) *National Service Framework for Older People*. HMSO, London

Department of Health (2005a) *National Service Framework for Long-Term Conditions*. HMSO, London

Department of Health (2005b) *Supporting People with Long-Term Conditions: An NHS and Social Care Model to Support Local Innovation and Integration*. HMSO, London

Dyck, I. and Jongbloed, L. (2000) Women with multiple sclerosis and employment issues: a focus on social and institutional environments. *Canadian Journal of Occupational Therapy*, **67**(5), 337–346

Eccles, M. and Mason, J. (2001) How to develop cost-conscious guidelines. *Health Technology Assessment*, **5**(16), 1–78

Edwards, S. (2003) *Neurological Physiotherapy a Problem-Solving Approach*. Churchill Livingstone, London

Finlayson, M. (2004) Concerns about the future among older adults with multiple sclerosis. *American Journal of Occupational Therapy*, **58**(1), 54–63

Finlayson, M., Van Denend, T. and DalMonte, J. (2005) Older adults' perspectives on the positive and negative aspects of living with multiple sclerosis. *British Journal of Occupational Therapy*, **68**(3), 117–124

Fischer, J.S., LaRocca, N.G., Miller, D.M., Ritvo, P.G., Andrews, H. and Paty, D. (1999) Recent developments in the assessment of quality of life in multiple sclerosis (MS). *Multiple Sclerosis*, **5**(4), 251–259

Fisher, A. (1998) Uniting practice and theory in an occupational framework. *American Journal of Occupational Therapy*, **52**(7), 509–521

Gillen, G. (2000) Improving mobility and communication in an adult with ataxia. *American Journal of Occupational Therapy*, **56**(4), 462–466

Giuffrida, C.G. (2003) Motor learning: an emerging frame of reference for occupational performance. In: *Willard and Spackman's Occupational Therapy*. Ed. Crepeau, E.B., Cohn, E. and Schell Boyt, B.A., pp. 267–275. Lippincott Williams & Wilkins, Philadelphia

Hakim, E.A., Bakheit, A.M.O., Bryant, T.N., Roberts, M.W.H., McIntosh-Michaelis, S.A., Spackman, A.J., Martin, J.P. and McLellan, D.L. (2000) The social impact of multiple sclerosis – a study of 305 patients and their relatives. *Disability and Rehabilitation*, **22**(6), 288–293

Hemmett, L., Holmes, L., Barnes, M. and Russell, N. (2004) What drives quality of life in multiple sclerosis? *QJM: An International Journal of Medicine*, **97**(10), 671–676

Higginson, C., Arnett, P.A. and Voss, W.D. (2000) The ecological validity of clinical tests of memory and attention in multiple sclerosis. *Archives of Clinical Neuropsychology*, **15**(3), 185–204

Hobart, J.C., Lamping, D.L. and Fitzpatrick, R. (2001) The Multiple Sclerosis Impact Scale (MSIS-29); a new patient-based outcome measure. *Brain*, **124**, 962–973

Hobart, J.C., Riazi, A., Lamping, D.L., Fitzpatrick, R. and Thomson, A.J. (2004) Improving the evaluation of therapeutic interventions in multiple sclerosis development of a patient-based measure of outcome. *Health Technology Assessment*, **8**(9), 45–46

Iriarte, J., Katsamakis, G. and De Castro, P. (1999) The fatigue descriptive scale (FDS): a useful tool to evaluate fatigue in multiple sclerosis. *Multiple Sclerosis*, **5**(1), 10–16

Jacobs, K. (1999) *Ergonomics for Therapists,* 2nd edn. Butterworth Heinemann, Boston

Langdon, D.W. and Thompson, A.J. (1999) Multiple sclerosis: a preliminary study of selected variables affecting rehabilitation outcome. *Multiple Sclerosis*, **5**(2), 94–100

Law, M., Cooper, B., Strong, S., Stewart, D., Rigby, P. and Letts, L. (1996) The Person-Environment-Occupation Model: a transactive approach to occupational performance. *Canadian Journal of Occupational Therapy*, **63**(1), 9–23

Lincoln, N.B., Dent, A., Harding, J., Weyman, N., Nicholl, C., Blumhardt, L.D. and Playford, E.D. (2002) Evaluation of cognitive assessment and cognitive intervention for people with multiple sclerosis. *Journal of Neurology, Neurosurgery, and Psychiatry*, **72**(1), 93–98

Mackie, C. and Brattle, S. (1999) *Me and My Shadow: Living with Multiple Sclerosis*. Aurum Press Ltd, London

Mallik, P.S., Finlayson, M., Mathiowetz, V. and Fogg, L. (2005) Psychometric evaluation of the Energy Conservation Strategies Survey. *Clinical Rehabilitation*, **19**(5), 538–543

Månsson, E. and Lexell, J. (2004) Performance of activities of daily living in multiple sclerosis. *Disability and Rehabilitation*, **26**(10), 576–585

Mathiowetz, G., Finlayson, M., Marcia, L., Matuska, K.M., Chen, H.Y. and Luo, P. (2005) Randomized controlled trial of an energy conservation course for persons with multiple sclerosis. *Multiple Sclerosis*, **11**(5), 592–601

McKeown, L., Porter-Armstrong, A. and Baxter, G. (2004) Caregivers of people with multiple sclerosis: evidence of support. *Multiple Sclerosis*, **10**(2), 219–230

MS Trust (2001) *Multiple Sclerosis Information for Health and Social Care Professionals*. Multiple Sclerosis Trust, Letchwood

National Collaborating Centre for Chronic Conditions (2003) *Multiple Sclerosis: Management of Multiple Sclerosis in Primary and Secondary Care: Clinical Guideline 8*. National Institute for Clinical Excellence (NICE), London

National Collaborating Centre for Chronic Conditions (2004) *Multiple Sclerosis: National Clinical Guideline for Diagnosis and Management in Primary and Secondary Care*. National Institute for Clinical Excellence (NICE), London

National Health Service (2005) *Expert patients programme*. http://www.expertpatients.nhs.uk/ (accessed 11 January 2006)

National Multiple Sclerosis Society (2000) *Multiple Sclerosis in 2000: A Model of Psychosocial Support*. http://www.mscare.org/pdf/mssp.pdf (accessed 9 December 2005)

National Multiple Sclerosis Society (2006) *Measuring Success*. http://www.mssociety.org.uk/ for_professionals/standards_of_care/health_care/measuringsuccess.html (accessed 11 January 2006)

Neufeld, P. and Kniepmann, K. (2001) Gateway to wellness: an occupational therapy collaboration with the National Multiple Sclerosis Society. *Community Occupational Therapy Education and Practice*, **13**, 67–84

Neurological Alliance (2003) *Neuro Numbers: a Brief Review of the Numbers of People in the UK with Neurological Conditions*. http://www.neural.org.uk/docs/neuro_numbers/NEURONUM.PDF (accessed 20 November 2005)

Nicholl, C., Lincoln, N. and Playford, E. (2002) The reliability and validity of the Nottingham Extended Activities of Daily Living Scale in patients with multiple sclerosis. *Multiple Sclerosis*, **8**(5), 372–376

Nichols, J.L. (1999) *Women Living with Multiple Sclerosis: Walking May Be Difficult, But Together We Fly.* Hunter House Inc, Alameda

O'Hara, L., Cadbury, H., De Souza, L. and Ide, L. (2002) Evaluation of the effectiveness of professionally guided self-care for people with multiple sclerosis living in the community: a randomized controlled trial. *Clinical Rehabilitation*, **16(2)**, 119–128

O'Hara, L., De Souza, L.H. and Ide, L. (2000) A Delphi study of self-care in a community population of people with multiple sclerosis. *Clinical Rehabilitation*, **14(1)**, 62–71

Patti, F., Ciancio, M.R., Reggio, E., Lopes, R., Palermo, F., Cacopardo M. and Reggio, A. (2002) The impact of outpatient rehabilitation on quality of life in multiple sclerosis. *Journal of Neurology*, **249(8)**, 1027–1033

Patti, F., Ciancio, M.R., Cacopardo, M., Reggio, E., Fiorilla, T., Palermo, F., Reggio, A. and Thompson, A.J. (2003) Effects of a short outpatient rehabilitation treatment on disability of multiple sclerosis patients-a randomised controlled trial. *Journal of Neurology*, **250(7)**, 861–866

Peachey-Hill, C. and Law, M. (2000) Impact of environmental sensitivity on occupational performance. *Canadian Journal of Occupational Therapy*, **67(5)**, 304–313

Polman, C. and Uitdehaag, B.M.J. (2000) Drug treatment of multiple sclerosis. *British Medical Journal*, **321**, 490–494

Power, M.J., Bullinger, M., Harper, A. and the WHOQOL Group (1999) The World Health Organization WHOQOL-100: Tests of the universality of quality of life in fifteen different cultural groups worldwide. *Health Psychology*, **18(5)**, 495–505

Primary Care Contracting (2004) National Enhanced Service for the Provision of More Specialised Services for Patients with Multiple Sclerosis. http://www.natpact.nhs.uk/uploads/MS.doc (accessed 16 January 2006)

Riazi, A., Hobart, J.C., Lamping, D.L., Fitzpatrick, R. and Thompson, A.J. (2002) Multiple Sclerosis Impact Scale (MSIS-29): reliability and validity in hospital based samples. *Journal of Neurology Neurosurgery and Psychiatry*, **73**, 701–704

Rijken, P. and Dekker, J. (1998) Clinical experience of rehabilitation therapists with chronic diseases: a quantitative approach. *Clinical Rehabilitation*, **12(2)**, 143–150

Ritvo, P.G., Fischer, J.S., Miller, D.M., Andrews, H., Paty, D.W. and LaRocca, N.G. (1997) *MSQLI – Multiple Sclerosis Quality of Life Inventory: a User's Manual.* National Multiple Sclerosis Society, New York

Rowles, G.D. (2003) The meaning of place as a component of self. In: *Willard and Spackman's Occupational Therapy.* Ed. Crepeau, E.B., Cohn, E., Boyt Schell B.A., pp. 111–119. Lippincott Williams & Wilkins, Philadelphia

Sackett, D., Richardson, W., Rosenberg, W. and Haynes, R. (1996) *Evidence-Based Medicine.* Churchill Livingstone, Edinburgh

Schwartz, C.E. (1999) Teaching coping skills enhances quality of life more than peer support: results of a randomized trial with multiple sclerosis patients. *Health Psychology*, **18(3)**, 211–220

Seidel, A.C. (2003) Rehabilitation perspectives. In: *Willard and Spackman's Occupational Therapy.* Ed. Crepeau, E.B., Cohn, E., Boyt Schell, B.A., pp. 235–242. Lippincott Williams & Wilkins, Philadelphia

Shumway-Cook, A. and Woollacott, M.H. (2001) *Motor Control: Theory and Practical Applications.* Lippincott Williams and Wilkins, Baltimore

Smith, M. (2002) Efficacy of specialist versus non specialist management of spinal cord injury within the UK. *Spinal Cord*, **40**, 11–16

Smith, M.M. and Arnett, P.A. (2005) Factors related to employment status changes in individuals with multiple sclerosis. *Multiple Sclerosis*, **11**(5), 602–609

Snell, R.S. (2001) *Clinical Neuroanatomy for Medical Students*. Lippincott Williams & Wilkins, Baltimore

Somerset, M., Campbell, R., Sharp, D.J. and Peters, T.J. (2001) What do people with MS want and expect from health-care services? *Health Expectations*, **4**(1), 29–37

Somerset, M., Sharp, D. and Campbell, R. (2002) Multiple sclerosis and quality of life: a qualitative investigation. *Journal of Health Services and Research Policy*, **7**, 151–159

Steultjens, E.M., Dekker, J., Bouter, L.M., Cardol, M., Van de Nes, J.C. and Van den Ende, C.H. (2003) Occupational therapy for multiple sclerosis. *The Cochrane Database of Systematic Reviews*. Issue 3; Art. No.: CD003608. DOI: 003610.001002/14651858. CD14003608

Stokes, M. (2002) *Neurological Physiotherapy*. Mosby, London

Strong, S. (1999) Application of the Person-Environment-Occupation Model: a practical tool. *Canadian Journal of Occupational Therapy*, **66**(3), 122–133

Tariot, P. (1985) How memory fails: a theoretical model. *Geriatric Nursing*, **6**(3), 144–147

Vanage, S.M., Gilbertson, K.K. and Mathiowetz, V. (2003) Effects of an energy conservation course on fatigue impact for persons with progressive multiple sclerosis. *American Journal of Occupational Therapy*, **57**(3), 315–323

Vaughan, R., Morrison, L. and Miller, E. (2003) The illness representation of multiple sclerosis and their relations to outcome. *British Journal of Health Psychology*, **8**, 287–301

Verza, R., Carvalho, M.L.L., Battaglia, M.A. and Uccelli, M.M. (2006) An interdisciplinary approach to evaluating the need for assistive technology reduces equipment abandonment. *Multiple Sclerosis*, **12**(1), 88–93

Wade, D. and Bareld, A. (2000) Recent advances in rehabilitation. *British Medical Journal*, **320**, 1385–1388

Ward, C.D., Turpin, G., Dewey, M.E., Fleming, S., Hurwitz, B., Ratib, S., von Fragstein, M. and Lymbery, M. (2004) Education for people with progressive neurological conditions can have negative effects: evidence from a randomized controlled trial. *Clinical Rehabilitation*, **18**(7), 717–725

Wollin, J., Dale, H., Spenser, N. and Walsh, A. (2000) What people with newly diagnosed MS (and their families and friends) need to know. *International Journal of MS Care*, **2**(3), 4

World Health Organization (2002) *Towards a Common Language for Functioning, Disability and Health*. World Health Organization, Geneva

Yahav, R., Vosburgh, J. and Miller, A. (2005) Emotional responses of children and adolescents to parents with multiple sclerosis. *Multiple Sclerosis*, **11**(4), 464–468

5: Protection and preservation: maintaining occupational independence in clients with rheumatoid arthritis

Ruth MacDonald and Kerry Sorby

Introduction

A wide range of comprehensive studies including systematic reviews (Egan *et al.*, 2001; Steultjens *et al.*, 2004), clinical trials (Stamm *et al.*, 2002; Hammond *et al.*, 2004) and national surveys (Cross *et al.*, 2006) supports the use of educational–behavioural joint protection strategies and the provision of assistive technology, including orthoses, when working with individuals who have rheumatoid arthritis. The evidence affirms the occupational therapist's position in supporting, educating and empowering clients to manage this often painful condition, in order to maintain their vocational capacity and existing life roles whilst reducing vocational disability (Nordmark *et al.*, 2006). This inspires the individual to maintain his/her locus of control and self-efficacy (Cross *et al.*, 2006). The evidence provides the rationale and justification for the use of energy conservation and joint protection principles whilst considering the appropriateness of splinting (Hammond and Jeffreson, 2002; Niedermann *et al.*, 2004), provision of assistive devices and expenditure on environmental modifications.

Rheumatoid arthritis is the most common form of inflammatory arthritis, affecting around 387000 adults in the UK (Arthritis and Musculoskeletal Alliance (AMA), 2004). Rheumatoid arthritis is a chronic autoimmune disease, characterised by an inflammatory process affecting the synovial joints (synovitis) and tendon sheaths (Phillips, 1995). It usually occurs between the ages of 25 and 55 years and is more common in women. This chapter will provide an overview of occupational therapy in rheumatology services, focusing on a person with rheumatoid arthritis, who, for the purpose of this text, will be named Tricia. The chapter will present information on rheumatoid arthritis before focusing on the occupational therapy process from the point of referral to discharge and will incorporate relevant treatment strategies. The chapter will show how the *'four core processes of occupational therapy'* (Creek, 2003, p. 29) can assist Tricia in *'maintain (ing). . . . a match . . . between the abilities of the person, the demands of her occupations and the demands of the environment'* (Creek, 2003, p. 14).

An occupational therapist may encounter a range of people with varied arthritic conditions. These may be inflammatory in nature, for instance rheumatoid arthritis and juvenile chronic inflammatory arthritis, connective tissue disorders, such as scleroderma or benign joint familial hypermobility syndrome (Beighton *et al.*, 1989), joint failure, such as osteoarthritis (OA), and soft tissue manifestations, such as fibromyalgia (for a summary of these conditions see Hill, 1998).

Although the range of conditions people present with may be broad, the core occupational therapy skills of *'enablement, problem solving and use of activity as a therapeutic tool'* (Creek, 2003, p. 36) are frequently used, as are the key intervention areas of joint protection, assistive device provision, energy conservation and splinting.

Rheumatology allows the occupational therapist to use evidenced-based interventions of a high standard, i.e. randomised controlled trials, in the specific areas of joint protection and energy conservation (Helewa *et al.*, 1991; Hammond and Freeman, 2001; Hammond *et al.*, 2004). The results of much research are incorporated in the National Association of Rheumatology Occupational Therapists (NAROT) guidelines (NAROT/College of Occupational Therapists, 2003a, b, c) and the Arthritis and Musculoskeletal Alliance (ARMA) Standards of Care (Arthritis and Musculoskeletal Alliance, 2004), which give clear and detailed suggestions for incorporating evidence into service delivery. Specific examples of these are included, for instance Standard 11 (ARMA, 2004), which identifies access to a nurse-led helpline and self-management training, i.e. expert patient programmes (Department of Health, 2001).

Explanation of rheumatoid arthritis

The clinical features of rheumatoid arthritis vary between individuals, but the course is characterised by unpredictable acute episodes of flare-ups and remissions. The clinical features can be divided into two groups:

▪ Articular: for a period, lasting weeks or months, there is pain, inflammation, warmth, stiffness or reduced range of movement at affected joints. The small joints of the hands and feet are most commonly affected, often in a symmetrical pattern. With repeated acute episodes of inflammation, there may be weakening of supporting joint structures, destruction of joint cartilage and erosion of bone. The inflammatory process eventually leads to muscle and tendon imbalance, joint instability and subluxation (joints can temporarily move out of alignment) or joint dislocation. Joint deformities, such as ulnar deviation, can develop in the hand at the metacarpophalangeal joint and swan neck and boutonniere deformity can be seen in the fingers (Melvin, 1989; Phillips, 1995).
▪ Systemic: anaemia, fatigue, general malaise, weight loss, lung or cardiac or, in some cases, neurological impairment.

Involvement of the joints of the hand is one of the earliest signs of rheumatoid arthritis (Blenkiron, 2005; Eberhardt *et al.*, 2001), with some deformities occurring within the first 2 years of diagnosis. It is therefore important that the occupational therapist has a good understanding of hand anatomy, how deformities of the hand occur and the possible impact on hand function. For example, ulnar drift (deformity at the metacarpophalangeal joints) occurs due to a combination of the active disease at these joints and the position of the hand in normal movement. When turning a tap, opening a jar or wringing out a face cloth, the metacarpal heads slope in an ulnar direction. The essential reason for using joint protection techniques is to teach compensation strategies to prevent these malalignment problems.

Management

The management of rheumatoid arthritis involves pharmacological and surgical interventions, and education coordinated by a multidisciplinary team (MDT).

The multidisciplinary team

The MDT is essential in helping manage rheumatoid arthritis (David and Lloyd, 1998; Scholten *et al.*, 1999; Sanford *et al.*, 2000). The team consists of Tricia and her husband and children, general practitioner (GP), rheumatologist, physiotherapist, occupational therapist, nurse and chiropodist, and can also include her orthopaedic consultant, social worker and dietician. The team may be hospital- or community-based or a combination of the two. Good liaison and communication are essential to ensure a smooth transition of care between primary and secondary care, dependent on Tricia's needs at any given time. The overall aim of the team is to control the disease activity, alleviate pain, maintain level of functioning and maintain quality of life (American College of Rheumatology, 2002). A particular focus of occupational therapy is in teaching joint protection and energy conservation principles in order to allow Tricia to manage her rheumatoid arthritis more satisfactorily.

Education

This is a vital component to enable Tricia to manage her condition and lifestyle. To make informed choices about her care, she needs to have a good understanding of the disease, its symptoms, how her medication works and how to adapt or modify tasks, behaviours and her environment in order to continue to engage in meaningful occupations.

Pharmacological management

Tricia may be prescribed a combination of types of medication to control her presenting symptoms. It is important that the occupational therapist understands the medication Tricia is taking and their possible implications on level of functioning. Below is a summary of the types of drugs that may be prescribed. Leaflets on individual drugs are available from www.arc.org.uk.

- Analgesics – reduce pain (e.g. co-proxamol, paracetamol).
- Non-steroidal anti-inflammatory drugs (NSAIDs) – relieve pain and inflammation. (e.g. aspirin, ibuprofen, diclofenac). These drugs are known to cause side effects of stomach ulcers or bleeding, so are used with supervision.
- Corticosteroids – these reduce inflammation and may have some disease-modifying effects. (e.g. prednisolone, prednisone). They can be administered by injection (directly into an inflamed joint, intramuscularly or intravenously) or orally.
- Disease-modifying anti-rheumatoid drugs (DMARDs) – often referred to as 'second-line agents' (Royal College of Nursing, 2003). These are used to reduce pain, swelling and stiffness (e.g. sulphasalazine, methotrexate). They are slow-acting drugs that have the potential to induce remission, reducing joint damage associated with severe rheumatoid arthritis.
- Biological/anti-tumour necrosis factor (anti-TNF) drugs (e.g. adalimumab, etanercept, infliximab). Tumour necrosis factor (TNF) is a polypeptide hormone (or cytokine) that promotes inflammation and is therefore believed to play a key role in rheumatoid arthritis. Anti-TNF drugs inhibit the action of TNF within the body. This is a new and expensive form of medication, therefore current Guidelines by the British Society for Rheumatology (2003) and National Institute for Clinical Effectiveness (2002) restrict their use to people who fail to respond to two or more DMARDs. There is an increasing number of people being treated with good effect; the long-term complications of these drugs are still not fully known (Royal College of Nursing, 2003).

Surgical management

Surgical intervention may be offered when a client presents with unacceptable levels of pain, significant loss of joint range of movement and/or limitation in their level of functioning (Kennedy et al., 2005). The range of procedures include carpal tunnel release, synovectomy (when the synovial fluid is removed), joint replacement and/or joint fusion. The results are difficult to predict as the disease can still affect the joints.

Tricia's experience

Referral

Twelve months after the diagnosis of rheumatoid arthritis was made, Tricia was referred by her consultant rheumatologist to an occupational therapist for full assessment. This highlighted problems at work and early morning joint stiffness.

Information gathering during the initial interview

During the initial interview, the occupational therapist gathered information about Tricia's medical history, occupations, needs and strengths and support networks (Creek, 2003). Tricia's consent to occupational therapy was obtained in order to meet the requirements of the Code of Ethics and Professional Conduct (College of Occupational Therapists, 2005 – section 2.1.2).

Tricia is a 49-year-old Caucasian woman who lives with her husband, Michael, and two children (aged 22 and 24). Her husband and their children work full-time. Tricia, until recently, used to work full-time in a busy wine bar. The family live in an owner-occupied, four-bedroom semi-detached house in a small town.

At home she is responsible for most domestic tasks and is able to ask for help from her daughter or husband when preparing vegetables and the laundry. She is finding meal preparation more painful, particularly after work, in terms of standing to prepare vegetables and to cook food at the cooker. She has morning joint stiffness of about 30 minutes which reduces her ability to dress herself and clean her teeth. Her sleep is interrupted approximately twice nightly due to pain in her joints.

Tricia recently changed jobs and now works part-time in a working man's club. Her shifts are Monday evening and 12–5 pm on Wednesday and Thursdays. Operating hand-pulled beer pumps is painful on a 'bad day', due to reduced grip, and she suffers hand and wrist joint pain when holding (frequently wet) pint glasses. She has pain in her feet due to standing still during quieter periods at work and tiredness immediately after work (lasting up to 2 hours) which continues into the following day. Her leisure time is spent either gardening or socialising at the pub with her family.

About a year ago she developed symptoms of painful and swollen toes, shoulders, elbows, wrists and hands, especially at the metacarpophalangeal joints. Her GP referred her to the local rheumatologist who confirmed the diagnosis of rheumatoid arthritis with blood tests and clinical examination. At this initial consultation she was given an intramuscular steroid injection and prescribed methotrexate (one of the DMARDs) at the lowest dose. After 6 weeks the initial symptom relief given by the steroid injection started to diminish and the dose of methotrexate was increased. Tricia is not pain-free but feels that her new dose is much more effective at controlling her symptoms. She is currently taking folic acid (to compensate for reduced levels of calcium caused by methotrexate) and ibuprofen (a NSAID) to control her symptoms. It was after this second consultant outpatient appointment that Tricia agreed to a referral to occupational therapy.

Detailed assessment

The initial assessment was carried out using the Canadian Occupational Performance Measure (COPM) (Canadian Association of Occupational Therapists, 1994). This is a semi-structured interview and self-rating assessment, led by the occupational therapist, whereby Tricia identifies problems in her occupational performance (**self-care**, **productivity** and **leisure**) which are rated in terms of importance to the individual on a scale of 1–10 (10 being the most important).

In the area of **self-care** Tricia identified the sub-section of **personal care** as a major area of frustration, identifying that she had difficulty with dressing and cleaning her teeth in the morning due to joint stiffness. She rated both of these as 10/10 in terms of importance.

In the area of **productivity** she identified two sub-sections of **paid work** and **household management** as areas of concern. In paid work she had difficulty in handling and carrying glasses (10/10) with high levels of tiredness after work (9/10). In household management she had difficulty in turning taps on and off (10/10) and preparing food (9/10).

In the last section, **leisure**, she identified areas of personal unease in the sub-sections of **quiet recreation** and **socialisation**. In quiet recreation she had difficulty with holding a book to read whilst seated and in bed (8/10) and, with socialisation, her levels of tiredness were such that she felt unable to socialise in the pub with her husband (Michael) after work, or on her days off (10/10).

The five areas which were rated the highest in terms of importance to Tricia were:

▨ Dressing herself and cleaning her teeth (10/10).
▨ Managing at work (10/10).
▨ Tiredness after work and its affect upon socialisation (10/10).
▨ Turning taps (10/10).
▨ Preparing food (9/10).

The occupational therapist then encouraged Tricia to rate these five problem areas in terms of her perceived performance of these occupations on a scale of 1–10 and her level of satisfaction with her performance on a scale of 1–10. A score of 1 reflects a low performance or low satisfaction score, whereas a score of 10 reflects a high performance or high satisfaction with performance (Tyrell and Burn, 1996). The results can be seen in Fig. 5.1.

These numerical scores allow the occupational therapist to calculate an **overall performance score** (by adding all the performance scores together and dividing

	Performance	Satisfaction
1. Dressing herself and cleaning her teeth	7	3
2. Managing at work	5	3
3. Tiredness after work and its affect on socialisation	5	2
4. Turning taps	3	2
5. Preparing food	3	2

Figure 5.1 Perceptions of performance and performance satisfaction.

by the number of problems, for example 23/5 = 4.6) and an **overall satisfaction score** (by adding all the satisfaction scores and dividing by the number of problems 12/5 = 2.4) (Canadian Association of Occupational Therapists, 1994).

The COPM can be used as an outcome measure allowing the re-measurement of Tricia's perception of her occupational performance over the course of occupational therapy (Canadian Association of Occupational Therapists, 1994; Finlay, 1997). Initial scores can be compared with the reassessment scores. These scores can be used to identify change in performance and change in satisfaction score (Canadian Association of Occupational Therapists, 1994).

The second part of the assessment involved the occupational therapist observing Tricia make a light snack (beans on toast) in the occupational therapy department's kitchen. The occupational therapist used a non-standardised kitchen assessment using detailed demand analysis (Foster and Pratt, 2002) to frame her observations. During the kitchen assessment Tricia also demonstrated how she carried a number of pint glasses. The results of this assessment are as follows:

▪ Physical skills – Tricia found the demands of standing for the whole task bearable, but commented that any meal preparation of a more complex task would be too tiring. She found the movements required to turn the taps and to open the can of beans painful. She was able to generalise that if the task had been putting jam on toast, she would have found opening the jar difficult and painful. The same concerns were raised if the task had been cheese on toast, as cutting food items (i.e. cheese or vegetables) was usually painful. The strength required to carry four empty glasses was tolerated within the assessment kitchen, but the endurance of the task required at work was currently too much for Tricia. In terms of hand function, Tricia could perform all hand grips, but her confidence in the strength required was reduced due to pain avoidance.
▪ Sensory and perceptual skills – Tricia presented with no problems in vision, auditory, olfactory and touch sensation.
▪ Cognitive skills – concrete thinking is required for this task; Tricia could show more creativity with meal preparation on a larger scale.
▪ Social interaction skills – generally this task is carried out in isolation, alone in the kitchen, although it could on a larger scale be a more sociable activity, i.e. cooking a meal with her husband.
▪ Emotional skills – the task observed provided little opportunity for choice of snack, but contains great value to Tricia as she sees herself as an independent person who can make a light snack for herself and her family.
▪ Cultural demands – the task was appropriate to Tricia's gender, class and age. The task has meaning as her role of mother and wife (based on Foster and Pratt, 2002, p. 151).

In order to assess Tricia's level of tiredness or fatigue, she was asked to complete an activity diary sheet which recorded her activities alongside her levels of tiredness (Strong *et al.*, 2002). A diary sheet consists of a grid with all the days of the week listed, and hour units of time. The sheet was given to Tricia with all the sections blank; the occupational therapist and Tricia decided that she would

Time	Monday	Tuesday	Wednesday	Thursday	Friday	Saturday	Sunday
6.00am							
7.00am							
8.00am							
9.00am							
10.00am							
11.00am							

Times continue until 12.00pm and could include during the night to record sleep patterns.

Key

Red pen – occupations carried out

Blue pen – medication taken

Yellow pen – energy levels (high, low or moderate)

Figure 5.2 Sample of an activity diary sheet.

record (in different colours) what she did in the hourly slots, what pain relief she had taken and how she felt in terms of energy levels. She would bring this to the second appointment, to allow the occupational therapist to look for patterns to Tricia's energy levels (Fig. 5.2).

The diary sheet showed that Tricia experienced more fatigue during a shift which was quiet, i.e. Monday evening, as she was required to stand at the bar and chat to customers. In addition she was tired after her shifts on Wednesdays and Thursdays for about 2 hours, which was exacerbated by needing to prepare and cook the family's evening meal. From these results the occupational therapist was able to apply the principles of energy conservation.

Goal setting

By choosing the COPM, the occupational therapist had chosen an outcome measure which is based on the Model of Occupational Performance (Townsend, 2002) which emphasises a client-centred approach (Sumison, 1999), and this concept is reflected throughout the occupational therapy process. Tricia has identified the five most important areas in occupational performance to her at this time and these form the basis of the treatment aims. After discussion the following treatment **aims** were agreed:

▫ Tricia will be able to wash herself and clean her teeth independently.
▫ Tricia will be able to continue her present employment.
▫ Tricia will be able to socialise with her family in the pub after work.
▫ Tricia will be able to prepare a meal for herself and her husband independently.

In order to achieve these aims, **goals** are established with outcomes to achieve during treatment. Goals can have short-, medium- and/or long-term timescales. In rheumatology, a review of treatment is common at 2 weeks, i.e. to discuss how a splint is useful in supporting Tricia's chosen occupations; this would be a short-term goal.

Short-term goals

In 2 weeks Tricia will:

- Wear a custom-made night resting splint during sleep for 2 weeks to reduce length of time she experiences morning stiffness from 30 minutes to 10 minutes.
- Take her NSAID (ibuprofen) medication 20 minutes prior to rising; this will involve Michael bringing her a cup of tea, with her medication, prior to her rising from bed.
- Use a built up handle on the toothbrush and a pump action toothpaste dispenser and be able to clean her own teeth independently 30 minutes after rising.
- Use a plastic drinks carrier when collecting glasses, and place the handle of the carrier on her forearm.
- Use two hands to reach and grasp clean glasses from shelves before carrying the glass to the pump.
- Wear a wrist brace on her right hand and use an industry-provided glass stand to hold the glass when pouring a pint.
- Use her own large-handled bottle opener to open all bottles.
- Use a perching stool during quieter periods at work on Mondays for up to 20 minutes at a time.

Long-term goals

Long-term goals are usually set when the therapist and client are in contact for a prolonged period of time (Creek, 2003). In rheumatology this can be for up to 2 months after the initial interview session and then cases may remain open for up to a year. The purpose of a long-term goal is for the client to 'achieve a satisfying performance and balance of occupations . . . that will support . . . health, wellbeing and social participation' (Creek, 2003, p. 32). The long-term goals set by the occupational therapist and Tricia focus on leisure activities, i.e. socialising at the pub, and applying strategies, such as joint protection and energy conservation, which will have long-term benefits for Tricia. The Canadian Model of Occupational Performance (Townsend, 2003) allows the occupational therapist to remain client-centred and the COPM (Canadian Association of Occupational Therapists, 1994) process means that Tricia's satisfaction with her performance is an integral part of the reassessment process. In 4 weeks Tricia will aim for these long-term goals:

- Socialise in the pub with Michael following her evening shift, once a week.
- Prepare and cook the family meal three times a week.
- Demonstrate three joint protection principles when making a cup of tea in 20 minutes, after completing reading and homework sheets.
- Show three energy conservation principles based on her original diary sheet in 20 minutes, after completing reading and homework sheets.

Models and approaches

Model

The model chosen to frame the intervention with Tricia was the Canadian Model of Occupational Performance (Townsend, 2002). It places the client at the centre of the occupational therapy process and has a clear focus on occupational performance. Rheumatology practice, by its definition, focuses on joints and joint pain, and using this model allows the occupational therapist to remain *'in tune with our professional philosophy . . . and our unique occupational therapy focus'* (Finlay, 1997, p. 27). The model places the person at the core, gives meaning to their occupations (namely, self-care, productivity and leisure) and this is influenced and surrounded by the environment (physical, institutional, cultural and social) (Foster, 2002). The interaction between these three components (person, occupations and the environment) is crucial to the model as is the concept of client-centred practice and occupational performance. Occupations are categorised as:

- Productivity – paid and unpaid work, household management.
- Leisure – quiet recreation, active recreation, socialising with others.
- Self-care – personal care (i.e. activities for daily living), functional mobility and community management (i.e. shopping).

The model can be used with a number of different approaches, assessments, such as the COPM outcome measure, and interventions (Foster, 2002). Using both the model (Canadian Model of Occupational Performance) and the accompanying outcome measure (COPM) (Canadian Association of Occupational Therapists, 1994) allows a seamless application of the model. The COPM is well suited to clients that have primarily practical rather than emotional difficulties (Finlay, 1997), as the requirement of self-rating one's own performance and satisfaction, with an area of occupational performance, could be too difficult for some clients. The occupational therapist has used her clinical reasoning when selecting outcome measures.

Frame of reference

Within this model, both the **learning** and **compensatory** frame of references can successfully be applied. Tricia's ability to learn about her condition, and to adapt and change to optimise her performance, is considered to be the core component of the learning frame of reference. The application of joint protection techniques and energy conservation techniques uses the learning frame of reference.

The compensatory frame of reference assumes that Tricia's ability to function, by utilising a number of compensatory techniques, is essential to her well-being (Foster, 2002). The uses of adaptive equipment and task modifications are examples of how this frame of reference can be applied. Historically, the compensatory frame of reference is linked to the medical model; the occupational therapist needs to consider Tricia's personal choice during this process, and not the quickest or cheapest option, and be aware that Tricia may find it difficult to accept compensatory techniques as they may reinforce the permanence of her loss of function.

In addition, the **biomechanical** frame of reference is used in the design of splinting. This frame of reference seeks to explain function and dysfunction in terms of anatomy and physiology and makes good use of tools, such as splinting materials, to promote physical function (Foster, 2002). The limitation of this frame of reference when used exclusively, is that the client risks becoming rather passive in the treatment process, as the therapist leads the treatment. This may be appropriate for many professionals and medical treatment, but is at odds with the core philosophy of occupational therapy (Creek, 2003).

Treatment approaches

One of the core components of managing rheumatoid arthritis is patient education. The occupational therapist will work collaboratively with Tricia and her family in order to enable Tricia to make informed decisions about how she would like to manage her clinical condition. An **educative approach** is used when providing information on joint protection and energy conservation. Education may be provided verbally and supported with written information booklets. These may be written by the department or national organisations (see www.arc.org.uk leaflets).

The **compensatory approach** is used to compensate for dysfunction in a variety of occupations, i.e. meal preparation, where the supply of assistive devices, such as an Ergonon knife (Fig. 5.3), compensates for the difficulty experienced with using a traditional knife handle. A change to the environment, such as in the layout of a kitchen and the provision of splints, also comes from this approach.

Using the **adaptive skills approach** (Foster, 2002) involves the therapist understanding the client's present skill level (from assessment) and being able to suggest alternatives ways of carrying out the chosen occupation. For example, using two hands to lift glasses off a shelf rather that one hand is using a different method to achieve the same goal.

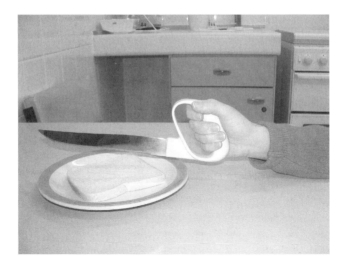

Figure 5.3 Ergonon knife.

Action/treatment

This section will outline the intervention based on the plan and goals and will incorporate the evidence base to support intervention. The main areas of involvement are joint protection, assistive devices, energy conservation and splinting. Each section will outline the basic principles of treatment and link to Tricia's short- and long-term goals.

Joint protection

The use of joint protection was first suggested by Cordery in 1965, who identified a number of principles which aimed to assist clients in protecting their joints from further damage by completing everyday tasks in a different way. Joint protection aims to:

▪ Manage and/or reduce pain during activities.
▪ Reduce local inflammation in joints which is caused by mechanical pressures on joints.
▪ Improve or maintain function.
▪ Help limit the development and/or progression of deformities (NAROT/College of Occupational Therapists, 2003d).

Research (cited by NAROT/College of Occupational Therapists, 2003d) has shown that joint protection principles are effective in reducing pain and morning stiffness, but there is little current evidence to substantiate the claim of reducing joint damage. The systematic review by Steultjens *et al.* (2004) states that there is '*strong evidence that instruction in joint protection leads to an improvement in functional ability*' but there is '*limited evidence for the efficacy of comprehensive occupational therapy on functional ability*' (Steultjens *et al.*, 2004).

The original eleven principles introduced by Cordery 1965 have been reduced to nine by Palmer and Simmons (1991) in an attempt to include those which are supported by evidence. The generally accepted principles are (Cordery, 1965, the latter two have been deleted by Palmer and Simmons 1991):

- Distribute strain over as many joints as possible.
- Use larger joints.
- Avoid gripping too tightly.
- Avoid holding one position for too long.
- Avoid forcing your joints into deforming positions.
- Balance between rest and activity.
- Exercise little and often.
- Find easier work methods.
- Wear your splints.
- *Listen to your body.*
- *Watch your weight.*

The principles of avoiding gripping too tightly and avoiding deforming positions are the reason why a toothbrush with a built up handle was suggested. (The handle can be widened by applying a short piece of plasterzote rubber tubing over the handle). The larger handle reduces the amount of finger flexion required at the metacarpophalangeal joints and fingers, and will help reduce pain, as excessive flexion on already swollen joints will be painful. The same principle applies to using a large handled bottle opener. The suggestion of a pump action toothpaste dispenser (commonly available at most supermarkets) encourages Tricia to use larger joints, i.e. the palm of the hand, to push on to the dispenser and avoids forcing her joints into deforming positions by not flexing the metacarpophalangeal and finger joints in a squeezing action in order to get the toothpaste out of the tube.

Some of Tricia's short-term goals relate to her work environment; when carrying the drinks carrier on her forearm, Tricia is using the principle of distributing the strain over as many joints as possible and using larger joints, i.e. the elbow joint, rather than the small joints of the hand. Stamm *et al.* (2002), using a randomised controlled trial, found that the application of such strategies, together with home hand exercises improved hand function in clients with arthritis.

Joint protection can be used by the occupational therapist to guide specific interventions and is offered in the form of teaching and learning sessions. This includes using good quality literature, such as the Arthritis Research Campaign leaflet, *Looking After your Joints* (Arthritis Research Campaign, 2001). Traditionally, teaching joint protection has been offered either individually or in a group setting lasting up to an hour (Hammond, 1997). However, research evaluating whether clients have adopted joint protection principles in the long term have found this traditional method (i.e. sessions lasting up to an hour) to be of limited value (Hammond and Freeman, 2001; Badamgarav *et al.*, 2003).

The most effective method of presenting information on joint protection, in terms of long-term change, is a 6-week educational–behavioural joint protection programme (Hammond and Freeman, 2001; Hammond *et al.*, 2002). This programme incorporates cognitive and behavioural learning techniques. In the programme, clients practice various kitchen tasks utilising joint protection principles in small groups, whilst including strategies such as mental rehearsal, goal setting and supervised practice with feedback. The course lasts 8 hours over four sessions, each session lasting 2 hours. In a randomised controlled trial Hammond and Freeman (2001) found that individuals demonstrated *'significant improvements in pain, disease status and functional ability'* (p. 1044). Previous studies by Helliwell *et al.* (1999), Lindroth *et al.* (1997) and Brus *et al.* (1998) support these findings.

The timing of joint protection education is very important. A randomised controlled trial study by Hammond *et al.* (2004) found that occupational therapy in the early months post-diagnosis (6, 12 and 18 months) was of limited benefit. This emphasises the importance of assessing an individual's responsiveness to receiving occupational therapy guidance and advice, which may vary according to the individual's circumstances (Hammond and Klompenhouwer, 2005). In Tricia's situation she was happy to accept help 12 months post-diagnosis.

Assistive devices

The term assistive device is now widely used (Pain *et al.*, 2003) and refers to specialist equipment, aids or assistive technology. Assistive devices can be described as *'any product . . . used by people with disabilities . . . to prevent, compensate, relieve . . . the impairment'* (Baldursdottir *et al.*, 2001). The prescription of assistive devices evolves from the compensatory frame of reference whereby the occupational therapist recommends a compensatory technique to alleviate dysfunction by *'supplying adapted tools'* (Foster, 2002, p. 78), such as an Ergonon/Reflex knife and perching stool.

Tricia identified that she has difficulties with chopping vegetables, opening jars and standing long enough to prepare a meal. The reason for suggesting an Ergonon/Reflex knife when chopping vegetables is that this activity usually requires the person to maintain a tight grip on the handle of the knife, whilst pushing the wrist into ulnar deviation in order to chop the vegetables. The Ergonon knife enables Tricia to apply joint protection principles by:

- Using a large handle which enables Tricia to avoid gripping the utensil too tightly.
- Using elbow and shoulder (larger joints) movements to create a sawing action to chop the vegetable. An ordinary knife requires a smaller joint (the wrist) to be used.
- Maintaining a sawing action for cutting, allows the wrist to be maintained in anatomical alignment. An ordinary knife encourages the wrist to be used in ulnar deviation.

Similar reasoning can be applied to using an electric can opener and a Dycem mat to open tins and jars or using a plastic glass carrier to carry several pint glasses. It was suggested that Tricia use the following assistive devices for some of her difficulties identified following the kitchen assessment:

- Problem: pouring and carrying drinks. Assistive devices recommended: glass carrier, large handled bottle opener, glass stand.
- Problem: turning taps on and off to wash and bathe. Assistive device: tap turners.
- Problem: opening jars. Assistive device: Dycem mat and jar opener.
- Problem: opening tins. Assistive device: electric can opener.
- Problem: standing for long periods of time. Assistive device: perching stool.

When identifying an assistive device for a client, often the local authority is unable to supply this free of charge. In some areas there may be a small charge or a means test or no provision. In many cases the client has to purchase items privately. In this situation the occupational therapist needs to recommend at least two independent suppliers (ideally a list of all suppliers in the region). This is in order to comply with the Code of Ethics and Professional Practice (College of Occupational Therapists 2005, section 4.5.1) in relation to avoiding personal profit or gain from commercial organisations.

Energy conservation

Energy conservation is the process whereby a client can *'save energy during daily tasks, giving greater control in distributing energy to more meaningful activities'* (Hammond and Jeffreson, 2002) It aims to *'reduce fatigue, reduce pain, and increase activity tolerance to achieve greater overall productivity and quality of life'* (NAROT/ College of Occupational Therapists, 2003b). Research cited in NAROT/College of Occupational Therapists (2003b) states that energy conservation does increase energy levels but does not contribute to reducing pain and fatigue levels. It consists of the following principles (Melvin, 1989):

- Pre-plan and organise the proposed activity.
- Ascertain priorities.
- Eliminate unnecessary tasks.
- Use good postures when performing the activity.
- Avoid unnecessary activity or energy expenditure.
- Organise the most ergonomic work environment.
- Use assistive devices where possible.
- Take frequent, planned rest periods.

The method of delivery is similar to that of joint protection, i.e. through discussion with Tricia. It is most effective when linked with personal examples. This is achieved through the initial interview and by using a diary sheet to identify those times when Tricia's energy levels are low and fatigue levels are high (Strong *et al.*,

2002). The diary sheet showed that Tricia experienced more fatigue during a working shift which was quiet, i.e. Monday evenings, as she was required to stand at the bar and chat to customers. In addition, she was tired after her shifts on Wednesday and Thursday for about 2 hours, which was exacerbated by needing to prepare and cook the family's evening meal. From these results, the occupational therapist is able to apply the principles of energy conservation.

Energy conservation advice

In relation to preparing food, Tricia was advised to rest for up to 45 minutes after coming home from work and accept offers of refreshments from family members. She was asked to discuss with the family the possibility of changing the family main meal to lunch time rather than at tea time. On days when this was not possible, Tricia agreed to make the family meals in advance (on her days off), freeze them and either reheat them herself or await the family's return from work. Tricia was asked to reflect on how she uses her time off and consider including periods of rest in order to 'bank' these for when she was at work.

Splinting

A night resting splint (or a static volar resting splint) was made for Tricia's left and right hands in an attempt to reduce morning stiffness in wrist and hand joints from 30 minutes to 10 minutes (see short-term goals) to make dressing and teeth cleaning easier (Fig. 5.4). Tricia will wear a splint on alternate hands on alternate nights, as both splints cannot be easily tolerated at the same time.

A night resting splint is provided to immobilise or rest the whole hand and forearm, often during acute periods of inflammation. The hand and forearm are supported in the splint in a resting position which is comfortable for sleep and this helps to reduce morning stiffness and joint swelling which can occur overnight (NAROT/College of Occupational Therapists, 2003d). When designing and fabricating a custom-made splint the occupational therapist needs to consider the purpose of the splint, the mechanical principles of a splint, the anatomy of the hand and forearm and the choice of material to be used.

The purpose of a night resting splint is to (NAROT/College of Occupational Therapists, 2003d):

- Rest and support painful joints in the correct position.
- Decrease pain, inflammation and swelling during exacerbations.
- Maintain structural and functional integrity.
- Reduce/prevent contracture.
- Prevent/minimise deformity.
- Decrease early morning stiffness.

There is inconsistency within the literature regarding a definition of the 'resting position' of the hand. In general there are some key points:

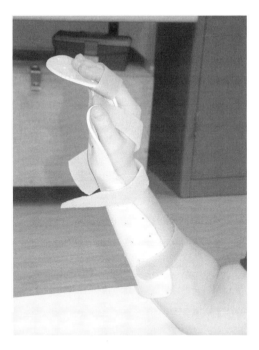

Figure 5.4 Night resting splint.

- The metacarpophalangeal joints should be supported in 25–30° of flexion (Falconer, 1991; Phillips, 1995; Wilton, 1997; Fess *et al.*, 2004).
- It is important to create an ulnar border on the splint to correct passively and support the metacarpophalangeal joints into anatomical alignment.
- The design of the strapping should enable the client to get the splint on and off easily. In addition, the occupational therapist is aware that Tricia is taking methotrexate, and is therefore prone to poor skin healing (Royal College of Nursing, 2003) and care needs to be taken that the straps do not cause undue pressure and potential skin breakdown.

(For a detailed summary see Coppard and Lohmann, 2001; Belkin, 2002; Fess *et al.*, 2004.)

Wrist immobilisation splint (wrist splint or brace)

A wrist splint or brace was provided to enhance Tricia's level of functioning when at work. The provision of such a working splint has recently been questioned by a systematic review undertaken by Niedermann *et al.* (2004), who stated that the short-term effects of their use are reasonable but long-term changes were not so convincingly demonstrated. They recommended that further research was needed in this area. As Tricia was only to use such a splint for limited periods each week, the short-term outcome justified its provision. A wrist brace supports/rests the affected wrist at the same time as allowing free movement of the metacarpopha-langeal and interphalangeal joints (Fig. 5.5). Prefabricated wrist braces are fre-quently used in the clinical setting as they are considered time effective. The time-consuming process of design and fabrication of the splint has already been undertaken by the manufacturers. In addition, they are easy to apply, do not require postgraduate training by the professional fitting them, and are therefore considered to be cost effective. There is a wide range of commercially available wrist braces, varying in materials used, design patterns and cost. In choosing the appropriate wrist brace, the occupational therapist needs to consider various factors.

The purpose of the splint

The purposes include some of the following:

- Rest and support painful joints in the correct position.
- Decrease pain (Nordenskiold, 1990; Kjeken et al., 1995; Haskett et al., 2004).
- Maintain structural and functional integrity.
- Improve grip strength (Nordenskiold, 1990; Kjeken et al., 1995) and enhance function.

Frequency of use

How often will the splint be worn? The wearing regime needs to be balanced to promote support and rest of the wrist but to avoid muscle wasting. Client educa-tion is vital, to ensure Tricia understands how this splint meets joint protection principles.

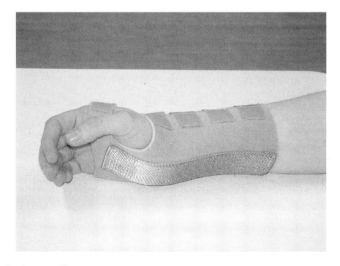

Figure 5.5 Wrist brace splint.

Fit and comfort

The splint should be correctly fitted and be comfortable to wear. Important ana-tomical landmarks to consider are:

- Distal palmar crease – the distal edge of the material should lie below this to allow full metacarpophalangeal joint flexion.
- Thenar eminence – the radial border of the splint should allow free movement of the thumb, particularly for opposing each digit for prehension.
- First web space – again to allow movement of the thumb, but also the soft tissue in this region is very thin and therefore prone to rubbing.
- Proximal fit at the forearm – the proximal edges should meet to reduce migra-tion and therefore ensure appropriate positioning at the wrist.

Ease of getting the splint on and off

Tricia should be able to put on and take off the splint independently. Tricia needs sufficient dexterity in her non-dominant hand to manipulate the straps on her right hand. It may be possible to modify the strapping to facilitate hand dexterity (e.g. oversewing the edges of the Velcro, adhering thermoplastic material to the trapping to facilitate hand dexterity).

Activities that will be undertaken whilst wearing the splint

McKee and Rivard (2004) give clear examples of how occupation-based splinting truly reflects a client-centred approach. The occupational therapist needs to con-sider the activities that Tricia will undertake that require a power grip (i.e. when preparing vegetables in her kitchen at home and when pulling pints at work).

Position of the splint

The angle of wrist extension should be approximately 30°, but this can be varied according to Tricia's needs and occupations to be done whilst wearing the brace (Medical Devices Directory, 1997).

Advice

For each splint provided for Tricia, the occupational therapist provides an information leaflet about the splint, including instructions on how and when to wear the splint, and a contact number for any enquiries. The splint will be regularly reviewed to evaluate if the splint provided is still meeting Tricia's needs.

Evaluation

After all treatment sessions were completed, the occupational therapist asked Tricia to review the original five most important areas of occupational performance that she identified at the assessment stage. Her new scores are as follows:

▪ Dressing herself and cleaning her teeth (10/10).
▪ Managing at work (10/10).
▪ Tiredness after work and its effect upon socialisation (9/10).
▪ Turning taps (10/10).
▪ Preparing food (9/10).

Tricia was asked to re-rate these areas in terms of her assessment of her performance (on a scale of 1–10) and her satisfaction with her performance of these tasks (on a scale of 1–10). The same method of calculation is carried out in order to obtain a reassessment performance score of 7.0 and a reassessment satisfaction score of 5.6. These reassessment scores are compared with the original score find a change in performance and change in satisfaction score (Canadian Association of Occupational Therapists, 1994).This can be shown as:

▪ Reassessment performance score (7.0) minus original performance score (4.6) = 2.4.
▪ Reassessment satisfaction score (5.6) minus original satisfaction score (2.6) = 3.0.

These figures are used to provide subjective feedback for both the occupational therapist and Tricia.

In addition the occupational therapist repeated the kitchen assessment using detailed demand analysis (Foster and Pratt, 2002) in order to ascertain whether there was a reduction in the nature of the difficulties that Tricia was experiencing. It would also enable the occupational therapist to determine if Tricia was using the joint protection principles (see long-term goals). On reassessment, Tricia found that she had minimal difficulties in the kitchen now as she was using the suggested assistive devices and found that she was starting to use joint protection techniques more frequently, but this took time. If the occupational therapist used the Educational–Behavioural Joint Protection Programme (Hammond and Freeman, 2001) she could have used outcome measures specifically designed to assess and reassess Tricia's knowledge of joint protection: the Joint Protection Knowledge Assessment (JPKA) (Hammond and Lincoln, 1999a). Also, in order to assess and reassess how well a client is able to incorporate joint protection principles in everyday kitchen tasks, the occupational therapist could have used the Joint Protection Behaviour Assessment (JPBA) (Hammond and Lincoln, 1999b). This does involve video recording a client performing a set kitchen task which might have been a little daunting for Tricia.

The low usage of standardised assessments within rheumatology has created some debate within the profession (Murray et al., 2000; Blenkiron, 2005). There are several standardised assessments available to the occupational therapist, although they do not appear to be widely used in this clinical area, with therapists preferring to use non-standardised assessments. This may be due to lack of resources within individual departments, lack of knowledge about the assessments available and/or lack of time within a busy clinical environment. Because rheumatoid arthritis is a complex, long-term and unpredictable condition, each person's presentation will be unique and therefore the choice of outcome measurement will vary from individual to individual.

In the Blenkiron (2005) study of 160 senior occupational therapists working in rheumatology the most commonly used instruments to assess task performance were:

▪ The Jebsen–Taylor Test of Hand Function (Jebsen *et al.*, 1969).
▪ The Nine Hole Peg Test (Mathiowetz *et al.*, 1985).
▪ The Purdue Pegboard (Mathiowetz *et al.*, 1986).
▪ Sequential Occupational Dexterity Assessment (van Lankveld *et al.*, 1999).
▪ The Sollerman Hand Function Test (Sollerman and Ejeskar, 1995).

Alternatively, the following assessments could have been used with Tricia, which could have also served as useful outcome measurements. These have been specifically designed for a patient with rheumatoid arthritis:

▪ Grip Ability Test (Dellhag and Bjelle, 1995). This test provides precise instructions for administration, is portable, the objects for the three tests are easily obtained and it only takes 5 minutes to administer (Simpson, 2005). However, it does only assess hand function and therefore sensory–motor components, such as pain, swelling and fatigue, would not be highlighted.
▪ Arthritis Impact Measure Scales (AIMS 1 and AIMS 2) (Meenan *et al.*, 1980; Meenan *et al.*, 1992). This is a self-reported questionnaire and takes 23 minutes on average to complete (Simpson, 2005). It covers a broad range of functional tasks, including functional mobility, upper limb functioning, self-care, domestic and work tasks and social influences. Unfortunately, it does not appear to be widely used by occupational therapists working in rheumatology (Hammond, 1996).
▪ The Disability of Arm, Shoulder and Hand (DASH) Outcome Measure (Hudak *et al.*, 1996). This was developed for use with people with a range of musculoskeletal conditions and focuses on the upper limb as a single functional unit. This assessment would not therefore identify the impact of Tricia's painful and swollen toes on her standing tolerance or fatigue.
▪ Joint Protection Knowledge Assessment (JPKA) (Hammond and Lincoln, 1999a) and Joint Protection Behaviour Assessment (JPBA) (Hammond and Lincoln, 1999b). Both of these two assessments focus on one aspect of intervention (joint protection) and are not recommended to be used in the early stages of occupational therapy intervention as they measure the effectiveness of intervention, not Tricia's current level of functioning.

Tricia did not present to the occupational therapist with any specified hand deformities and grip function/dexterity was not identified as a key presenting feature of her rheumatoid arthritis at this particular stage of her condition. However, Tricia did state that her condition was affecting a broad range of domestic and work tasks; the COPM was therefore selected to evaluate this impact at the present time, and would be repeated over the course of Tricia's occupational therapy intervention. Although the COPM has not been specifically designed for those with rheumatoid arthritis, it is a useful tool to identify Tricia's perception of how her rheumatoid arthritis is affecting her lifestyle; it encourages Tricia to identify her priorities for occupational therapy intervention and hence take an active role in any future decision-making processes.

Challenges to the reader

This chapter has provided an overview of occupational therapy for a client with rheumatoid arthritis and has shown how the occupational therapy process can assist a client in *'maintain(in g) . . . a match between the abilities of the person, the demands of her occupations and the demands of the environment'* (Creek, 2003, p. 14) There are several points that this chapter raises in terms of practice and service development:

- Key national documents cited within the text promote vocational rehabilitation. How would you help Tricia to maintain her work role, potentially until retirement?
- The NAROT clinical guidelines identify that occupational therapy intervention, in particular self-management education should be *'provided in a timely fashion when the person is ready to act'* (NAROT/College of Occupational Therapists, 2003a), based partly upon the study by Hammond et al. (2004), which found that occupational therapy intervention was not effective with patients with a diagnosis of less than 2 years. Consider how, and with what tools, the occupational therapist could ascertain the person's 'readiness for change' and therefore how the service could accommodate this need in order to be more effective.
- What is the prevalence of rheumatoid arthritis within the Asian community? What strategies are in place in order to incorporate cultural competence (MacDonald, 1998) and meet the demands of the Code of Ethics and Professional Conduct (College of Occupational Therapists, 2005)? There is currently only one patient ARC leaflet (www.arc.org.uk) in a language other than English.
- How are the psychological needs of those with rheumatoid arthritis provided for within a rheumatology services? Do individuals have access to a nurse-led helpline, as recommended by the Arthritis and Musculoskeletal Alliance (2004)? How could a local community mental health trust (i.e. pain management team) assist?

References

American College of Rheumatology (2002) Guidelines for the management of rheumatoid arthritis. *Arthritis and Rheumatism*, **46**(2), 328–346

Arthritis and Musculoskeletal Alliance (2004) *Standards for People with Inflammatory Arthritis.* Arthritis and Musculoskeletal Alliance, London

Arthritis Research Campaign (2001) *Looking After your Joints when you have Rheumatoid Arthritis.* Arthritis Research Campaign, Derbyshire

Badamgarav, E., Croft Jr, J.D., Hohlbauch, A., Louie, J.S., O'Dell, J., Ofman, J.J., Suarez Almazor, M.E., Weaver, A., White, P. and Katz, P. (2003) Effects of disease management programs on functional status of patients with rheumatoid arthritis. *Arthritis Care and Research*, **49**(3), 377–387

Baldursdottir, R., Flo, R., Hurnasti, T., Jensen, L. and Sandberg, K. (2001) User involvement in the development of assistive technology in the Nordic countries (USDAT). In: *Assistive Technology – Added Value to the Quality of Life*. Ed. Marincek, C., Buhler, C., Knops, H. and Andrich, R., pp. 95–98. IOS Press, Amsterdam

Beighton, P.H., Grahame, R. and Bird, H. (1989) *Hypermobility of Joints*, 2nd edn. Springer-Verlag, Heidelberg

Belkin, J. (2002) Orthotics. Hand splinting: principles, practice and decision making. In: *Occupational Therapy Practice Skills for Physical Dysfunction*. Ed. Pedretti, L. and Early, M, pp. 529–558. Mosby, St. Louis

Blenkiron, E. (2005) Uptake of standardised hand assessments in rheumatology. Why is it so low? *British Journal of Occupational Therapy*, **68**(4), 148–163

British Society for Rheumatology (2003) *Annual Report*. www.rheumatology.org.uk

Brus, H.L., Van de Laar, M.A., Taal, E., Rasker, J. and Weigman, O. (1998) Effects of patient education on compliance with basic treatment regimes and health in recent onset active rheumatoid arthritis. *Annals of Rheumatic Diseases*, **57**(3), 146–151

Canadian Association of Occupational Therapists (1994) *Canadian Occupational Performance Measure*, 2nd edn. Canadian Association of Occupational Therapists, Toronto

College of Occupational Therapists (2005) *Code of Ethics and Professional Conduct*. College of Occupational Therapists, London

Coppard, B. and Lohman, H. (2001) *Introduction to Splintmaking. A clinical reasoning and problem solving approach*. Mosby, London

Cordery, J.C. (1965) Joint protection: a responsibility of the occupational therapist. *American Journal of Occupational Therapy*, **19**, 285–294

Creek, J. (2003) *Occupational Therapy Defined as a Complex Intervention*. College of Occupational Therapists, London

Cross, M.J., March, L.M., Lapsley, H.M., Byrne, E. and Brooks, P.M. (2006) Patient self-efficacy and health locus of control: relationships with health status and arthritis-related expenditure. *Rheumatology*, **45**(1), 92–96

David, C. and Lloyd, J. (1998) *Rheumatological Physiotherapy*. Mosby, London

Dellhag, B. and Bjelle, A. (1995) A grip ability test for use in rheumatology practice. *Journal of Rheumatology*, **22**(8), 1559–1565

Department of Health (2001) *The Expert Patient. A New Approach to Chronic Disease*. HMSO, London

Eberhardt, K., Markus Johnson, P., Rydrgen, L. (1991) The occurrence and significance of hand deformities in early rheumatoid arthritis. *British Journal of Rheumatology*, **30**, 211–213

Egan, M., Brosseau, L., Farmer, M., Ouimet, M.A., Rees, S., Wells, G. and Tugwell, P. (2001) Splints and orthoses in the treatment of rheumatoid arthritis. *The Cochrane Database of Systematic Reviews*, Issue 4, No CD004018. DOI: 004010.001002/14651858. CD 14004018

Falconer, J. (1991) Hand splinting in rheumatoid arthritis: a perspective on current knowledge and directions for research. *Arthritis Care and Research*, **4**(2), 81–86

Fess, E., Philips, C., Gettle, K. and Janson, R. (2004) *Splinting the Hand and Upper Extremity: Principles and Methods*. Mosby, London

Finlay, L. (1997) *The Practice of Psychosocial Occupational Therapy*, 2nd edn. Stanley Thornes, Cheltenham

Foster, M. (2002) Theoretical frameworks. In: *Occupational Therapy and Physical Dysfunction*, 5th edn. Ed. Turner, A., Foster, M. and Johnson, S.E., pp. 47–84. Churchill Livingstone, Edinburgh

Foster, M. and Pratt, J. (2002) Activity analysis. In: *Occupational Therapy and Physical Dysfunction*, 5th edn. Ed. Turner, A., Foster, M. and Johnson, S.E., pp. 145–164. Churchill Livingstone, Edinburgh

Hammond, A. (1996) Functional and health assessments used in rheumatology occupational therapy. A review and United Kingdom survey. *British Journal of Occupational Therapy*, **59**(6), 254–259

Hammond, A. (1997) Joint protection education: what are we doing? *British Journal of Occupational Therapy*, **60**(9), 401–406

Hammond, A. and Freeman, K. (2001) One-year outcomes of a randomized controlled trial of an educational–behavioural joint protection programme for people with rheumatoid arthritis. *Rheumatology*, **40**, 1044–1051

Hammond, A. and Jeffreson, P. (2002) Rheumatoid arthritis. In: *Occupational Therapy and Physical Dysfunction*, 5th edn. Ed. Turner, A., Foster, M. and Johnson, S.E., pp. 543–564. Churchill Livingstone, Edinburgh

Hammond, A. and Klompenhouwer, P. (2005) Getting evidence into practice: implementing a behavioural joint protection education programme for people with arthritis. *British Journal of Occupational Therapy*, **68**(1), 25–34

Hammond, A. and Lincoln, N. (1999a) The Joint Protection Knowledge Assessment (JPKA). *British Journal of Occupational Therapy*, **62**(3), 117–123

Hammond, A. and Lincoln, N. (1999b) The Joint Protection Behavioural Assessment (JPBA). *Arthritis Care and Research*, **12**(3), 200–207

Hammond, A., Jeffreson, P., Jones, N., Gallagher, J. and Jones, T. (2002) Clinical applicability of an educational-behavioural joint protection programme for people with rheumatoid arthritis. *British Journal of Occupational Therapy*, **65**(9), 405–412

Hammond, A., Young, A. and Kidao, R. (2004) A randomised controlled trial of occupational therapy for people with early rheumatoid arthritis. *Annals of Rheumatic Disease*, **63**(1), 23–30

Haskett, S., Backman, C., Porter, B., Govert, J. and Palejko, G. (2004) A crossover trial of custom-made and commercially available wrist splints in adults with inflammatory arthritis. *Arthritis Care and Research*, **51**(5), 792–799

Helewa, A., Goldsmith, C.H., Lee, P., Bombardier, C., Hanes, B., Smythe, H.A. and Tugwell, P. (1991) A randomised controlled trial of home exercise on the rheumatoid hand. *Lancet*, **337**, 1453–1456

Helliwell, P., O'Hara, M., Holdsworth, J., Hesselden, A., King, T. and Evans, P. (1999) A 12-month randomised controlled trial of patient education on radiographic changes and quality of life in early rheumatoid arthritis. *Rheumatology*, **38**(4), 303–308

Hill, J. (1998) *Rheumatology Nursing. A Creative Approach*. Churchill Livingstone, Edinburgh

Hudak, P., Amadio, P. and Bombardier, C. (1996) Development of an upper extremity measure of the DASH (disability of the arm, shoulder, hand). *American Journal of Industrial Medicines*, **29**, 6002–6008

Jebsen, R., Taylor, N., Trieschmann, R., Trotter, M. and Howard, L. (1969) An objective and standardised test of hand function. *Archive of Physical Medicine and Rehabilitation*, 311–319

Kennedy, T., McCabe, C., Struthers, G., Sinclair, H., Chakravaty, K., Bax, D., Shipley, M., Abernethy, R., Palferman, T. and Hull, R. (2005) BSR guidelines on standards of care for persons with rheumatoid arthritis. *Rheumatology*, **44**, 553–556

Kjeken, I., Moller, G. and Kvien, T. (1995) Use of commercially produced elastic wrist orthoses in chronic arthritis: a controlled study. *Arthritis Care and Research*, **8(20)**, 82–87

Lindroth, Y., Brattstrom, M., Bellman, I., Ekestaf, G., Olofsson, Y., Strombeck, B., Stenshed, B., Wikstrom, I., Nilsson, J.A. and Wollheim, F.A. (1997) A problem-based education program for patients with rheumatoid arthritis: evaluation after three and twelve months. *Arthritis Care and Research*, **10(5)**, 325–332

MacDonald, R. (1998) What is cultural competency? *British Journal of Occupational Therapy*, **61**, 325–329

Mathiowetz, V., Rogers, S.L., Dowe-Keval, M., Donahoe, L. and Rennells, C. (1986) The Purdue Pegboard: norms for 14- to 19-year-olds. *American Journal of Occupational Therapy*, **40(3)**, 174–179

Mathiowetz, V., Weber, K., Kashman, N. and Volland, G. (1985) Adult norms for the Nine Hole Peg Test. *Occupational Therapy Journal of Research*, **5(1)**, 24–38

McKee, P. and Rivard, A. (2004) Orthoses as enablers of occupation: client-centred splinting for better outcomes. *Canadian Journal of Occupational Therapy*, **71(5)**, 306–314

Medical Devices Directory (1997) *Wrist Splints for People with Rheumatological disease – A comparative evaluation*. Medical Devices Agency, Norwich

Meenan, R., Gertman, P. and Mason, J. (1980) Measuring health status in arthritis: impact measurement scales. *Arthritis and Rheumatism*, **23**, 146–152

Meenan, R., Mason, J., Anderson, J., Guccione, A. and Kazis, L. (1992) AIMS2. The content and properties of a revised and expanded arthritis impact measurement scales health status questionnaire. *Arthritis and Rheumatism*, **35(1)**, 1–10

Melvin, J.L. (1989) *Rheumatic Disease in the Adult and Child*, 3rd edn. FA Davis, Philadelphia

Murray, K., Topping, M. and Simpson, C. (2000) Investigation of the hand assessment techniques used within the United Kingdom. *British Journal of Hand Therapy*, **5(4)**, 125

National Association of Rheumatology Occupational Therapists/College of Occupational Therapists (2003a) *Clinical Guidelines 1 Occupational Therapy in the Management of Inflammatory Rheumatic Diseases*. NAROT/COT, London

National Association of Rheumatology Occupational Therapists/College of Occupational Therapists (2003b) *Clinical Guidelines 2 Joint Protection and Energy Conservation*. NAROT/COT, London

National Association of Rheumatology Occupational Therapists/College of Occupational Therapists (2003c) *Clinical Guidelines 3 Psychological Well-being and Self Management*. NAROT/COT, London

National Association of Rheumatology Occupational Therapists/College of Occupational Therapists (2003d) *Occupational Therapy Clinical Guidelines for Rheumatology – Splinting.* College of Occupational Therapists/NAROT, London

National Institute for Clinical Effectiveness (2002) *The Clinical Effectiveness and Cost Effectiveness of Etanercept and Infliximab for Rheumatoid Arthritis and Juvenile Poly-articular Idiopathic Arthritis.* London, HMSO

Niedermann, K., Fransen, J., Knols, R. and Uebelhart, D. (2004) Gap between short- and long-term effects of patient education in rheumatoid arthritis patients: a systematic review. *Arthritis and Rheumatism,* **51**(3), 388–398

Nordenskiold, U. (1990) Reduction of pain and increase in grip force for women with rheumatoid arthritis. *Arthritis Care and Research,* **3**(3), 158–162

Nordmark, B., Blomqvist, P., Andersson, B., Hägerström, M., Nordh Grate, K., Rönnqvist, R., Svensson, H. and Klareskog, L. (2006) A two year follow up of work capacity in early rheumatoid arthritis: a study of multidisciplinary team care with emphasis on vocational support. *Scandinavian Journal of Rheumatology,* **35**(1), 7–14

Pain, H., McLellan, L. and Gore, S. (2003) *Choosing Assistive Devices.* Jessica Kingsley Publishers, London

Palmer, P. and Simmons, J. (1991*)* Joint protection: a critical review. *British Journal of Occupational Therapy,* **54**(12), 453–457

Phillips, C.A. (1995) Therapists' management of patients with rheumatoid arthritis. In: *Rehabilitation of the Hand, Surgery and Therapy,* 4th edn. Ed. Hunter, J., Mackin, E. and Callaghan, A., pp. 1345–1350. Mosby: St Louis

Royal College of Nursing (2003) *Assessing, Managing and Monitoring Biologic Therapies for Inflammatory Arthritis. Guidance for Rheumatology Practitioners.* Royal College of Nursing, London

Sanford, M. and Wolfe, T. (2000) Rheumatoid arthritis. In: *Rheumatologic Rehabilitation Series: Volume 2. Adult Rheumatic Diseases.* Ed. Melvin, J.L. and Ferrell, K.M., pp. 161–204. American Occupational Therapy Association, Bethesda

Scholten, C., Brodowicz, T., Graninger, W., Gardavsky, I., Pils, K., Pesau, B., Eggl-Tyl, E., Wanivenhaus, A. and Zielinski, C. (1999) Persistent functional and social benefit 5 years after a multidisciplinary arthritis training program. *Archives of Physical Medicine and Rehabilitation,* **80**(10), 1282–1287

Simpson, C. (2005) *Hand Assessment. A clinical guide for therapists,* 2nd edn. APS Publishing, Wiltshire

Sollerman, C. and Ejeskar, A. (1995) Sollerman hand function test. *Scandinavian Journal of Plastic and Reconstructive Surgery,* **29**, 167–176

Stamm, T.A., Machold, K.P., Smolen, J.S., Fischer, S., Redlich, K., Graninger, W., Ebner, W. and Erlacher, L. (2002) Joint protection and home hand excercises improve hand function in patients with hand osteoarthritis: a randomised controlled trial. *Arthritis and Rheumatism,* **47**(1), 44–49

Steultjens, E.E.M.J., Bouter, L.L.M., Deckker, J.J., Kujk, M.M.A.H., Schaardenburg, D.D. and Van den Ende, E.C.H.M. (2004*) Occupational Therapy for Rheumatoid Arthritis.* The Cochrane Database of systematic Reviews Issue 1 Art. No. CD 003114.PUB2.DOI : 10. 1002/14651858.CD003114.pub2

Strong, J., Sturgess, J., Unrah, A. and Vincenzio, B. (2002) Pain assessment and measurement. In: *Pain. A textbook for therapists.* Ed. Strong, J., Unrah, A., Wright, A. and Baxter, G., pp. 123–147. Churchill Livingstone, London

Sumison, T. (1999) The client-centred approach. In: *Client-centred Practice in Occupational Therapy: A guide to implementation*. Ed. Sumison, T. Churchill Livingstone, Edinburgh

Tyrell, J. and Burn, A. (1996) Evaluating primary care occupational therapy results from a London primary health care centre. *British Journal of Therapy and Rehabilitation*, **3(7)**, 380–385

Van Lankveld, W., Graff, M. and van't Pad Bosch, P. (1999) The short version of the sequential occupational dexterity assessment based on individual's sensitivity to change. *Arthritis Care and Research*, **12(6)**, 417–423

Wilton, J. (1997) *Hand Splinting. Principles of Design and Fabrication*. WB Saunders Company Ltd, Cheltenham

6: Individual support for a person with motor neurone disease

Amanda Richardson

Introduction

The efficacy of palliative care provides a contentious and emotional challenge to those seeking to base their practice on a secure evidence base. This chapter emphasises the fact that the psychosocial and spiritual concerns experienced by those who have neurodegenerative conditions cannot easily be evaluated using systematised methodology; rather, best practice must be based on the clients' direct experience. This will necessitate the use of case reports, interviews and interactive observations. The occupational therapist, as part of the multidisciplinary palliative care team, seeks to minimise the effects of disability and contribute to quality of life for both the individual and his/her family. Best available evidence is therefore sought to support the diverse interventions offered by the palliative care team. These include:

- The provision of assistive devices (Agree, 1999).
- Carer support (Goldstein *et al.*, 1998; Brown, 2003).
- Facets concerning quality of life (Foley, 2004).
- Provision of home adaptations (Heywood, 2001; Hawkins and Stewart, 2002).
- Identification and strategies for addressing cognitive changes (Neary *et al.*, 2000)
- Provision of timely, accurate and honest information (O'Brien, 2004).
- Health promotion (vanderPloeg, 2001).
- Consideration of the unique spiritual needs of the individual at varying stages of the disease process (Prochnau *et al.*, 2003).

The National Service Framework for Long-Term Conditions (Department of Health, 2005) describes four groups of long-term neurological conditions, including progressive diseases such as motor neurone disease. It acknowledges the considerable challenge that these neurodegenerative conditions pose for individuals, their families and health and social care providers.

Motor neurone disease is a rapidly progressing and unpredictable neurodegenerative disease causing wasting and atrophy of muscles. There is an incidence of 1:100 000, and prevalence of 5:100 000, with males being more at risk than females, with a ratio of 1.5:1. Onset usually occurs after the age of 50. The mean survival rate of people diagnosed with this condition is 14 months from diagnosis (2–5 years from the onset of symptoms) (Ringel *et al.*, 1993). The speed with which motor neurone disease strips away the ability of the individual to perform many, if not all, occupations, can result in professionals and carers involved feeling impotent to do anything to really help. For the occupational therapist, physical and psychosocial issues share an equal importance and need to be addressed to minimise the effects of disability and contribute to quality of life for the individual and his/her family.

With the 1990s (the so-called 'decade of the brain') came a new surge in research and literature about the causes, drug therapy and management of motor neurone disease. Unfortunately, few of these relate directly to the role of occupational therapy. Those that do, tend to constitute mainly of expert opinion taken from experience in this and related fields. There is emerging evidence that a coordinated approach to care may, in itself, prolong survival and need not be costly (Corr *et al.*, 1998) To be truly effective, occupational therapy services must always sit within a multidisciplinary or interdisciplinary model and a clear understanding of the overall management and the roles of other team members is essential (Miller *et al.*, 1999; Oliver and Webb, 2000; Higginson *et al.*, 2003). The terminal nature of motor neurone disease also supports a palliative care approach to management (Oliver, 2002) and a great deal of literature can be found in the palliative care journals.

In the following sections, just over 2 years in the life of Angela (pseudonym), will be presented. The *Standards for Practice for Occupational Therapists Working with People having Chronic and/or Progressive Neurological Disorders* (College of Occupational Therapists, 2002) provides a framework to inform occupational therapy intervention. Service development is a dynamic process incorporating new evidence and clinical guidelines as they emerge. It is hoped that this chapter will add to the reader's knowledge and skill base in what is a varied and challenging field.

Motor neurone disease – an outline

Motor neurone disease was first described by in 1869 as a disease characterised by rapid degeneration of the motor neurones. Its cause is as yet unknown, although there are theories linked to diet (Ludolph and Spencer, 1996), environmental poisons (Howlett *et al.*, 1990), autoimmune factors (Meucci *et al.*, 1996) and viruses (Berger *et al.*, 2000). There are certain forms of motor neurone disease where there is a clear link between familial genetics and the condition (Rosen *et al.*, 1993). The term motor neurone disease is used in the UK to encompass a number of clinical subgroups.

Clinical subgroups

Amyotrophic lateral sclerosis

Amyotrophic lateral sclerosis (ALS) is by far the most common subgroup, comprising 85% of the estimated 5000–6000 people in the UK living with the disease. ALS most commonly strikes people between 40 and 60 years of age, but younger and older people also can develop the disease. Men are affected more often than women. ALS can be distinguished from other conditions of the motor system by the presence of both upper and lower motor neurone involvement (Mitsumoto *et al.*, 1998).

Upper motor neurone cell bodies reside in the motor cortex of the cerebrum. Their axons descend to make contact with the lower motor neurones. Lower motor neurone cell bodies are situated in the brainstem and anterior horns of the spinal cord and their axons make contact with muscle fibres. These are the motor pathways or corticospinal tracts which allow movement through selective control of muscles.

Symptoms of upper motor neurone damage include stiffness, spasticity (increased muscle tone), hyperreflexia (exaggerated reflex responses) and emotional lability (uncontrollable laughing or crying). Symptoms of lower motor neurone degeneration include weakness, atrophy (wasting) and fasciculation (involuntary twitching movements of muscle fibres, often visible under the skin) (Purves *et al.*, 2001).

Onset is insidious. People generally visit their doctor complaining of muscle weakness and thinning in the small muscles of one hand, or foot drop causing them to trip or fall. Symptoms tend to be asymmetrical initially, progressing to the opposite limb within a short space of time. Mobility is often quickly affected and associated with muscle cramps. Falls become frequent, necessitating the use of mobility aids, such as wheeled walking frames and wheelchairs, and environmental adaptations, such as grab rails and stair lifts. Loss of grip, stability and strength in the joints of the upper limbs may result in the inability to carry out personal care, feeding and drinking, domestic activities, employment and leisure activities (Eisen and Krieger, 1998).

Eventually all limbs and trunk musculature may be affected, resulting in difficulty maintaining or altering posture. Mobility in bed and in sitting may only be safely possible through the use of powered equipment, such as profiling beds, chairs and hoists. The diaphragm and intercostal muscles, responsible for breathing, weaken, causing symptoms of dyspnoea (shortness of breath), hypoventilation, fatigue and sleep disturbance. Respiratory issues have a large bearing on survival. Early onset and rapid progression of respiratory impairment will usually result in early death. Assisted ventilation is increasingly being offered to manage symptoms but brings with it ethical and financial considerations.

Progressive bulbar palsy

Progressive bulbar palsy (PBP) is a form of ALS which manifests in the bulbar muscles which control speech and swallowing; it comprises approximately 25% of all cases of motor neurone disease. Degeneration of the cranial nerves is responsible for loss of muscular control of the palate, pharynx and larynx. Fasciculation and wasting of the tongue may be evident (Motor Neurone Disease Association, 2000).

Nutritional issues arise early, and feeding via a gastrostomy is often recommended to assist the individual to maintain well-being and quality of life. Fear of choking can be ameliorated with education and good management by a speech and language therapist. The muscles of the face may be impaired, affecting expression (Lapiedra *et al.*, 2002).

PBP is associated with early-onset respiratory muscle impairment and individuals with this form tend to respond poorly to non-invasive ventilation (Gelinas *et al.*, 1998; Bradley *et al.*, 2002). Early weakening of the muscles of the neck and shoulder girdle is also associated with bulbar onset. Collars and tilt-in-space/reclining chairs can be useful. Survival in this group is 18 months to 2 years from the onset of symptoms (Shaw and Strong, 2003).

Progressive muscular atrophy

Progressive muscular atrophy (PMA) is a more slowly progressing form of motor neurone disease, which predominantly affects the lower motor neurones (Gouveia *et al.*, 2004).

Primary lateral sclerosis

Primary lateral sclerosis (PLS) is a condition characterised by purely upper motor neurone degeneration. Survival may be 30+ years (Swash *et al.*, 1999).

Familial motor neurone disease

Familial motor neurone disease (FALS) occurs in an estimated 5% of diagnosed cases. The identification of a specific gene, superoxide dismutase (SOD1) was found to be responsible for the development of the disease in 20% of FALS, which sparked a flurry of research (Garofalo, 1995).

Symptoms

Although the onset and progression of the disease may indicate a particular subtype of motor neurone disease, symptoms will nearly always progress to encompass some if not all symptoms of ALS. In 90% of people, bulbar muscles may eventually become involved, affecting the ability to speak and chew and swallow food safely. By the time motor neurone disease begins to manifest itself as any of the symptoms described, it is thought that the vast majority of motor neurones have already been destroyed. Currently Rilutek (riluzole) is the only licensed drug available that is believed to have a moderate effect on delaying the progression of the disease (Dib, 2003)

The cranial nerves controlling ocular movements are spared, as is the smooth muscle of the heart, gastrointestinal tract and sphincter muscles of bladder and bowel (autonomic nervous system). Sensation generally remains intact, although some clients may report changes in temperature regulation and altered smell and taste. Physical responses to intimacy remain.

At one time it was thought that intellect remained intact. Recent research, however, suggests that as many as 30–40% of people affected may experience some frontotemporal involvement, with symptoms ranging from poor concentration and inability to make complex decisions to full blown dementia with associated memory loss and socially inappropriate behaviour (Barson *et al.*, 2000; Neary *et al.*, 2000) People with PBP often develop literacy and language problems which further compound communication issues (Cobble, 1998; Murphy, 2004). Mood disturbances are a further feature (Moore *et al.*, 1998).

Psychological impact

It is not possible to overestimate the psychological distress caused by being given a diagnosis of motor neurone disease and the subsequent frustrations of living with increasing disability until death (Goldstein *et al.*, 1998). Most people will experience strong grief reactions, such as numbness, shock, anger, denial, guilt, fear, anxiety, sadness and depression. These symptoms will often present for several weeks after the diagnosis, and can resurface at any point as the disease progresses. Acceptance and a degree of equilibrium are sometimes achieved only to be lost again following the loss of another valued aspect of independence. Identification and management of psychological issues, which are impacting on the individual's ability to engage in everyday life, are important.

Psychological status correlates strongly with survival (Johnston *et al.*, 1999). Low self-esteem, worthlessness and feeling that there is no purpose left to life will hasten the progress of the disease. Promoting (realistic) hope cannot be over-emphasised (Carter *et al.*, 1998). Herth (1990) described seven factors that promote hope. These are factors which occupational therapists can encourage throughout their involvement:

- Interpersonal connectedness.
- Achievable goals.
- Spiritual base.
- Personal attributes.
- Humour/light-heartedness.
- Uplifting memories.
- Affirmation of worth.

Government directives

There are several government directives which have influenced the clinical reasoning of occupational therapists working with those who have motor neurone disease. The following were particularly relevant when working with Angela.

The National Service Framework for People with Long-Term Conditions was published in 2005 with comprehensive quality standards expected for those working with clients such as Angela, who are living with a long-term condition (Department of Health, 2005). The first standard refers to the need to provide a **person-centred service**. This is an essential human right which involves the individual being provided with as much information as possible in order to help him/her make informed decisions about his/her care and treatment, and if possible how to manage his/her condition personally. This is conducive to good occupational therapy practice. It is important, however, that the timing of information is considered; too much, too early can have serious consequences on the individual's attitude to their condition and their psychological well-being (Goldstein *et al.*, 1998). The information provided also must be true and accurate, based on evidence. This may be particularly difficult when the client wishes to discuss issues relating to death and dying (Foster, 2005).

Quality requirement 5 of the National Service Framework for People with Long-Term Conditions (Department of Health, 2005) recommends that those who have conditions such as motor neurone disease should have **ongoing** access to a *'comprehensive range of rehabilitation, advice and support, to meet their continuing and changing needs, to increase their independence and autonomy and help them to live as they wish'* (Department of Health, 2005). The location of where rehabilitation is provided should be directed by the individual, be this at home, in a hospice or in a palliative care unit. This promotes an ongoing involvement by the occupational therapist which, in Angela's situation, covered a duration of 2 years.

Quality requirement 7 recommends that people who have motor neurone disease should *'receive timely, appropriate **assistive technology/equipment and adaptations** to accommodation to support them to live independently; help them with their care; maintain their health and improve their quality of life'* (Department of Health, 2005). This suggests that funding should be freely available to pay for these adaptations and devices. The reality is, however, that the NHS and Social Services budgets are not finite and towards the end of the financial year funding is extremely limited; several charitable organisations have, therefore, helped in the provision of certain items of reusable equipment, such as the King's Fund and Motor Neurone Disease Association (MNDA).

The importance of a comprehensive **palliative care** service is emphasised in quality requirement 9 of the National Service Framework (Department of Health, 2005). This should focus on help to control symptoms, offer pain relief and meet needs for personal, social, psychological and spiritual support, in line with the principles of palliative care. The spiritual care of the client is often neglected in many aspects of occupational therapy but its importance for those with a limited life cannot be underestimated. It is, therefore, important that the occupational therapist is sensitive to individuals' personal perceptions of spirituality, taking care not to impose personal beliefs at a susceptible time.

In addition to the National Service Framework quality standards for those with long-term conditions, the Disability Discrimination Act passed in 1995 adds credence to the human rights of those with motor neurone disease. Since October 1999 community services, such as access in shops, portable ramps for use in taxis or public buildings, have to make **reasonable adjustments** for those who may have to use a wheelchair or other mobility aid. This was extended in October 2004 so all new buildings and current public buildings are accessible to those who have a physical limitation. The latest edition (Disability Discrimination Act 2005) places a duty on all public bodies to promote equality of opportunity to all disabled people. This will not only include environmental access, but also work and leisure facilities.

As the person with motor neurone disease becomes increasingly dependent on others due to the degenerative nature of the disease, an appreciation of the Carers Recognition and Services Act 1995 is valuable (Harding and Higginson, 2003). A carer is defined in the Act as someone who provides substantial amounts of care on a regular basis to another person. It refers to a family member or unpaid volunteer who is supported and financially rewarded for their care. The Act applies only to these 'informal carers', that is carers who are not providing care under a contract and who are not volunteers for a voluntary organisation. The importance of carers' support was highlighted in a Scottish study of carers by van Teijlingen *et al.* (2001) who found that four out of ten carers have their sleep disturbed regularly, and a quarter of the 153 people involved longed for more support in their caring role. A recent ethnographic study of caregivers by Ray and Street (2005) reiterates these findings.

On 26 December 2003, the Secretary of State introduced a scheme to improve care for people coming to the end of their lives. This reinforces the National Service Framework quality standards by ensuring that all those individuals nearing the end of life will have access to high quality specialist palliative care to be able to live and die in the place of their choice. The Preferred Place of Care (PPC) is an empowering scheme intended to be managed by the individual through his/her path of care into the variety of differing health and social care settings. The document provides an opportunity to record:

▦ A family profile and carer's needs.
▦ The person's thoughts about his/her care, their choices and preferences.
▦ The services that are available in a locality and being accessed by the individual.
▦ Any changes in care needs.

The scheme is very important; a retrospective study by Chaudri *et al.* (2003) of patterns of mortality in clients with motor neurone disease determined that 36% of the 179 clients involved in the study died in hospital (either intensive care unit or accident and emergency department). They concluded that this number could have been reduced further as a number of those who died on hospital wards could have been cared for conservatively at home, the preferred place for the individual, with the support of the palliative care team.

Frames of reference and associated approaches

Occupational therapists working with clients with motor neurone disease need to be aware of the neuroanatomy of this complex, degenerative condition, in addition to the government directives which relate to the individual human rights of those with such a debilitating condition. They also need to be aware of the various frames of reference and associated approaches pertinent to palliative care (Hagedorn, 2001). The following are those employed by the occupational therapist working with Angela.

The **humanistic** frame of reference is essential when working with individuals who have terminal or progressive conditions like motor neurone disease. It is strongly holistic and considers the individual as a whole within the context of his/her social and physical environment. The individual has the right to personal choice and autonomy, and is capable of controlling his/her life events. It is supported by current clinical guidelines for the overall management of the disease and evidence for best practice (Brown, 2003).

The **client-centred approach** (Sumsion, 1999) sits within the humanistic frame of reference and requires that the therapist give control to the client. The therapist facilitates the provision of information and opportunities about which the client can make decisions. The therapist then arranges the resources or intervention to achieve the client's desired outcomes (Cott, 2004).

The **physiological** frame of reference (Hagedorn, 2001) is concerned with the body's ability to maintain a stable physiological state. From an occupational therapy perspective, two approaches sit within this frame of reference: the biomechanical approach and the neuro-developmental approach. Interventions from both approaches may form part of the occupational therapist's 'toolkit'.

When using the **biomechanical approach** (Pedretti and Early, 2001), the use of orthoses and mobile arm supports can promote fine motor function and prevent flexor contractures at the wrist in individuals with motor neurone disease. The use of assistive devices to **compensate** for a lack of motor control, such as tilt-in-space chairs and cushioning, can promote good posture through positioning, which in turn will assist with respiration, feeding and control of lower limb oedema. Adaptive equipment can maintain the ability to participate in self-care and domestic activities.

The **neuro-developmental approach** (Hagedorn, 2001) can be applied in the early stages of the disease when the principles of normal movement can be demonstrated in order to educate the individual in understanding how to move from one postural set to another (i.e. sitting to standing) most effectively. Later, correct positioning and handling, taught to carers, can help to inhibit abnormal reflexes and normalise muscle tone. It is therefore very important that the occupational therapist is familiar with moving and handling procedures.

The **palliative care approach** is defined as: *'The active total care of patients whose disease is not responsive to curative treatment. Control of pain, of other symptoms, and of psychological, social and spiritual problems is paramount. The goal of palliative care is the achievement of the best possible quality of life for patients and their families'* (World Health Organization, 2002). This approach requires the occupational therapist to be aware of information and research pertaining to the condition, and to offer this at a time determined by the client. Therefore an **educative approach** is also adopted. The value of occupational therapy in promoting the quality of life in those with life-limiting conditions is increasingly being recognised (Dawson and Barker, 1995; Higginson *et al.*, 2000; Ewer-Smith and Patterson, 2002; O'Brien, 2001).

The **multidisciplinary approach** refers to a comprehensive multidisciplinary team approach to management, often comprising of a 'core' team of neurologist, general practitioner (GP), physiotherapist, specialist nurse, speech and language therapist, dietician, occupational therapist and clinical psychologist (Young, 1998; Corr *et al.*, 1998; Higginson *et al.*, 2003). In reality, a dedicated team for such a relatively small group of clients is unrealistic and services may vary widely in the resources and skills available.

In the case study to follow, the occupational therapist fulfils this role within a multidisciplinary team of professionals dedicated to providing a fast-track, evidence-based, key worker-led model of care. Angela will remain on the team's caseload until she dies.

Angela's experience

Angela was 57 years old when diagnosed with motor neurone disease. She is an educated woman who started work at 16 years of age. She enjoyed various jobs but the last 20 years of her working life she felt had been the most fulfilling, working as a carer for people with learning difficulties. She married but later divorced, bringing up two children, her daughter, Carol, and son, Ian, both now married with children of their own. Angela never remarried and states that she enjoys her own space and independence.

From the outset, Angela was assertive about her need to remain in control of her own life. She lives in a one-bedroom flat, to which she is attached, and enjoys choosing colours and fabrics to decorate it. She used to enjoy activities and holidays involving the local church and long-term friends, in particular, flower arranging and walking holidays.

At the age of 54, Angela was diagnosed with breast cancer which was a serious blow to her independent lifestyle as she felt that she should resign from her job. Following a mastectomy, Angela was treated with the drug tamoxifen and was nearing the 5-year 'all clear' when she suffered a set-back. Angela began to notice that her legs felt more tired than usual after routine shopping trips. She also noticed that the muscles around the thumb of her right hand seemed thinner. She began to drop things and could not get a good grip on zip tabs and small buttons.

Her GP knew her well and was quick to refer her for a private consultation with a local neurologist. There is no specific diagnostic test for motor neurone disease; the diagnosis was made following careful clinical assessment over time, supported by blood tests, magnetic resonance imaging and electromyography to eliminate other conditions.

Finally, at the age of 57, with her walking becoming more unstable, Angela was told her 'probable' diagnosis of motor neurone disease. It was a text book delivery of the diagnosis: in a private room, in the presence of her daughter, with sufficient time for questions. They did not ask about the prognosis and left knowing that this disease affects the nerve supply to muscles and would get worse over time. They had been told about the specialist multidisciplinary motor neurone disease clinic, held once a month and that she would be invited to attend the next available appointment.

At this time Angela presented with weakness of both lower limb muscles with the more significant problem of proprioceptive loss, resulting in an unsteady gait and fear of falling. There was evidence of wasting and weakness of the thenar eminence of her right hand. Fortunately, she is left hand dominant. She stated that she was having difficulties getting in and out of the bath and was feeling tired all the time.

Assessment

Initial multidisciplinary assessment

During her first clinic appointment it was made clear by Angela that she wanted to be in control of her disease and any decisions regarding the management of symptoms. Her presenting problems were:

- Impaired balance whilst mobilising, which had caused two falls outdoors.
- Difficulty controlling the actions of sitting and rising in her bath.
- Difficulty with fastening buttons.
- Difficulty with holding and manipulating a knife in her right hand.
- Lack of confidence in carrying items up and down stairs.

The physiotherapist identified loss of proprioception in foot placement, foot-drop in the left foot and mild muscle weakness in her lower limbs as causes of her impaired balance and falls, and prescribed a walking stick and right ankle/ foot orthosis. The occupational therapist arranged a visit at a time to suit Angela to assess the other occupations in her home environment. Angela was reluctant to commit to an early appointment with the occupational therapist as she was still processing the reality of her diagnosis. She set the appointment at 1 month from her clinic date.

Initial occupational therapy assessment

The initial occupational therapy assessment took place in Angela's home. The first part of the assessment involved inviting Angela to give a narrative account of her life using open questions. Use of narrative reinforces self-worth and client-centredness and elicits information regarding a person's past and present interests, occupations and values, family and social life and understanding of their disease history to that point. Following this, clarification was sought about what seemed to be important to her to maintain quality of life. The occupational therapist then addressed the issues Angela had raised in the multidisciplinary team clinic, attended previously. A functional assessment of each of the activities was carried out, during which fatigue was identified as having a major effect on Angela's ability to maintain the range of activities in her life. The occupational therapist suggested that a further session could be arranged to discuss fatigue management.

With a rapidly progressing condition, preparation is essential. Although a formal assessment of joint range of movement and muscle strength was not carried out in clinic, Angela had described her current symptoms in terms of what she found difficult to do. Angela had asymmetrical weakness in her upper and lower limbs which rendered her unable to raise herself from the bottom of the bath. The occupational therapist then gauged the value placed on the activity of 'bathing'. Angela enjoyed a daily relaxing 'soak' in the bath which provided her with thinking time. She enjoyed using aromatherapy oils and candles to enhance the experience. This information allowed the occupational therapist to save time on her first visit by arriving with assessment equipment that might prove useful, such as a powered reclining bathlift. Gooch (2003) recommends that bathing assessments should be carried out in the context of the person's own home, taking into account their individual bathing habits. Gooch (2003) also recommends that bathing assessments should be undertaken with the bath *full of water* as this is certainly a more realistic situation.

Environmental assessment

During the home visit, the occupational therapist was able to carry out an informal assessment of the environment using structured observation. A short, steep communal driveway led to a side gate. Five rustic stone steps of uneven height and tread led to a short path and a two step action into the property. The kitchen was compact with minimal floor space. A narrow staircase with two 90° turns led from the open plan dining/living area to two doorways off a small landing on the first floor. The first entered the bathroom, the second the bedroom.

Key-worker assessment

Within the multidisciplinary model of care which supports Angela, the occupational therapist not only has to assess the individual from an occupational perspective, but, as key worker, considering other possible ramifications of the disease process in order to refer appropriately to other services (Jain *et al.*, 2005). A non-standardised screening tool was devised to assist the key worker (and other members of the multidisciplinary team) in the home setting (Fig. 6.1). It was not designed to cover every possible symptom and professional intervention but to prompt observation and awareness.

The assessment was designed to be used informally and in conjunction with clinical observation. The aim is to screen at least monthly if the condition is progressing quickly and to refer on to other team members promptly if changes are noted by the client. The client should always agree to the referral being made and liaison between team members will help to prevent duplication of assessment and visits.

Further assessment

Angela did not wish to undertake any formal evaluation of her occupational skills as she was fearful that it would highlight more issues than she could currently cope with. Therefore the occupational therapist agreed to establish specific goals in collaboration with Angela at a time determined by herself. Had Angela been willing, the Canadian Occupational Performance Measure (COPM) (Law *et al.*, 1994) would have served as a useful monitor of Angela's level of functioning. The COPM is a client-centred assessment tool which incorporates the client's perception of both performance ability and satisfaction with achieving valued activities prior to and following intervention. It allows the occupational therapist to choose the most appropriate treatment approach or technique and also serves as a useful outcome measure. In order for the COPM to work for someone with a rapidly progressing condition it needs to be used in a dynamic way and the goals need to be stated in such a way as to reflect the nature of the condition. If a person is unwilling to grasp the consequences of his/her diagnosis, goals may prove to be short term and therefore impractical to evaluate within a very short timeframe.

Further assessments could have been used to determine Angela's emotional state and cognitive ability. For example the Hospital Anxiety and Depression Scale (HADS) (Zigmond and Snaith, 1983) was found to be useful in determining significant mood disturbance and support the use of antidepressants or anxiety management/counselling intervention. Its reliability has been validated by literature collated by Bjelland *et al.* (2002). The Cognitive Assessment of Minnesota (CAM) (Rustad *et al.*, 1993) or Behavioural Assessment of Dysexecutive Syndrome (BADS) (Wilson *et al.*, 1996) could also have been used, with the client's permission, to identify difficulties around information processing, problem solving and behavioural organisation (Beresford, 2002). Foley and Neeley (2003) encourage occupational therapists to consider the impact that cognitive dysfunction has on the everyday living skills of a person with motor neurone disease. They cite a study by Barson *et al.* (2000) who used a modified version of the Dysexecutive

Name of Client _____ Date of Visit _____

Speech and language therapist

1. Has the client experienced any difficulty chewing?
2. Is there evidence of an impaired swallow, e.g. coughing, choking, regurgitating fluids or drooling saliva?
3. Has there been any change in speech such as a change in volume, tone or slurring?

Dietitian

4. Has the client or carer noticed a change in weight or appetite?

    Present weight _____

Occupational therapist

5. Is the client experiencing/likely to experience difficulties getting around his/her home or out and about?
6. Has there been any deterioration in lower or upper limb function resulting in difficulties with personal, domestic, work or leisure activities?
7. Is the client experiencing disabling fatigue?

Physiotherapist

8. Has the client had any falls or stumbles?

9. Has there been any neck or shoulder pain, problems holding head up?

10. Have there been any alterations in muscle tone or cramps?

Liaison nurse/specialist respiratory nurse

11. Has the client experienced any morning headache, alterations to sleeping pattern, shortness of breath when lying or sitting or excessive daytime sleepiness?
12. Have there been any issues with medication or side effects?
13. Has the client experienced any continence issues?

Medical physics

14. If the client has impaired mobility or upper limb function can he/she access the TV, entertainment systems, telephone, let carers in or alert carers if required, change position of riser, recliner, chair or bed independently?
15. Have there been any difficulties with an existing environmental control system?

Regional care adviser

16. Does the individual have an interest in knowing more about the support offered by Motor Neurone Disease Association?
17. Do they or their carer feel the need to speak to other people with MND or caring for someone?

Pschosocial issues

18. Is the client/carer experiencing persistent low mood or anxiety?
19. Is there evidence of severe emotional lability, cognitive/behavioural changes?
20. Has there been a significant change in financial circumstances?

Figure 6.1 Multidisciplinary screening assessment tool.

Questionnaire (DEX) (Burgess *et al.*, 1996) to determine the incidence of cognitive dysfunction on those with motor neurone disease and found that this had important implications for individuals' care and support services. Goldstein and Leigh (1999) also stress the importance of identifying the effects of cognitive dysfunction on coping behaviour, with the subsequent effects on quality of life.

The information gleaned from the initial assessment, the multidisciplinary screening assessment and the environmental observation helped the occupational therapist to consider the possibilities for helping Angela come to terms with her condition and provide her with the best quality of life possible. This informed her clinical goal setting over the 2 years which followed.

Clinical reasoning and goal setting

Clinical reasoning within a client-centred approach is a dynamic process. The occupational therapist must be led by the client and yet also be aware that the client may not be aware of therapeutic interventions and social support available to them. The rapidity of the disease process means that the occupational therapist must be constantly thinking ahead and working to prepare the client for decision making, which is often painful. It requires the therapist to be sensitive and knowledgeable about referral processes and local resources so as not to lead people to have unrealistic expectations which can 'hijack' hope. An ongoing working relationship, which is based on trust and honesty, can help to ease someone through difficult life transitions where time is of the essence. Crisis management should be avoided if at all possible but is sometimes inevitable and should not be seen as failure but as an opportunity for reflection and learning (Billinghurst, 2001).

Angela had already faced a life-threatening illness and learnt from the experience. She was determined to maintain a positive outlook and did not want to look too far ahead. Goal setting took place on two levels – an insightful and evolving awareness of what quality of life actually meant for her enabled her to cope with short-term practical solutions and interventions which facilitated the achievement of her long-term goals. For example, her desire to remain in her own home helped her to accept adaptations, equipment and care services which enable her to do so. Her wish to be able to continue to attend her local church service most Sundays created a positive response to using first a scooter and later a personal assistant to push her there in a wheelchair. Her desire to remain usefully engaged in 'mental' activity despite her deteriorating physical condition meant that she was quite easily persuaded (despite her initial reservations) to learn how to use a computer. This now allows her to purchase presents, shop for groceries and engage in 'virtual travel'.

Rather than present individual occupational therapy episodes of care which were timed according to Angela's needs, examples of a range of solutions to issues identified by Angela will be presented. Evidence justifying the occupational therapist's course of action will also be offered. This will demonstrate the implementation of an educative, palliative care and compensatory approach.

Intervention

Over a period of 2 years, Angela identified a number of functional difficulties which were affecting her quality of life. These included impaired fine motor skills in her right hand, difficulties transferring in and out of her bath safely and a high level of fatigue influencing her ability to carry out domestic chores and engage in leisure activities.

She also admitted to a high level of anxiety about how quickly the disease might progress and a fear of falling again. She asked a number of questions about the cause and nature of motor neurone disease and what research was presently being carried out into a cure. She made it clear that she did not want too much information immediately about what might happen to her as the disease progressed but was accepting of the occupational therapist's offer to assess regularly and offer information and advice as it was thought necessary. It was agreed that a **problem-solving, compensatory approach** would be adopted with the aim of maintaining her independence and autonomy within her own home and enabling her to continue to engage in meaningful spiritual and leisure activities (Foster, 2001). As motor neurone disease affects everyone differently in the context of their social and physical environment, Angela would be accepted as the 'expert' in her disease process and would orchestrate team intervention.

Personal care

This included continual assessment and advice regarding small items of equipment to facilitate independence in personal care and domestic tasks, for example, a button hook and key ring loops placed on zips assisted with fastenings. Later velcro replaced trouser buttons. The reclining powered bathlift proved invaluable in maintaining a valued leisure pursuit and safety in transfers until a level access shower could be provided. It was also less tiring for her to take a daily bath than attempt a strip wash. Agree (1999) supports this use of assistive devices and technology in enabling indivduals to continue to live as independently as possible.

Domestic tasks

A kitchen workstation with vegetable clamp, ergonomic knife, Dycem mat and jar opener maintained her kitchen skills for a period of 4 months. Angela purchased these along with a one-handed non-slip tray to continue to take items up and down stairs in her right hand and was advised to consider a left descending stair rail for safety. This she declined until a near fall a month later. The importance of ongoing domiciliary support for those with a degenerative condition was highlighted in a recent study by Kealey and McIntyre (2005), who used structured interviews to obtain both client and carers' views to evaluate domiciliary occupational therapy services. Although the focus was on those clients with cancer, the application is true for people with motor neurone disease. Both clients and carers reported high levels of satisfaction with the service offered although consistency of provision was sporadic; they recommended that further resources were needed if a consistent level of care were to be provided throughout the UK.

Fatigue management

An educational approach was used to help Angela prioritise her daily activities according to how much they contributed to her quality of life and how essential it was for her to be able to do activities in terms of satisfaction and enjoyment. A discussion then followed about how she would choose to spend her daily 'package' of energy without having to borrow energy from the following day. As a result of this she willingly engaged in suggestions that would help to reduce the amount of energy expended during the day without compromising her quality of life and decided to employ some domestic help with her disability living allowance to free up energy to continue attending a flower arranging class and a church counselling course.

The importance of fatigue management is supported by Kralik *et al.* (2005) who stress that it is vital for health care workers to give their clients opportunities to talk about their fatigue levels, validate their experiences and provide support with self-care. They encourage health professionals to *'challenge their own meanings and expectations surrounding a person's report of fatigue so that opportunities for therapeutic intervention can be facilitated'*.

To further reduce Angela's fatigue levels, a raised toilet seat was provided to maintain independence in toilet transfers with reduced effort. Two perching stools were provided for use in the bathroom and kitchen to preserve energy and assist with balance whilst focusing on dual tasks.

Angela identified feelings of anxiety and tiredness on rising each morning with 'a churning stomach'. She did not feel like she was waking refreshed. This raised concerns regarding her respiratory function. Angela decided to talk to her GP about her low mood and started to take anti-depressants as part of a coping strategy. She agreed to an assessment by the specialist respiratory nurse and subsequently attended an out patient clinic to see the respiratory consultant. During deep REM (rapid eye movement) sleep she was found to be experiencing dips in her oxygen levels interrupting her normal sleep cycle and resulting in tiredness. Non-invasive ventilation was discussed and Angela agreed to a trial to see if it helped her to obtain a better quality of sleep. This proved to be the case and she soon adjusted to having an oxygen mask on during the night. She woke with more energy and was less fatigued during the day. (Respiratory assessments are now carried out routinely in the motor neurone disease clinic from diagnosis.)

Information needs

The educational approach was also used to meet Angela's information needs. The MNDA's Personal Guide was provided, as well as information about the care and research centres at her request. Angela was encouraged to talk to her neurologist about the possibility of a referral to a specialist neurologist and participation in research trials. The importance of timely information was highlighted in a study by O'Brien (2004), who used semi-structured interviews to question seven people with motor neurone disease about their experiences in seeking and obtaining information on their condition. Three distinctive information-seeking categories emerged: active seekers, selective seekers and information avoiders. Angela adopted the selective seeking role, only asking for information which she deemed appropriate at a given time. What was evident from this research was that exposure to unsolicited information, for example through television documentaries and media coverage, had a negative effect on the individual's psychological well-being.

Leisure

Angela perceives herself as a physical, mental and spiritual being. She was concerned that she would not be able to participate in her physical interests for much longer. These included walking holidays and flower arranging. She also enjoyed writing a journal. With this in mind, the therapist explored the idea of using a computer. Angela stated that she had never been interested in using computers but when the occupational therapist described how one could be used to keep a journal, photographs of family, carry out on-line shopping and travel the globe in a virtual way, she gained interest. She was provided with information about Learn Direct, a library scheme encouraging the use of information technology skills and agreed to have a trial at her local library. She was so excited about learning this new skill that she completed the course and subsequently agreed to the occupational therapist approaching the local branch of the MNDA for a financial grant to purchase a laptop computer. She teamed up with a lady in her flower arranging class who provided the 'legs' to fetch and carry while she provided some creative advice.

Mobility

Angela's physiotherapist provided her with ankle/foot orthoses, which prevented her from catching her toes and falling forward. Evidence from a systematic review by Bakker *et al.* (2000) emphasises that the use of such orthoses in clients with neurodegenerative diseases can prolong assisted walking and standing, but it is uncertain whether it can prolong functional walking. Needless to say, Angela was determined to maintain her mobility and purchased her own fashionable height-adjustable walking stick in order to get into town to do her shopping. Over a 6-month period this was replaced by a weekly trip with her daughter and son-in-law because of increasingly impaired balance and a fear of falling. As part of an energy saving exercise she agreed to a wheelchair assessment and when her self-propelling wheelchair arrived, she agreed to have it with them in the car 'just in case'. In her own time she began to use the wheelchair more frequently as it allowed her to go further afield. At the same time she organised a scooter assessment with a local agent and purchased a reconditioned scooter to enable her to go to church independently.

Major adaptations

Perhaps the most daunting task for the occupational therapist was to approach a home loving Angela with the idea that her home would not be suitable for future wheelchair access at a time when she was still mobile with a stick! Fortunately, Angela provided the opportunity to discuss this by asking if anything could be done to make her external steps safer. A request was made to social services to assess whether a half step and rail could be provided. The therapist took the opportunity to ask Angela whether she had considered what she would do should she need to use her wheelchair more frequently, perhaps even in the house. It was explained that major adaptations, such as ramps and lifts, could take some time to arrange. In the interests of remaining in control and being informed about the process, Angela agreed to the social services occupational therapist assessing her property for future wheelchair access and having the Disabled Facilities Grant explained to her by an expert.

Towards the end of the first 6 months Angela had had time to consider the implications of major adaptations and had embraced the grant process in order to remain in her own home. An external wheelchair step-lift, through floor lift and wet floor shower had been recommended as being both necessary and appropriate.

There is clear evidence that housing adaptations work (Heywood, 2001), but the importance of being sensitive to the meaning of the home to the client cannot be underestimated. Hawkins and Stewart (2002) suggest that there are times when, in the process of recommending adaptations to the home environment, the significance of the home to the individual or his/her family can be overlooked and compromised by the changes that occur to it. They recommend that a social model of disability should be applied to the assessment process to provide a holistic view of the environmental barriers as perceived by the person, while gaining insight into the meanings the person places on the home.

Palliative care

There is a variety of palliative care models provided to those with motor neurone disease (Oliver *et al.*, 2000). Higginson *et al.* (2000) surveyed over 40 palliative care centres in the North and South Thames region. They identified that the most common activities provided in these centres were review of individuals' symptoms or needs, monitoring symptoms, bathing, physiotherapy, hairdressing and aromatherapy. Other activities developed creativity, music and carer-managed outings. Occupational therapy was provided but this was not consistent across centres, although the importance of this role was acknowledged. Further evidence highlights the importance of the occupational therapist teaching relaxation techniques to those with life-limiting conditions (Ewer-Smith and Patterson, 2002), while vanderPloeg (2001) refers to the occupational therapist's role in health promotion. Oliver and Webb (2000) recommend the involvement of an occupational therapist in specialist care services for people with motor neurone disease, although the small geographical numbers may make this financially untenable. On the other hand, Higginson *et al.* (2003) question whether palliative care teams alter end-of-life experiences of the client and their caregivers at all!

The occupational therapist was extremely frustrated by Angela's absolute refusal to discuss end-of-life issues. This conflicted strongly with her coping strategy of 'thinking positively'. Consequently, Angela did not want to be educated about the role of the hospice and palliative care services which could be invaluable in supporting both herself and her family in an emotional and spiritual way. Angela became agitated whenever the subject was raised, however sensitively, by a member of the team. This is not uncommon in those with motor neurone disease (Young *et al.*, 1995) She had, however, written a living will which stated that, should she develop a chest infection or become unable to breathe on the non-invasive ventilator, she would want to have a tracheotomy to enable her to continue to breathe artificially (Dimond, 2004). She had previously discussed this with the respiratory team. This measure could have serious ramifications for her remaining in her own home and achieving her long-term goal. Ventilator dependency does not prevent the disease from progressing eventually leading to 'locked in' syndrome, requiring 24-hour care. Locked-in syndrome is characterised by complete paralysis except for voluntary eye movements. It is usually caused by lesions in the nerve centres that control muscle contractions, or a blood clot that blocks circulation of oxygen to the brain stem (NINDs, accessed on-line 2006). In the USA and Japan, this situation is not uncommon. It is happening more frequently in the UK and places a large financial responsibility on health and social services, not to mention the human resource issue. Whilst some individuals have managed to obtain support to continue living in their own homes, others have found their local services unable or unwilling to support their personal choice to remain at home and have found themselves in long-term care homes. As key worker, Angela's occupational therapist has to work closely with the respiratory nurses, respiratory consultant and physiotherapist to plan an educative approach which will enable Angela to make a fully informed decision (Littlechild, 2004). Ultimately, her decision may challenge the motor neurone disease team considerably.

Quality of life

In many ways motor neurone disease confounds the fundamental principle that the science of occupational therapy is often defined by. How does someone who can neither move a muscle nor speak participate in purposeful activity in order to maintain or promote their own well-being? And yet, people do survive, and often with a perception of quality of life which might easily be questioned by observers. Others will choose to end life, even when the ability to mobilise and manage aspects of personal care is still possible. If this is the case, then quality of life, as a concept, must be much broader than the ability to *physically* (at some level) participate in an occupation. Quality of life then is important to define on an individual basis and sits neatly within a client-centred approach. If an approach or model is to be of use in working with people affected by motor neurone disease, it must be client centred and assist in defining quality of life for the individual in terms of, not just physical aspects of occupational performance, but spiritual well-being.

Occupational therapists may not be altogether comfortable addressing issues of spirituality. Rose (1999) considered the attitudes of 44 occupational therapists working within palliative care and only 8% stated that they consistently addressed spirituality within assessment or treatment. It was felt by 32% that their under-graduate education had not prepared them to deal with these needs and 64% wanted further training in spiritual care. Findings were similar in more recent studies by Hoyland and Mayers (2005) and Johnston and Mayers (2005).

People with an openly existential perspective, for whom discussing and living the experience of motor neurone disease is seen as a spiritual and psychological challenge, are often able to set treatment goals that span the remainder of their life. People, who measure quality of life in a more physical sense, may choose to 'fight' or 'give up' and goals may be much more practical and evolve as the disease progresses (Green *et al.*, 2003). The occupational therapist's sensitivity to these varying perspectives is vital in order for any intervention to be successful.

Outcome measurement

In evaluating the success of occupational therapy provision and the value of the multidisciplinary team, we are again challenged by the progression of the disease itself. Interventions provided by the occupational therapist and the rest of the multidisciplinary team, in collaboration with Angela, were successful in improv-ing her quality of life and maintaining her independence within the parameters of her condition. The palliative care service was active in continually appraising whether it had been appropriate in meeting Angela's individual needs. This is essential, as Hughes *et al.* (2005) stress the fact that care services cannot be estab-lished unless the experiences of the services are constantly evaluated. An inflexi-ble package of care cannot reflect the individuality of those coping with such a profound condition. Outcome measures used with Angela were based on her identifying a specific problem, and the occupational therapist addressing this through the timely provision of education, support, an assistive device or environmental adaptation.

A more formal method of evaluating the occupational therapy intervention could have considered the impact of occupational therapy on Angela's quality of life. Heffernan and Jenkinson (2005) identified 76 descriptive and cross-sectional studies which supported the use of health-related quality-of-life measures in measuring the impact of treatment and interventions on clients with long-term neurological disorders, including motor neurone disease. However, they recommend that further work is needed to ensure that measures are responsive enough to measure change.

Clarke *et al.* (2001) used the Schedule for the Evaluation of Individual Quality of Life (SEIQoL) (Hickey *et al.*, 1996) as a measure in ALS. Twenty-six clients with ALS were involved in the evaluation of this measure, which validated the internal consistency, reliability and validity of this tool. However they did acknowledge that those severely disabled by motor neurone disease would not be able to complete the measure. Further studies have also considered this measure with clients with motor neurone disease (Neudert *et al.*, 2001).

The COPM could also have been used to rate individual performance and satisfaction. Norris (1999) found this to be an effective means to determine issues important to the individual; however the self-rating scale proved difficult to use in practice. Norris felt that the final scores were somewhat subjective and interpretation could prove difficult.

An ongoing commitment

Angela continues to be seen by the occupational therapist on her own volition. The relationship established between her and the occupational therapist has provided a genuine basis from which issues can be openly shared and discussed as Angela's health continues to deteriorate.

Challenges to the reader

- How would you protect yourself from the emotional impact of working with someone who is going to die?
- How do we maintain a client-centred approach when someone appears unable to plan ahead and courts a crisis management approach to controlling life events?
- How do you use voluntary associations to support your role, educative or otherwise?

References

Agree, E.M. (1999) The influence of personal care and assistive devices on the measurement of disability. *Social Sciences and Medicine*, **48(4)**, 427–443

Bakker, J.P.J., de Groot, I.J.M., Beckerman, H., de Jong, B.A. and Lankhorst, G.J. (2000) The effects of knee-ankle-foot orthoses in the treatment of Duchenne muscular dystrophy: review of the literature. *Clinical Rehabilitation*, **14**, 343–359

Barson, F.P., Kinsella, G.J., Ong, B. and Mathers, S.E. (2000) A neurophysiological investigation of dementia in motor neurone disease (MND). *Journal of Neurological Sciences*, **180**, 107–113

Beresford, S.A. (2002) Focus on research . . . An exploration of the unconscious processes used by people with motor neurone disease in coping with the effects of their illness. *British Journal of Occupational Therapy*, **65(2)**, 64

Berger, M.M., Kopp, N. and Vital, C. (2000) Detection and cellular localization of enterovirus RNA sequences in spinal cord of patients with ALS. *Neurology*, **54**, 20–25

Billinghurst, B. (2001) Enabling communication and enhancing services for people with motor neurone disease. *Managing Community Care*, **9(3)**, 31–34

Bjelland, I., Dahl, A.A., Tangen Haug, T. and Neckelmann, D. (2002) The validity of the Hospital Anxiety and Depression Scale: an updated literature review. *Journal of Psychosomatic Research*, 52, 69–77

Bradley, M.D., Orrell, R.W. and Clarke, J. (2002) Outcome of ventilatory support for acute respiratory failure in motor neurone disease. *Journal of Neurology, Neurosurgery and Psychiatry*, **72(6)**, 752–756

Brown, J.B. (2003) User, carer and professional experiences of care in motor neurone disease. *Primary Health Care Research and Development*, **4(7)**, 207–217

Burgess, P.W., Alderman, N., Wilson, B.A., Evans, J.J. and Elmslie, H. (1996) The dysexecutive questionnaire. In: *Behavioural Assessment of the Dysexecutive Syndrome*. Ed. Wilson, B.A., Alderman, N., Burgess, P.W., Emslie, H. and Evans, J.J. Thomas Valley Test Company, Bury St. Edmunds

Carter, H., McKenna, C., MacLeod, R. and Green, R. (1998) Health professionals' responses to multiple sclerosis and motor neurone disease. *Palliative Medicine*, **12(5)**, 383–394

Chaudri, M.B., Kinnear, W.J.M. and Jefferson, D. (2003) Patterns of mortality in patients with motor neurone disease. *Acta Neurologica Scandinavica*, **107**, 50–53

Clarke, S., Hickey, A., O'Boyle, C. and Hardiman, O. (2001) Assessing individual quality of life in amyotrophic lateral sclerosis. *Quality of Life Research*, **10(2)**, 149–158

Cobble, M. (1998) Language impairment in motor neurone disease. *Journal of the Neurological Sciences*, **160(Supp1)**, 47–52

College of Occupational Therapists (2002*) National Association of Neurological Occupational Therapists: Minimum Standards of Practice for Chronic and Progressive Neurological Disorders*. College of Occupational Therapists, London

Corr, B., Frost, E., Traynor, B.J. and Hardiman, O. (1998) Service provision for patients with ALS/MND: A cost-effective multidisciplinary approach. *Journal of Neurological Sciences*, **160(Supp1)**, 141–145

Cott, C. (2004) Client-centred rehabilitation: client perspectives. *Disability and Rehabilitation*, **26(24)**, 1411–1422

Dawson, S. and Barker, J. (1995) Hospice and palliative care: a Delphi survey of occupational therapists' roles and training needs. *Australian Occupational Therapy Journal*, **42**(3), 119–127

Department of Health (2005) *National Service Framework for Long-Term Conditions*. Department of Health, London: Available at *ttp://www.dh.gov.uk/ Policy And Guidance/ Health And Social Care Topics*

Dib, M. (2003) Amyotrophic lateral sclerosis: progress and prospects for treatment. *Drugs*, **63**(3), 289–310

Dimond, B. (2004) The refusal of treatment: living wills and the current law in the UK. *British Journal of Nursing*, **13**(18), 1104–1106

Eisen, A. and Krieger, C. (1998) *Amyotrophic Lateral Sclerosis: A Synthesis of Research and Clinical Practice*. Cambridge University Press, Cambridge

Ewer-Smith, C. and Patterson, S. (2002) The use of an occupational therapy programme within a palliative care setting. *European Journal of Palliative Care*, **9**(1), 30–33

Foley, G. (2004) Quality of life for people with motor neurone disease: a consideration for occupational therapists. *The British Journal of Occupational Therapy*, **67**(12), 551–553

Foley, G. and Neeley, F. (2003) Cognitive impairment in amyotrophic lateral sclerosis: a consideration for occupational performance. *British Journal of Occupational Therapy*, **66**(9), 414–418

Foster, C. (2005) Misrepresentations about palliative options and prognosis in motor neurone disease: some legal considerations. *Journal of Evaluation in Clinical Practice*, **11**(1), 21–25

Foster, M. (2001) The role of physical, occupational and speech therapy in hospice: patient empowerment. *The American Journal of Hospice and Palliative Care*, **18**(6), 397–402

Garofalo, O., Figlewicz, D.A., Thomas, S.M., Butler, R., Lebuis, L., Rouleau, G., Meininger, V. and Leigh, P.N. (1995) Superoxide dismutase activity in lymphoblastoid cells from motor neurone disease/amyotrophic lateral sclerosis (MND/ALS) patients. *Journal of Neurological Sciences*, **129**, 90–92

Gelinas, D.F., O'Connor, P. and Miller, R.G. (1998) Quality of life for ventilator-dependent ALS patients and their caregivers. *Journal of Neurological Sciences*, **160**(supp1), 134–136

Goldstein, L.H. and Leigh, P.N. (1999) Motor neurone disease: a review of its emotional and cognitive consequences for patients and its impact on carers. *British Journal of Health Psychology*, **4**(3), 193–208

Goldstein, L.H., Adamson, M., Jeffrey, L., Down, K., Barby, T., Wilson, C. and Leigh, P.N. (1998) The psychological impact of MND on patients and carers. *Journal of Neurological Sciences*, **160**(Supp1), 114–121

Gooch, H. (2003) Assessment of bathing in occupational therapy. *British Journal of Occupational Therapy*, **66**(90), 402–408

Gouveia, R., Evangelista, T., Conceição, I., Pinto, A. and de Carvalho, M. (2004) Abrupt onset of progressive muscular atrophy. *Amyotrophic Lateral Sclerosis*, **5**(1), 61–62

Green, C., Kiebert, G., Murphy, C., Mitchell, J.D., O'Brien, M., Burrell, A. and Leigh, P.N. (2003) Patients' health-related quality-of-life and health state values for motor neurone disease/amyotrophic lateral sclerosis. *Quality of Life Research*, **12**(5), 565–574

Hagedorn, R. (2001) *Foundations of Practice in Occupational Therapy*. Churchill Livingstone, Edinburgh

Harding, R. and Higginson, I.J. (2003) What is the best way to help caregivers in cancer and palliative care? A systematic literature review of interventions and their effectiveness. *Palliative Medicine*, **17(1)**, 63–74

Hawkins, R. and Stewart, S. (2002) Changing rooms: the impact of adaptations on the meaning of home for a disabled person and the role of occupational therapists in the process. *British Journal of Occupational Therapy*, **65(2)**, 81–87

Heffernan, C. and Jenkinson, C. (2005) Measuring outcomes for neurological disorders: a review of disease-specific health status instruments for three degenerative neurological conditions. *Chronic Illness*, **1(2)**, 131–142

Herth, K. (1990) Fostering hope in terminally-ill people. *Journal of Advanced Nursing*, **15**, 1250–1259

Heywood, F. (2001) Housing adaptations: understanding their worth. *Housing Care Support*, **4(4)**, 20–23

Hickey, A.M., Bury, G. and O'Boyle, C.A. (1996) A new short form individual quality of life measure (SEIQoL-DW): application in a cohort of individuals with HIV/AIDS. *British Medical Journal*, **313**, 29–33

Higginson, I.J., Finlay, I.G., Goodwin, D.M., Hood, K., Edwards, A.G.K., Cook, A., Douglas, H.R. and Normand, C.E. (2003) Is there evidence that palliative care teams alter end-of-life experiences of patients and their caregivers? *Journal of Pain and Symptom Management*, **25(2)**, 150–168

Higginson, I., Hearn, J., Myers, K. and Naysmith, A. (2000) Palliative day care: what do services do? *Palliative Medicine*, **14(4)**, 277–286

Howlett, W.P., Brubaker, G.R. and Mlingi, N. (1990) Konzo, an epidemic upper motor neuron disease studied in Tanzania. *Brain*, **113(1)**, 223–235

Hoyland, M. and Mayers, C. (2005) Is meeting spiritual need within the occupational therapy domain? *British Journal of Occupational Therapy*, **68(4)**, 177–181

Hughes, R.A., Sinha, A., Higginson, I., Down, K. and Leigh, P.N. (2005) Living with motor neurone disease: lives, experiences of services and suggestions for change. *Health and Social Care in the Community*, **13(1)**, 64–74

Jain, S., Kings, J. and Playfor, E.D. (2005) Occupational therapy for people with progressive neurological disorders: unpacking the black box. *British Journal of Occupational Therapy*, **68(3)**, 125–130

Johnston, D. and Mayers, C. (2005) Spirituality: a review of how occupational therapists acknowledge, assess and meet spiritual needs. *British Journal of Occupational Therapy*, **68(9)**, 386–393

Johnston, M., Earll, L., Giles, M., Mcclenahan, R., Stevens, D. and Morrison, V. (1999) Mood as a predictor of disability and survival in patients newly diagnosed with ALS/MND. *British Journal of Health Psychology*, **4(2)**, 127–136

Kealey, P. and McIntyre, I. (2005) An evaluation of the domiciliary occupational therapy service in palliative cancer care in a community trust: a patient and carers perspective. *European Journal of Cancer Care*, **14(3)**, 232–243

Kralik, D. Telford, K., Price, K. and Koch, T. (2005) Women's experiences of fatigue in chronic illness. *Journal of Advanced Nursing*, **52(4)**, 372–380

Lapiedra, C.R., López, M.L.A. and Gómez. E.G.C. (2002) Progressive bulbar palsy: a case report diagnosed by lingual symptoms *Journal of Oral Pathology and Medicine*, **31(5)**, 277–279

Law, M., Baptiste, S., Carswell, A., Mc Coll, M., Polatajko, H. and Pollock, N. (1994) *The Canadian Occupational Performance Measure,* 2nd edn. Canadian Association of Occupational Therapists, Toronto

Littlechild, B. (2004) Occupational therapy in a hospice in-patient unit. *European Journal of Palliative Care,* **11(5)**, 193–196

Ludolph, A.C. and Spencer, P.S. (1996) Toxic models of upper motor neuron disease. *Journal of Neurological Sciences,* **139(suppl)**, 53–59

Meucci, N., Nobile-Orazio, E. and Scarlato, G. (1996) Intravenous immunoglobulin therapy in amyotrophic lateral sclerosis. *Journal of Neurology,* **243**, 117–120

Miller, R.G., Rosenberg, J.A. and Gelinas, D.F. (1999) Practice parameter: the care of the patient with amyotrophic lateral sclerosis (an evidence-based review). Neurology, **52**, 1311–1323

Mitsumoto, H., Chad, D.A. and Pioro, E.P. (1998) *Amyotrophic Lateral Sclerosis.* Davis, Philadelphia

Moore, M.J., Moore, P.B. and Shaw, P.J. (1998) Mood disturbances in motor neurone disease. *Journal of Neurological Sciences,* 160(Supp1), 53–56

Motor Neurone Disease Association (2000) *Motor Neurone Disease: a Problem-Solving Approach.* Motor Neurone Disease Association, Northampton

Murphy, J. (2004) 'I prefer contact this close': perceptions of AAC by people with motor neurone disease and their communication partners. *Augmentative and Alternative Communication,* **20(4)**, 259–271

National Institute of Neurological Disorders and Stroke http://www.ninds.nih.gov/disorders/ motor_neuron_diseases/motor_neuron_diseases.htm#Publications

Neary, D., Snowden, J.S. and Mann, D.M.A. (2000) Cognitive change in motor neurone disease/amyotrophic lateral sclerosis (MND/ALS). *Journal of Neurological Sciences,* **180(1)**, 15–20

Neudert, C., Wasner, M. and Borasio, G.D. (2001) Patients' assessment of quality of life instruments: a randomised study of SIP, SF-36 and SEIQoL-DW in patients with amyotrophic lateral sclerosis. *Journal of Neurological Sciences,* **191(15)**, 103–109

Norris, A. (1999) Occupational therapy. A pilot study of an outcome measure in palliative care. *International Journal of Palliative Nursing,* **5(1)**, 40–45

O'Brien, M.R. (2004) Information-seeking behaviour among people with motor neurone disease. *British Journal of Nursing,* **13(16)**, 964–968

O'Brien, T. (2001) Neurodegenerative disease. In: *Palliative Care for Non-Cancer Patients.* Ed. Addington-Hall, J. and Higginson, I.J., pp. 44–53. Oxford University Press, Oxford

Oliver, D. (2002) Palliative care for motor neurone disease. *Practical Neurology,* **2(2)**, 68–79

Oliver, D. and Webb, S. (2000) The involvement of specialist palliative care in the care of people with motor neurone disease. *Palliative Medicine,* **14(5)**, 427–428

Oliver, D., Borasio, G.D. and Walsh, D. (2000) *Palliative Care in Amyotrophic Lateral Sclerosis.* Oxford University Press, Oxford

Pedretti, L. and Early, M.B. (2001) *Occupational Therapy: Practical Skills for Physical Dysfunction,* 5th edn. Mosby, London

Prochnau, C., Liu, L. and Boman, J. (2003) Personal-professional connections in palliative care occupational therapy. *The American Journal of Occupational Therapy,* **2**, 196–204

Purves, D., Augustine, G.J., Fitzpatrick, D., Katz, L.C., La Mantia, A.S., McNamara, J.O. and Williams, S.M. (2001) *Neuroscience.* Sinauer Associates, MA

Ray, R.A. and Street, A.F. (2005) Who's there and who cares: age as an indicator of social support networks for caregivers among people living with motor neurone disease. *Health and Social Care in the Community,* **13**(6), 542–552

Ringel, S.P., Murphy, J.R. and Alderson, M.K. (1993) The natural history of amyotrophic lateral sclerosis. *Neurology,* **43**, 1316–1322

Rose, A. (1999) Spirituality and palliative care: the attitudes of occupational therapists. *British Journal of Occupational Therapy,* **62**, 307–312

Rosen, D.R., Siddique, T. and Patterson, D. (1993) Mutations in Cu/Zn superoxide dismutase gene are associated with familial amyotrophic lateral sclerosis. *Nature,* **362**, 59–62

Rustad, R.A., DeGroot, T.L., Jungkunz, M.L., Freeberg, K.S., Borowick, L.G. and Wanttie, A.M. (1993) *Cognitive Assessment of Minnesota.* Psychological Corporation, London

Shaw, P.J. and Strong, M.J. (2003) *Motor Neurone Disorders.* Butterworth Heinemann, Oxford

Sumsion, T. (1999) *Client Centered Practice in Occupational Therapy: A Guide to Implementation.* Churchill Livingstone, Oxford

Swash, M., Desai, J. and Misra, V.P. (1999) What is primary lateral sclerosis? *Journal of the Neurological Sciences,* **170**(1), 5–10

vanderPloeg, W. (2001) Viewpoint. Health promotion in palliative care: an occupational perspective. *Australian Occupational Therapy Journal,* **48**(1), 45–48

van Teijlingen, E.R., Friend, E. and Kamal, A.D. (2001) Service use and needs of people with motor neurone disease and their carers in Scotland. *Health and Social Care in the Community,* **9**(6), 397–403

Wilson, B.A., Alderman N., Burgess P., Emslie H. and Evans J.J. (1996) *Behavioural Assessment of the Dysexecutive Syndrome.* Thames Valley Test Company, Bury St Edmunds

World Health Organization. Palliative care (2002) Available at: www.who.int/hiv/topics/palliative/PalliativeCare/en/ (accessed January 2006)

Young, C.A. (1998) Building a care and research team. *Journal of Neurological Sciences,* **160**(**Supp1**), 137–140

Young, C.A., Tedman, B.M. and Williams, I.R. (1995) Disease progression and perceptions of health in patients with motor neurone disease. *Journal of Neurological Sciences,* **129**, 50–53

Zigmond, A.S. and Snaith, P.R. (1983) The Hospital Anxiety and Depression Scale. *Acta Psychiatrica Scandinavica,* 67, 361–370.

7: Travelling the integrated pathway: the experience of a total hip replacement

Kerry Sorby

Introduction

The effectiveness of a comprehensive integrated care pathway provides the focus for identifying best practice when addressing the needs of those who experience total hip replacement. This is now a common and effective procedure for reducing pain and maintaining function in a large population struggling with progressive osteoarthritis. However the Government's emphasis on reducing waiting lists has impacted on the average length of hospital stay following surgery; as a consequence most integrated care pathways now indicate a 5–7-day hospital admission. The economic justifications for rapid throughput may appear to steer occupational therapists into accepting seemingly reductionist ideology and practice. However, the value of the multidisciplinary team adopting an integrated pathway which combines pre-operative education, including a preliminary home visit (Rivard *et al.*, 2003; Gursen and Ahrens, 2004; McDonald *et al.*, 2005), post-operative in-patient rehabilitation (Tribe *et al.*, 2005) and post-operative discharge procedures (Roberts, 2003; Sharma *et al.*, 2005), is evident in the literature. Rigorous randomised controlled trials and systematic reviews complement qualitative evidence to present the impact on hospital expenditure, i.e. shorter length of hospital stay (Crowe and Henderson, 2003; Siggeirsdottir *et al.*, 2005) and client experience (Spalding, 2000).

A total hip replacement is now considered to be an effective orthopaedic surgical procedure to reduce discomfort and immobility in a population presenting with physical limitations as a result of degenerative joint disease of the hip, and is available in most NHS and independent hospitals (British Orthopaedic Association, 1999). In 2005, over 58 000 total hip replacements procedures alone were carried out in the UK (National Joint Registry, 2005). The numbers reflect the evidence that this procedure is effective in reducing pain and improving function, and that these positive results remain for a considerable period of time (Fitzpatrick *et al.*, 2000). A systematic review by Faulkner *et al.* (1998) of 17 randomised controlled trials and 61 observational studies found that 70% of people who had undertaken this operation rated their pain and function levels as 'good/excellent' 10 years after their original operation. Occupational therapists are participants in this procedure and work both pre- and post-operatively to ensure that individuals return to their former roles and occupations, through education and the carefully graded and adapted use of meaningful occupations.

For professionals working with individuals who will undertake this procedure there are several published guidelines to identify and define best practice (British Orthopaedic Association, 1999; National Institute for Clinical Excellence, 2000; National Health Service Modernisation Agency, 2002) however many of these focus on the **medical management** of the individuals' experience, offering little guidance for rehabilitation. It is therefore not surprising that occupational therapy intervention varies from one hospital to another and appears to be related to the surgeon's personal preferences and availability of rehabilitation resources, rather than evidence-based practice (McMurray *et al.*, 2000; Occupational Therapy Orthopaedic and Trauma Annual Conference, November 2005).

Many hospitals have developed local integrated care pathways to ensure that the rehabilitation service provides a comprehensive service, based on available evidence and best practice, to address the needs of individuals both before and after surgery. An integrated pathway is defined by Middleton and Roberts (2000) as *'a multidisciplinary outline of anticipated care, placed in an appropriate timeframe, to help an* individual *with a specific condition or set of conditions move progressively through a clinical experience to positive outcomes'*. This is the focus for occupational therapy in this context.

This chapter will follow Mr. Tony Stansfield, a 63-year-old man with osteoarthritis in both hips, on his journey through an identified integrated care pathway; from pre-assessment screening to admission to the ward and post-operative rehabilitation. This will reflect one of the newest challenges to service provision for allied health professions, nurses and medical staff, which is the Department of Health's introduction to the 'Choose and Book' Scheme (Department of Health, 2003) whereby from December 2005 individuals who require any elective referral will be offered a choice of four to five hospitals for their surgery. In this scheme a client may be offered his/her elective surgery at a local hospital, a hospital within the region or even a hospital at some distance from his/her home. Aftercare and rehabilitation following their hospital admission will be delivered locally. This will encourage the establishment of national rehabilitation protocols which will, in turn, challenge the occupational therapist as he/she balances person-centred practice with agreed standards of care.

Osteoarthritis of the hip

Osteoarthritis is the most common cause of disability in the UK (Arthritis and Musculoskeletal Alliance, 2004; Hammond, 2005). It is estimated that 44–70% of people aged over 55 years have radiological evidence of osteoarthritis (Arthritis and Musculoskeletal Alliance, 2004); this rises to 85% in people aged over 85 years (Grant, 2005). In a population survey by Frankel *et al.* (1999) 15.2 people per 1000 aged 35–85 years had hip disease severe enough to warrant surgery; this equates to a potential 760000 people within England and Wales. It is therefore somewhat disappointing that the government has not targeted this clinical condition specifically within any national service frameworks. Due to the degenerative and progressive nature of this condition, the National Service Framework for Long-Term Conditions (Department of Health, 2005) would have been a primary forum for outlining clinical guidelines and standards for best practice.

Osteoarthritis affects more women than men, and tends to affect people as they get older, but is also common amongst people of working age (Northmore-Ball, 1997; Woolf and Pfleger, 2003). Occupational therapists are treating more individuals with osteoarthritis, partly due to an aging population, but also due to this population being more active, engaging in leisure and work pursuits that are physically demanding beyond the recognised age of retirement (Moran, 2001). Osteoarthritis can also develop as a condition secondary to an abnormality in the biomechanics of a joint, for example, as a result of trauma, obesity or restricted range of normal movement (Cooper *et al.*, 1998).

It is the degeneration of the joint which is the primary cause of pain and immobility for those who have osteoarthritis of the hip. The hip joint consists of a ball (the head of the femur) and socket (the acetabulum) joint, which permits a wide range of movement (flexion, extension, abduction, adduction, internal and external rotation). It also provides a stable base for functioning and mobility of the whole leg. Everyday activities, such as getting up from a chair, using the toilet or bending down to put on a sock or shoe, all require stability and a wide range of movement at the hip joint. In a healthy joint, both the ball and socket are covered in hyaline cartilage allowing smooth movement. A capsule of dense fibrous tissue surrounds the joint, strengthened by ligaments on all sides, allowing movement to occur at the hip joint. The inside of the capsule produces synovial fluid; this lubricates the joint and facilitates movement. The onset of osteoarthritis is precipitated when the flow of the synovial fluid is restricted to an articular (joint) surface.

The onset of osteoarthritis causes a progressive loss of the articular cartilage in the weightbearing joints (i.e. hips, knees, spine). The roughened bony surfaces of the femur and the acetabulum rub against each other causing pain, stiffness and deformity (Fig. 7.1). Bony outgrowths can occur, further aggravating these presenting symptoms. This is likely to impact directly on a client's level of functioning and quality of life.

Treatment can involve the use of the following:

▪ Medication such as analgesics and anti-inflammatory drugs to alleviate pain (Superio Cabuslay *et al.*, 1996).
▪ Thermotherapy (Brosseau *et al.*, 2003).
▪ Balneotherapy (hydrotherapy or spa therapy) (Verhagen *et al.*, 2004).
▪ Exercise (Fransen *et al.*, 2001).

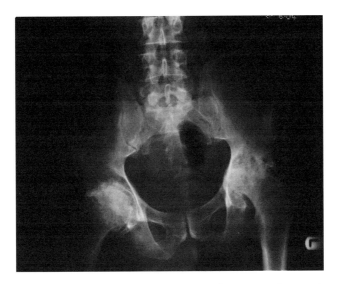

Figure 7.1 Hips affected by osteoarthritis. Image Courtesy of Mr L.M. Koch, Consultant Orthopaedic and Trauma Surgeon, Dewsbury and District Hospital, UK.

- Diet (Messier *et al.*, 2004).
- Education (Hopman Rock and Westhoff, 2000).
- Energy conservation, task modification and use of adaptive equipment (Moran 2001; Grant 2005).

A total hip replacement is only offered when conservative treatment has been unsuccessful (Fig. 7.2). This operation involves the surgical replacement of the damaged surfaces of the joint with a smooth alternative surface, allowing a return of smooth, friction-free movement, correction of deformity and, in almost all individuals, pain relief (Fig. 7.3).

Government directives

Government directives have had a huge impact on the service delivery of integrated care pathways for individuals undergoing total hip replacement in recent years. For example, reducing waiting times has been a national priority for the National Health Service since 2000 (Appleby, 2005; Department of Health, 2005). A collaborative study by the the Royal College of Surgeons of England and the British Orthopaedic Association (2000) found substantial variation in waiting times for a first appointment and timing of surgery. These two factors were foci for the Government initiating waiting list targets in 2000/2001. The main impact of waiting list targets has been to reduce the average length of hospital stay in order to increase throughput; as a consequence most integrated care pathways now indicate a 5–7-day hospital admission. Length of stay is often determined as

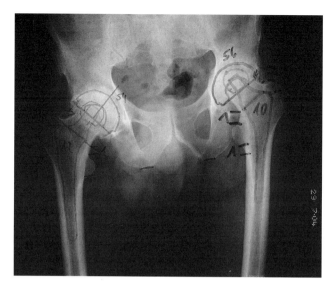

Figure 7.2 Surgical planning prior to total hip replacements. Image Courtesy of Mr L.M. Koch, Consultant Orthopaedic and Trauma Surgeon, Dewsbury and District Hospital, UK.

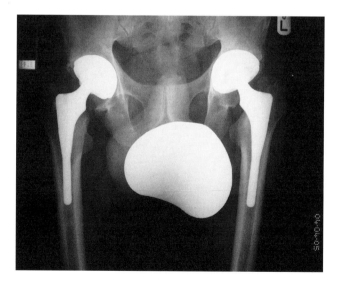

Figure 7.3 Hip replacements following surgery. Image Courtesy of Mr L.M. Koch, Consultant Orthopaedic and Trauma Surgeon, Dewsbury and District Hospital, UK.

an outcome measure for this surgical procedure, however the validity of this must be questioned as the prime focus should be on individual quality of life, not numerical targets. This UK study did report that following a total hip replacement, symptoms and functional status improved substantially, with results continuing to improve during the first year after the operation. This national study used the Oxford Hip Score (Dawson *et al.*, 1996) to measure functional status. This appears to be a widely used and effective outcome measure (McMurray *et al.*, 1999; Dawson *et al.*, 2000; Fitzpatrick *et al.*, 2000; Field *et al.*, 2005) and will be described later in this chapter.

Action on Orthopaedics and the Orthopaedics Services Collaborative (AOOSC) developed two major programmes, 'Action On Orthopaedics' and 'Collaborative', to improve and standardise trauma and orthopaedic services in England. These led to the publication of *Improving Orthopaedic Services* (AOOSC, 2002) which was intended as a guide to help clinicians, managers and service commissioners improve services for their clients (NHS Modernisation Agency, 2002). This focuses on the medical management of the individual and offers little guidance for rehabilitation or occupational therapy intervention. However, it does identify that *'any appliances or adaptations required by the patient after the operation should be sorted out in good time. (Sometimes simply providing the necessary equipment can meet the patient's needs and then they decide not to have the surgery).'* (p. 14). The document emphasises the importance of pre-operative education classes and multidisciplinary working.

In 2003, following the Department of Health's publication, *Building on the Best Choice, Responsiveness and Equity in the NHS: A Summary*, the Choose and Book scheme was introduced (Department of Health, 2004). This appears to be a stark contrast to the philosophy of integrated care pathways, as it places the individual at the epicentre of the episode of care by giving each person the choice as to where his/her surgery is delivered. By December 2005, those who require surgery will be offered a choice of four to five hospitals and a choice of time and date for their booked appointment. The intention is that aftercare and rehabilitation services will be delivered locally. The success of this scheme is unpredictable and offers some challenges for service delivery (Ciampolini and Hubble, 2005). It would appear that the Government perceives that individual choice will be based solely upon (objective) average waiting times. The fact that many clients will make this choice based upon their relationship with his/her consultant orthopaedic surgeon and the accompanying multidisciplinary team, appears to have been underestimated. The information given to the individual and/or his/her general practitioner does not yet appear to be standardised; anecdotal evidence from those who have been offered a choice suggests that individuals are not aware that rehabilitation may vary from hospital to hospital. Ciampolini and Hubble (2005) reiterate the concern that clients may not be empowered to make an *informed* choice about the package of care offered. It is acknowledged that this scheme is still in an embryonic stage; in the author's experience to date, individuals are most likely to choose their local hospital for convenience.

Another challenge that may occur is communication between service providers. For example, if an individual has their inpatient treatment at hospital A (in another region) and their outpatient treatment at hospital B (local hospital), the person's journey may travel along two very different care pathways, and difficulties may arise if a collaboration of services is not facilitated. For example, who will deliver pre-operative assessment and education? Which service provider will provide and fit the equipment required to facilitate an effective and timely discharge home? At the time of writing, the service used by the client described was at the early stage of introducing this controversial scheme.

Tony's circumstances

Tony is a 63-year-old gentleman who lives with his wife, Linda, in an owner-occupied three-bedroom semi-detached house. They have lived here throughout their married life and have two children, Samuel and Rebecca. Rebecca is married with three children, aged 5, 7 and 10, and lives locally. Samuel lives away from his home town and is divorced. Tony and Linda have an active childcare role with their grandchildren.

Tony owns his own building company but has taken a less active/managerial role for the past 3–5 years due to pain and deformity in his hips, particularly his right hip. His wife continues to work part-time as a dental receptionist.

Tony can walk outdoors with a walking stick. He finds his necessity to use a stick quite uncomfortable as it reminds him of his increasingly deteriorating level of function. He particularly finds it uncomfortable when walking on uneven ground, this is apparent when he goes 'on site' to see building work in progress. Tony's GP discussed his care with him, recommending that Tony was referred to a consultant orthopaedic surgeon. Under the 'Book and Choose' scheme, his GP offered him five options. Tony chose his local hospital as he felt it would be convenient to attend for hospital appointments and rehabilitation as required; and that he could fit in these with his current work and family commitments.

Six months later, Tony attended his local hospital for an initial consultation. Tony reported to the consultant that he feels less able-bodied, and the pain in his hip is now not only impacting on his work role but also on his leisure pursuits: golf and walking. In the past, he has successfully used these leisure pursuits to close business deals. Tony feels that the pain and limited movements of both his hips is now impacting on both his physical and psychological well-being, as well as on his valued roles as breadwinner, husband, business owner, parent and grandparent. His wife stated that Tony was now avoiding playing with his grandchildren during floor play or physically demanding activities and she had observed that he tended to be *more grumpy nowadays*'. Tony completed the Oxford Hip Score (Dawson *et al.*, 1996); this is a self-reporting questionnaire which is often used as an outcome measure to monitor the progress of a individual following a total hip replacement. This highlighted several areas of functional impairment:

- Nocturnal pain affecting sleep pattern.
- Mobility (for example, moderate difficulty climbing the stairs).
- Moderate difficulty with activities of daily living (for example, rising from a chair, putting on socks and shoes, getting in/out of a car).

His overall score was 42; this indicated severe osteoarthritis and therefore Tony should be considered for surgical intervention (Dawson *et al.*, 1996). Radiographs and physical examination confirmed Tony's story; the bony joint surfaces have narrowed, particularly on his right hip, resulting in pain, deformity (shortening of his leg) and limited range of movement in both of his hips. Following discussion with Tony and his wife, it was decided that Tony would benefit from a total hip replacement in both hips, and was placed on the consultant's waiting list for primary arthroplasty (hip replacement).

Tony's occupational therapy intervention was initiated when he attended the pre-assessment screening clinic at his local hospital, 4 weeks prior to his planned date of surgery.

Theoretical models and approaches

As already identified, osteoarthritis is a long-term condition. Due to the nature of this elective orthopaedic surgery, Tony is only likely to be working with the occupational therapist during this episode of care, which may only be one session prior to admission, approximately 5 days during his admission on the ward, with optional follow-up post-discharge. Therefore the model chosen was Reed and Sanderson's (1999) **Model of Adaptation through Occupations** (MAO), as it focuses on wellness not illness. The model is represented by three overlapping circles: physical environment, sociocultural environment and psychobiological environment. Central to these is Tony's ability to learn and adapt/adjust to his new hip by modifying or adapting his occupations during the post-operative phase of his rehabilitation; a period of 12 weeks. This is important as Tony has identified that he wished to regain his functional independence and satisfaction in self-care, leisure and work roles (Foster, 2002). This also reflects the goals of the multidisciplinary team, of which Tony will be an active participant.

This model does tend to focus on the physical aspects of Tony's level of functioning, which Tony highlighted as his priority on his initial appointment. Alternatively, if Tony had voiced concerns regarding the psychological influences of his condition, such as anxiety, depression, loss of role, body image, impact on personal relationships and/or low mood, a more client-centred model, such as the Canadian Occupational Performance Model (Law *et al.*, 1994) would have been used.

Within the MAO model both the **learning** and **compensatory** frame of references can successfully be applied. Tony's abilities to learn about his surgery, to follow precautions and to adapt and change to optimise his performance are considered to be the core components of the learning frame of reference. The application of joint protection techniques and energy conservation techniques uses the learning frame of reference. The compensatory frame of reference assumes that Tony's ability to function, by utilising a number of compensatory techniques, is essential to his well-being (Foster, 2002). The use of adaptive equipment and task modifications are examples of how this frame of reference can be successfully applied. Historically the compensatory frame of reference is linked to the medical model; one must remember that all occupational therapy intervention for this surgical intervention involves the application of post-operative precautions. The occupational therapist needs to consider Tony's personal choice during this process, and not the quickest or cheapest option, and be aware that Tony may find it difficult to accept compensatory techniques as they may remind him of his loss of function in the early stages of rehabilitation. Tony's compliance and engagement in his rehabilitation are key foci for successful outcomes.

Education is the key to ensuring that Tony successfully applies the post-operative precautions in order to return to his valued occupations. Hagedorn (2001) identified education as a core skill of occupational therapy; it follows, therefore, that the occupational therapist should be involved in Tony's education from pre-operative sessions, to post-operative and post-discharge sessions, to enable Tony to progress his level of functioning and return to independence. The occupational therapist will work collaboratively with Tony and his family to identify a range of problem-solving options, to enable Tony to make informed decisions about how he would like to manage his period of rehabilitation. An **educative approach** is used by the whole multidisciplinary team and is considered to be the focus of all interventions used when working with Tony. Education may be provided verbally and supported with written information booklets: these may be written by the local multidisciplinary team or national organisations, for example the Arthritis and Rheumatism Council. Within occupational therapy, individual education may be offered either in a group situation or on a one-to-one basis. The following sections will demonstrate this by presenting the occupational therapist's involvement with Tony at these stages:

- Pre-operative.
- Post-operative, in hospital.
- Post-operative, following discharge.

Pre-operative occupational therapy

Prior to his surgery, Tony and his wife were invited to attend the pre-operative assessment clinic, run at his local hospital, to obtain further information regarding his operation and collate final assessment details. McMurray *et al.* (2000) highlighted the fact that 89% of NHS Trusts in the United Kingdom routinely invite over half of those who will undertake a primary elective total hip replacement to attend a pre-admission clinic for the purposes of medical assessment and/or information provision. Clinics are often managed by a nurse but the education sessions are delivered by a multidisciplinary team of a nurse, doctor, physiotherapist and occupational therapist. The education programme is structured to reflect the journey the individual will experience through the integrated care pathway (Spalding, 1995).

The aims of the clinic are to:

- Prevent last minute surgery cancellations by checking that individuals are medically fit for the surgical procedure.

▓ Prevent, where possible, post-operative complications.

▓ Assist the individual and their family in identifying appropriate discharge arrangements.

▓ To enhance post-operative compliance by informing the individual of the surgical and rehabilitation procedures that they will undertake.

▓ Familiarise the client with the ward environment and the staff they will be working with in order to alleviate anxieties about the surgery.

Tony received comprehensive information presented in written, visual and verbal form within a pre-operative group. The creation of an informal atmosphere and use of humour were used to engage Tony in the group; he was encouraged to ask questions throughout the occasion, thus achieving maximum benefit from the session. A written educational booklet was also given to reinforce/complement the information provided.

This approach is very successful, as several studies have shown that educating clients about their planned hospital care before admission reduces both their anxiety and their length of stay post-operatively (Beddows, 1997; Spalding, 2000, 2003; MacDonald et al., 2005). Crowe and Henderson (2003) and Siggeirsdottir et al. (2005) found that the best outcomes (shorter length of stay) were achieved when combining pre-operative education with individually tailored rehabilitation programmes and Heaton et al. (2000) and Rivard et al. (2003) found that group education sessions were cost effective and appropriate for the majority of individuals, particularly with regard to professional time. However, they express caution that this approach needs to be flexible, as individuals with more multifaceted needs will need to be seen individually. It is also important to recognise that as length of stay in hospital increasingly shortens, pre-operative education becomes more central to the role of occupational therapy; it provides the individual with the opportunity to be well prepared for their surgery and engaged in their rehabilitation and return to independence. The principles of pre-operative education serve to empower the individual. This is an integral part of client-centred practice (Sumsion, 1999) and has been made explicit within government White Papers, for example, The New NHS: Modern, Dependable (Department of Health, 1997).

During the group education session, Tony was provided with general information from the occupational therapist regarding how to modify everyday tasks, such as dressing, getting into or out of bed and rising from a chair. Following his surgery Tony would need to adhere to 'hip precautions' for a period of 12 weeks, to allow bone and soft tissue to heal in order to provide joint stability and movement, and perhaps more importantly to prevent the dislocation of his new prosthesis. The 'hip precautions' may vary from surgeon to surgeon and from hospital to hospital. Regardless of surgical technique, however, the three basic precautions are:

▓ Do not flex the operated hip beyond 90° hip flexion.

▓ Do not adduct the operated hip beyond the midline.

▓ Do not rotate the hip (internal or external rotation).

Dressing aids were demonstrated to the group as an example of how to apply these surgical precautions to a functional task (i.e. putting on lower limb garments). Participants were provided with the aids and advised to familiarise themselves with the technique demonstrated and practice at home in preparation for their impending hospital stay.

To reinforce the techniques discussed and demonstrated during this session, and to apply them to Tony's individual circumstances, the occupational therapist carried out a non-standardised assessment in Tony's own home. The aims of this visit were to:

▒ Reinforce post-operative precautions, by giving practical individual-centred examples.
▒ Assess and modify, or adapt where appropriate, Tony's home environment to accommodate the post-operative precautions.
▒ Assist Tony, and his family, in identifying appropriate discharge arrangements.
▒ Set individually tailored goals for Tony's individual stay in hospital.

There is evidence that the information gained from one pre-operative visit can reduce the number of post-operative visits, which in turn reduces home health expenditures without a significant change in client outcomes (Gursen and Ahrens, 2004). In preparation for the visit, the occupational therapist needed to have a good understanding of hip anatomy, the surgery to be undertaken and hence the potential implications of the surgery on Tony's level of functioning and lifestyle.

Post-operative, hospital-based intervention

The home visit carried out prior to admission provided the occupational therapists with information from which goals could be identified and agreed to be addressed following the surgical procedure and prior to Tony's discharge home, a period of approximately 5 days (the numbering of days commences after the day of surgery, therefore the day of surgery = day 0).

Goal 1: Tony will be able to transfer and lift his operated leg in order to get into and out of bed independently

During the pre-operative visit, Tony stated that he normally slept with his wife in their double bed. He usually slept on the left-hand side of the bed (left side as one lies in the bed). This indicates that he currently gets into bed, using his 'affected' leg first. This is opposite to the technique that will be taught to him post-operatively. Tony had previously agreed to swap sides of the bed with his wife, so that he could practise getting into bed with his good leg first and out with his operated leg first, prior to surgery, to avoid hip adduction.

This goal will be achieved by day 4.

Goal 2: Tony will be able to dress himself independently using the equipment previously provided

An easireach, sock aid and long-handled shoe horn were provided during his attendance at the pre-assessment clinic. Independent dressing would be achieved by day 2 (post surgery).

Goal 3: to wash independently

Tony usually has a shower which is positioned over his bath. This manoeuvre is contraindicated post-surgery, and therefore Tony will need to be shown how to have a strip-wash at the bathroom sink. This will be taught by the end of day 2. He will need to continue this approach for a period of 12 weeks.

Goal 4: to enable Tony to transfer from a chair that is no lower than 50 cm (20 inches)

Rising from a chair, bed, toilet or car seat is an important precursor to functional mobility and engagement in meaningful occupations. Normally, when Tony moves from a sitting position into a standing position, he will bring his upper body forward by flexion of his hip and trunk during the initial (flexion–momentum) stage of this movement. The reader is encouraged to explore the two papers by Chan *et al.* (1999) and Laporte *et al.* (1999) for a detailed analysis of rising from sitting. This, potentially, may compromise the surgical precautions if the seating is too low. The recommended height of a seat is 5 cm (2 inches) above the height of his popliteal height (this height is measured from the anatomical landmark of Tony's popliteal fossa to the ground whilst wearing his normal footwear). Tony's popliteal height is 45 cm (18 inches) and therefore his recommended seat height will be a minimum of 50 cm (20 inches). This permits some hip flexion as Tony rises out of the chair, off a bed or toilet. Tony will be taught how to rise safely and independently from an appropriate chair by the end of day 3.

During the pre-operative visit, all seating heights were measured and advice was given about their suitability to facilitate safe post-operative transfers. These chairs included his comfy armchair in the lounge, a dining chair used to have meals and an office chair used to access his computer and maintain his business interests.

Goal 5: to enable Tony to safely rise from the toilet

The standard height of a toilet is only 40 cm (16 inches); therefore in a sitting position Tony's hips will be lower than his knees, thus will compromise the surgical precautions. At the pre-operative visit, a 10 cm (4 inch) raised toilet seat and free-standing toilet frame were issued and fitted by the occupational therapist. On observation Tony was noted to lean forward and slightly rotate his hips, in order to reach the radiator in front to assist him transfer on and off the toilet. The provision of the equipment demonstrated how he should be position himself in anticipation for his restricted movement. Independent toilet transfers will be achieved by day 5.

Goal 6: Tony will be able to walk safely and independently, with aids provided, from his bed to the ward bathroom

He will be able to toilet himself independently by the end of day 4.

Goal 7: Tony will be able to safely and independently get into and out of the passenger seat of a car

Due to the nature of Tony's surgery he will not be able to drive during the 12-week period, but he will be able to travel as a passenger in a car. Tony will be able to get in/out car seat by the end of day 5.

Achievement of goals

In order for Tony to achieve his agreed goals, the occupational therapist focused on applying the surgical precautions to, and practising, self-maintenance tasks on the ward. During the pre-operative visit, the occupational therapist did not foresee any problems and identified that Tony's rehabilitation should follow the hospital's integrated care pathway. Service delivery in this clinical area continues to be influenced by increased demands for productivity, reduced timeframes and increased complexity of problems presented by patients (Sands, 2003). Therefore, in order to strive to continue to deliver client-centred care, innovative and creative practices are sought. The development of the role of the occupational therapy assistant/technical instructor, to work in collaboration with qualified staff, has been effectively used in some hospitals to manage service delivery.

Tony was well motivated and keen to return home. He was seen daily by the occupational therapy technical instructor who monitored his performance and fed information back to the occupational therapist. His treatment programme was graded to enable Tony to regain independence in self-maintenance tasks incorporating the following elements:

- Altering the task method (for example, Tony will be taught a new *technique* to get in to and out of bed and rise out of a chair).
- Modify the environment (for example, provision of toileting equipment to facilitate safe transfers).

▪ Adapt the task object (for example, using assistive devices to facilitate independence in dressing).
▪ Education – integral to the delivery of all interventions.

By day 5 all his goals were achieved successfully and he was discharged home
as planned.

Intervention post-discharge

In the hospital which Tony attended, the episode of care was completed on the
day of discharge home; this appears to be common practice (Occupational Therapy
Orthopaedic and Trauma Annual Conference, November 2005). However, only
the areas of self-maintenance were addressed during this intervention. Therefore,
it is important to consider whether the occupational therapists *should* be involved
in addressing other areas of occupational performance on discharge.

Tony's role as breadwinner and grandparent needs consideration. To enable
Tony to return to this valued occupation, guidance would be needed during the
12-week healing and rehabilitation period. It was unlikely that Tony would be
able to return to his work as a builder during this period as it would be considered
to be too physically demanding (and compromise the surgical precautions).
However, Tony could have been guided to structure his day by pursuing (light)
gardening activities or playing with his grandchildren, in such a way that his
strength and range of movement improved gradually, reducing the possible negative effects of over- or under-inertia.

Due to limitations in resources and speed of throughput, little follow-up may
be available. The occupational therapist should be creative in identifying methods
by which the client's progress is evaluated; this is particularly important in a
society where legal action against hospital services is increasing. There is a debate
whether rehabilitation following total hip replacement should occur within an
in-patient rehabilitation service, to ensure that the client is indeed safe to return
home. The results of such services have demonstrated improvements in long-term
outcomes, more significantly amongst older clients (over 74 years) (Lawlor *et al.*,
2005). However, this expensive option has been cautioned by Tribe *et al.*, (2005)
who suggest that selected criteria should be adopted to determine those clients
who are vulnerable and need in-patient rehabilitation, and those who can be
safely discharged home.

Aware of the concerns relating to direct discharge, Sharma *et al.* (2005) highlight the benefits of post-operative telephone interviews to determine clients'
levels of well-being, this being a cost-effective use of professional time. An endeavour to reinforce post-operative precautions at home led to the creation of a post-
operative video as an educational resource for selected clients (Roberts, 2003).

What is evident is that the Government's directives and targets are a source of
frustration to occupational therapists who would like to ensure that there is adequate follow-up to those clients who have undergone such extensive surgery, to

ensure that procedures, precautions and equipment are all being implemented with maximum efficiency to the satisfaction of the occupational therapist and benefit to the individual.

Outcome measurement

In an acute hospital setting, outcome measures are sought that are simple, quick and easy to administer. The effectiveness of Tony's inpatient stay was measured by the multidisciplinary team by evaluating whether Tony had followed the identified integrated care pathway within the given timeframe (5–7 days). A second outcome measure that was used with Tony was the Oxford Hip Score. This was not undertaken by the occupational therapist but was re-administered by the consultant orthopaedic surgeon when Tony was reviewed at 3 months post-surgery in the out-patient clinic. Three months is considered to be an appropriate timeframe as this reflects the timeframe of the normal healing process from the surgery undertaken. Most published studies support the re-administration of the Oxford Hip Score at 12 months (McMurray *et al.*, 1999; Dawson *et al.*, 2000; Fitzpatrick *et al.*, 2000; Field *et al.*, 2005). In some hospitals, this clinic review may be undertaken by an extended scope practitioner, who may be an occupational therapist.

Another outcome measure that can be successfully used is the Mayers Lifestyle Questionnaire (available free of charge from w.w.w.MayersLQ). This is also a self-reported questionnaire which could have been administered as Tony was placed on the waiting list for his surgery. The main issues that led Tony to consider this surgery were pain, instability of the hip and loss of movement at the hip joint; as previously stated these had functional implications. If Tony had completed the Mayers Lifestyle Questionaire the functional problems and problem-solving solutions would have been identified at an earlier date with the occupational therapist. This would have enabled Tony to manage his presenting symptoms more effectively for the 6 months whilst waiting for his operation and potentially delay further deterioration to his painful hip joints. In addition, it is likely that Tony has osteoarthritis in other joints (for example his knees or carpometacarpal joint of his thumb) which affect his overall level of functioning; these would also be addressed. This is supported by the Arthritis and Musculoskeletal Alliance (2004), who recommend that when joint pain limits a person's capacity to carry out activities of daily life – in their work, hobbies or social activities – people should have access to a multidisciplinary team to assess them and refer them for treatment or other services to help restore their independence.

Critical reflection

One of the main disadvantages of using an integrated care pathway with an individual undergoing a total hip replacement is that all occupational therapy intervention is led by the imposed surgical precautions. This, and ever-increasing reduced timescales, lead to a restricted choice in the selection of activities used. Self-maintenance occupations become central to the delivery of care, as they are a priority for a safe and timely discharge to the individual's home environment. However, if Tony lived alone further consideration would need to be given to kitchen and domestic activities; potentially this could increase his length of stay, albeit by perhaps only 1 day. In this scenario, Tony's wife had agreed to compensate for Tony's temporary dysfunction by solely undertaking the domestic role; it would be anticipated that Tony would share this role as his level of functioning improved with time. It could be argued that the client has consented to a 'reductionist' care pathway as the components of the care pathway would be made explicit during the pre-admission education sessions.

The benefits of following an integrated care pathway outweigh the disadvantages cited and are frequently used to improve the quality, consistency and efficiency of care. Integrated care pathways should (NHS Modernisation Agency, 2004):

▩ Provide a clear and structured plan for delivery of care on a daily basis.
▩ Promote the use of evidence-based practice.
▩ Provide a focus for interdisciplinary team working.
▩ Empower patients and carers to exercise choice and to participate in their own care.

The challenge for the occupational therapist is, therefore, to tailor the locally agreed integrated care pathway to the individual needs of the client within a tight timeframe. In addition to this, he/she needs to have a comprehensive understanding of the resources available within the local areas to support the identified care package. The occupational therapist needs to have a good understanding of the individual surgeon's precautions and be able to analyse an individual's occupation and roles in order to incorporate these. For example, an individual may ask if they can go to the local theatre, or visit their favourite restaurant, or travel out of the local area to visit friends and family.

In the future, modern advancements in technology and medicine may render the surgical precautions invalid; this will be an exciting, yet challenging time for the occupational therapist as intervention may move away from being led by the integrated care pathway towards a more person-centred approach to care.

Challenges to the reader

▩ The Arthritis and Musculoskeletal Alliance (2004) recommends that individuals should be empowered to manage their condition effectively. If a person presents with early stages of osteoarthritis, and surgical intervention was not yet indicated, what joint protection advice may you offer?

▦ Increasingly, younger people, even in their thirties, are now undergoing hip replacements. What advice may you offer an individual, aged 35, in order to maintain his/her work and leisure roles over the next 30 years?

▦ A large amount of verbal information was given to Tony during his pre-operative home visit and the 5 days during his admission. This was reinforced by a written education booklet. Consider what information that you would include in the booklet.

▦ How would you apply the surgical precautions to Tony's work role? What facilities and resources are available in your local area to support Tony in his work role?

▦ Tony decided to have his treatment at his local hospital. Consider the implications of service delivery if Tony had chosen to have his surgery at a hospital some distance from his home.

▦ What methods would you put in place to balance delivering integrated care pathways with individually tailored treatment programmes?

▦ Frequently in practice, the occupational therapist needs to be able to balance elective and trauma caseloads. The pace of work is often fast and focused on effective and timely discharges from an acute ward. One method of addressing this is to allow technical instructors to deliver the occupational therapy intervention for identified integrated care pathways. Consider the implications for supervision, service competencies and collaboration between the qualified occupational therapist and technical instructor.

References

Action on Orthopaedics and Orthopaedic Services Collaborative (2002) *Improving Orthopaedic Services.* HMSO: London

Appelby, J. (2005) Sustaining reductions in waiting times: identifying successful strategies. The Research Findings register. Summary number 1337. http://www.eFeR.nhs.uk/viewRecordasp?ID=1337 (Accessed 19 November 2005)

Arthritis and Musculoskeletal Alliance (2004*) Standards for People with Osteoarthritis.* ARMA, London

Beddows, J. (1997) Alleviating pre-operative anxiety in individuals: a study. *Nursing Standard,* **11(37)**, 35–38

British Orthopaedic Association (1999) *Total Hip Replacement: A Guide to Best Practice.* British Orthopaedic Association, London

Brosseau, L., Judd, M.G., Marchand, S., Robinson, V.A., Tugwell, P., Wells, G. and Yonge, K. (2003) Thermotherapy for treatment of osteoarthritis. *The Cochrane Database of Systematic Reviews,* Issue 4. Art. No.: CD004522. DOI: 10.1002/14651858.CD004522

Chan, D., Laporte, D. and Sveistrup, H. (1999) Rising from sitting in elderly people, part 2: strategies to facilitate rising. *British Journal of Occupational Therapy,* **62(2)**, 64–68

Ciampolini, J. and Hubble, M.J.W. (2005) Early failure of total hip replacements implanted at distant hospitals to reduce waiting lists. *Annals of the Royal College of Surgeons of England,* **87(1)**, 31–35

Cooper, C., Inskip, H., Croft, P., Campbell, L., Smith G., McLaren, M. and Coggon, D. (1998) Individual risk factors for hip osteoarthritis: obesity, hip injury, and physical activity. *American Journal of Epidemiology,* **147(6)**, 516–522

Crowe, J. and Henderson, J. (2003) Prearthroplasty rehabilitation is effective in reducing hospital stay. *The Canadian Journal of Occupational Therapy,* **70(2)**, 88–96

Dawson, J., Fitzpatrick, R., Carr, A. and Murray, D. (1996) Questionnaire on the perceptions of individuals about total hip replacement. *The Journal of Bone and Joint Surgery,* **78**, 185–190

Dawson, J., Fitzpatrick, R., Frost, S., Gundle, R., McLardy-Smith, P. and Murray, D. (2000) Evidence for the validity of a patient-based instrument for assessment of outcome after revision hip replacement. *The Journal of Bone and Joint Surgery,* **83**, 1125–1129

Department of Health (1997) *The New NHS Modern, Dependable.* HMSO, London

Department of Health (2000) *National Total Hip Replacement Outcome Study.* HMSO, London

Department of Health (2003) *Building on the Best Choice, Responsiveness and Equity in the NHS: A Summary.* HMSO, London

Department of Health (2004) *Choose and Book Scheme.* HMSO, London

Department of Health (2005) *National Service Framework for Long-Term Conditions.* HMSO, London

Faulkner, A., Kennedy, L.G. and Baxter, K. (1998) Effectiveness of hip prostheses in primary total hip replacement: a critical review of evidence and an economic model. *Health Technology Assessment,* **2**, 1–33

Field, R., Cronin, M. and Singh, P. (2005) The Oxford hip scores for primary and revision hip replacement. *Journal of Bone and Joint Surgery,* **87(5)**, 618–622

Fitzpatrick, R., Morris, R., Hajat, S., Reeves, B., Murray, D., Hannen, D., Rigge, M., Williams, O. and Gregg, P. (2000) The value of short and simple measures to assess outcomes for patients of total hip replacement surgery. *Quality in Health Care,* **9**, 146–150

Foster, M. (2002) Theoretical frameworks. In: *Occupational Therapy and Physical Dysfunction,* 5th edn. Ed. Turner, A., Foster, M. and Johnson, S.E., pp. 47–84. Chapter 3. Churchill Livingstone, Edinburgh

Frankel, S., Eachus, J., Paerson, N., Greenwood, R., Chan, P., Peters, T., Donovan, J., Davey Smith, G. and Dieppe, P. (1999) Population requirement for primary hip-replacement surgery: a cross-sectional study. *Lancet,* **353**, 1304–1309

Fransen, M., McConnell, S. and Bell, M. (2001) Exercise for osteoarthritis of the hip or knee. *The Cochrane Database of Systematic Reviews,* Issue 2; Pages Art. No.: CD004376. DOI: 004310.001002/14651858.CD14004376

Grant, M. (2005) Occupational therapy for people with osteoarthritis: scope of practice and evidence base. *International Journal of Therapy and Rehabilitation,* **12(1)**, 7–12

Gursen, M.D. and Ahrens, J. (2004) Research. The key to a new home care protocol: prospective visits. *Caring,* **23(1)**, 40–44

Hagedorn, R. (2001) *Foundations for Practice in Occupational Therapy.* Churchill Livingstone, Edinburgh

Hammond, A. (2005) Editorial comment. *International Journal of Therapy and Rehabilitation,* **12(1)**, 13

Heaton, J., McMurray, R., Sloper, P. and Nettleton, S. (2000) Rehabilitation and total hip replacement: patient perspectives on provision. *International Journal of Rehabilitation and Research,* **23**(4), 253–259

Hopman Rock, M. and Westhoff, M.H. (2000) The effects of a health education and exercise program for older adults with osteoarthritis of the hip or knee. *Journal of Rheumatology,* **27**(8), 1947–1954

Laporte, D., Chan, D. and Sveistrup (1999) Rising from sitting in elderly people, part 1: implications of biomechanics and physiology. *British Journal of Occupational Therapy,* **62**(1), 36–42

Law, M., Baptiste, S., Carswell, A., Mc Coll, M., Polatajko, H. and Pollock, N. (1994) *The Canadian Occupational Performance Measure,* 2nd edn. Canadian Association of Occupational Therapists, Toronto

Lawlor, M., Humphreys, P., Morrow, E., Ogonda, L., Bennett, D., Elliott, D. and Beverland, D. (2005) Comparison of early postoperative functional levels following total hip replacement using minimally invasive versus standard incisions. A prospective randomized blinded trial. *Clinical Rehabilitation,* **19**(5), 465–474

McDonald, S., Green, S. and Hetrick, S. (2005) *Preoperative Education for Hip or Knee Replacement.* (A Cochrane Review). Wiley and Sons, London

McMurray, R., Heaton, J., Sloper, P. and Nettleton. (1999) Measurement of patient perceptions of pain and disability in relation to total hip replacement: the place of the Oxford hip score in mixed methods. *Quality in Health Care,* **8**, 228–233

McMurray, R., Heaton, J., Sloper, P. and Nettleton, S. (2000) Variations in the provision of occupational therapy for patients undergoing primary elective total hip replacement in the United Kingdom. *British Journal of Occupational Therapy,* **63**(9), 451–455

Messier, S.P., Loeser, R.F., Miller, G.D., Morgan, T.M., Rejeski, W.J., Sevick, M.A., Ettinger, W.H., Pahor, M. and Williamson, J.D. (2004) Exercise and dietary weight loss in overweight and obese older adults with knee osteoarthritis: the arthritis, diet, and activity promotion trial. *Arthritis and Rheumatism,* **50**(5), 1501–1510

Middleton, S. and Roberts, A. (2000) *Integrated Care Pathways: A practical approach to implementation.* Butterworth Heinemann, Oxford

Moran, M. (2001) Osteoarthritis and occupational therapy intervention. *Physical Medicine and Rehabilitation,* **15**(1), 65–81

National Health Service Modernisation Agency (2002) *Improving Orthopaedic Services.* HMSO, London

National Health Service Modernisation Agency (2004) *Orthopaedic Learning Network. Bulletin No 3.* HMSO, London

National Institute for Clinical Excellence (2000) *Guidance on Selection of Prostheses for Primary Total Hip Replacement.* NICE, London

National Joint Registry (2005) *Joint Approach.* HMSO, London

Northmore-Ball, M.D. (1997) Young adults with arthritic hips. *British Medical Journal,* **315**, 265–266

Occupational Therapy Orthopaedic and Trauma Annual Conference, November (2005) Birmingham

Reed and Sanderson (1999) *Concepts of Occupational Therapy.* Lipincott Williams and Wilkins, Baltimore

Rivard, A., Warren, S., Voaklander, D. and Jones, A. (2003) The efficacy of preoperative home visits for total hip replacements clients. *Canadian Journal of Occupational Therapy,* **70**(4), 226–232

Roberts, K. (2003) Occupational therapy postoperative management: total hip replacement: Janet Fricke and Rachel Elliott (Scriptwriters). Produced by COMET, La Trobe University. *Australian Occupational Therapy Journal,* **50**(3), 191

Royal College of Surgeons of England and the British Orthopaedic Association (2000) *National Total Hip Replacement Outcome Study.* Royal College of Surgeons of England, London.

Sands, M. (2003) Practioners' perspectives on the occupational therapist and occupational therapy assistant partnership. In: *Willard and Spackman's Occupational Therapy.* Ed. Crepeau, E.B., Cohn, E.S. and Boyt Schell, B.M., pp. 147–153. Lippincott Williams and Wilkins, Philadelphia

Sharma, S., Shah, R., Draviraj, K.P. and Bhamra, M.S. (2005) Use of telephone interviews to follow up patients after total hip replacement. *Journal of Telemedicine and Telecare,* **11**(4), 211–214

Siggeirsdottir, K., Olafsson, O., Jonsson, H., Iwarsson, S., Gudnason, V. and Jonsson, B. (2005) Short hospital stay augmented with education and homebased rehabilitation improves function and quality of life after hip replacement: randomised study of 50 patients with 6 month follow-up. *Acta Orthopaedics,* **76**(4), 555–562

Spalding, N. (1995) A comparative study of the effectiveness of a preoperative education programme for total hip replacement patients. *British Journal of Occupational Therapy,* **58**(12), 526–531

Spalding, N. (2000) The empowerment of clients through preoperative education. *British Journal of Occupational Therapy,* **63**(4), 148–154

Spalding, N. (2003) Reducing anxiety by preoperative education: make the future familiar. *Occupational Therapy International,* **10**(4), 278–293

Superio Cabuslay, E., Ward, M.M. and Lorig K.R. (1996) Individual education interventions in osteoarthritis and rheumatoid arthritis: a meta-analytic comparison with nonsteroidal antiinflammatory drug treatment. *Arthritis Care and Research,* **9**(4), 292–301

Sumsion, T. (1999) A study to determine a British occupational therapy definition of client-centred practice. *British Journal of Occupational Therapy,* **62**(2), 52–58

Tribe, K.L., Lapsley, H.M., Cross, M.J., Courtenay, B.G., Brooks, P.M. and March, L.M. (2005) Selection of patients for inpatient rehabilitation or direct home discharge following total joint replacement surgery: a comparison of health status and out-of-pocket expenditure of patients undergoing hip and knee arthroplasty for osteoarthritis. *Chronic Illness,* **1**(4), 289–302

Verhagen, A.P., de Vet, H.C., de Bie, R.A., Kessels, A.G., Boers, M. and Knipschild, P.G. (2004) Balneotherapy for rheumatoid arthritis and osteoarthritis. *The Cochrane Database of Systematic Reviews* Issue 1; Pages Art. No. CD000518. DOI: 10.1002/14651858.CD000518

Woolf, A. and Pfleger, B. (2003) Burden of major musculoskeletal conditions. *Bulletin of the World Health Organization,* **8**, 646–656

8: Managing risk in the older person who has fallen

Maria Parks

Introduction

Increased life expectancy in the UK population may demonstrate a healthier life-style, but for the older population longevity also brings risks. One such threat is that of falling, this being the major cause of death and disability in older people (Millward *et al.*, 2003). The National Service Framework and National Institute of Health and Clinical Excellence Guideline 21 (Department of Health, 2001a; NICE, 2004) provides the evidence base and ideal standards to guide clinical practice in reducing the risk of falling in the older population. This emphasises the importance of both a multifactorial risk assessment and home hazard assessment in evaluating the home environment and personal circumstances, and helps to determine the interventions selected by the community-based multidisciplinary team, which includes the occupational therapist. Falls prevention programmes, which focus on exercise, home hazard management and home modifications, have been found to be an effective mode of reducing risk of falling. The evidence is based on systematic reviews (Chang *et al.*, 2004; McClure *et al.*, 2005), component-led clinical trials, i.e. home hazard management (Day *et al.*, 2002), exercise evaluation (Sherrington *et al.*, 2004), surveys regarding environmental modifications (Tse, 2005) and qualitative evaluations of psychological outcomes (Jørstad *et al.*, 2005).

In 2001 the Government published the National Service Framework for Older People (Department of Health, 2001a) setting out an ambitious agenda of modernising health and social care to improve services for older people. Standard 6 of the framework concentrates on falls, and sets specific milestones to reduce the number of falls by older people and to develop effective services in the prevention of falls and treatment of people who have fallen. In the White Paper, *Saving Lives – Our Healthier Nation* (Department of Health, 2001b), the Government also set a target of reducing death rates from accidents (including falls) by at least a fifth and reducing serious injuries from accidents by at least a tenth by 2010.

This chapter will present the experience of Samuel (pseudonym), a 71-year-old gentleman, to illustrate the contribution of community-based occupational therapy in falls prevention programmes working within the direction of the National

Service Framework and subsequent National Institute of Health and Clinical Excellence Clinical Guideline 21: *Falls: the assessment and prevention of falls in older people* (NICE, 2004).

Samuel is a retired greengrocer who is widowed and lives alone in his own house in a large city in the south of England. Originally from the Caribbean, Samuel moved to the United Kingdom in the late 1950s. His wife, Flora, died suddenly from a stroke 5 years ago and his three children, who are all in their late 40s, keep in touch but live too far away to visit regularly. Samuel recently had a fall on the stairs inside his house rushing to answer the telephone downstairs.

This chapter will follow Samuel's experience from hospital admission through to home discharge via the intermediate care team and falls service. This episode of care will include a multidisciplinary assessment of Samuel's risk of falling and the relevant occupational therapy interventions to reduce the risk of Samuel falling in the future. Information relating to Samuel presented in the figures relates to information obtained from a range of assessments and home visits.

Aging population

The example of an older person with a history of falls was selected because the United Kingdom has an aging population. In the middle of 2004, 16% were aged 65 or above (Office for National Statistics, 2005). By 2031, the Government Actuary Department has projected that 23% of the population will be aged ≥65 years and the number of very old people, of ≥80 years, is projected to reach 4.3 million by 2031 (Health Promotion England, 2001). Although improved life expectancy may indicate that the general population is healthier than ever before, the situation is not as positive for older people. In the last General Household Survey in 2002, 72% of people aged 75 and over reported themselves to be living with a longstanding illness, of which musculoskeletal and heart and circulatory conditions were the most common (Office for National Statistics, 2002). These figures are collated through self-reporting rather than objective data from general practitioners and are therefore likely to show an under-reporting of the real picture. Commentary from the General Household Survey suggests that some older people viewed their limitations in daily activities as a normal part of the aging process rather than a consequence of a specific medical condition.

Like Samuel, there is evidence that as people get older, more are living alone. The General Household Survey in 1998 found that 59% of women and 29% of men in the 75 and over age group were living alone (Office for National Statistics, 2000a and b). The decline of the extended family and the trend for younger generations to move out of their home towns to seek employment has also increased the number of older people like Samuel who do not have regular contact with their families. To summarise, the population in the United Kingdom, as elsewhere in the world, is aging.

Definition of a 'fall'

For many years the Kellogg International Working group's definition of a fall has been adopted in research studies (Lord, 2001):

> Unintentional coming to the ground or some lower level and other than as a consequence of sustaining a violent blow, loss of consciousness, sudden onset of paralysis as in stroke or an epileptic seizure (Gibson et al., 1987).

This definition allowed researchers to be consistent in the types of incidents they were investigating. More recently Tinnetti has added an alternative definition which complements the occupational therapist's understanding of person–environment fit (Letts et al., 1994):

> Falls occur when the environmental hazards or demands exceed the individual's ability to maintain postural control (Tinnetti, 2001).

Incidence of falls and older people

People of all ages experience slips, trips and minor falls, for example children playing or adults participating in sport. In general though, younger and healthy people will be able to recover their balance before falling to the ground and so there are less serious consequences resulting from such trips and falls. Only 5% of the total numbers of fatalities resulting from accidental injury are found in people aged ≤40 years. Both the incidence of falls and the consequence of falls in the older person are much more frequent and serious.

The Royal Society for the Prevention of Accidents estimates that 135 000 falls occur each year among those aged 75 years and over, and that approximately 30% of those aged 65 and over experience a fall at least once a year, rising to 50% among people aged 80 years and over (Health Education Authority, 1999). In the UK, there are over 4000 fatal accidents which occur inside the home each year and 46% of these are falls (Department of Trade and Industry, 1999). Millward et al. (2003) report that falls are a major cause of death and disability in older people and that 50% of all deaths in the UK resulting from accidental injury occur in the over 65 age group. Cryer (2001) reported to the Health Development Agency that for people aged 65 years or more, falls account for 71% of serious injuries resulting in hospital admission of 4 days or more. In people aged 85 years and over, falls account for 78% of accidental injuries resulting in death. All age groups are known to experience falls in the home, however people over 65 years account for 80% of these fatalities compared with only 5% of people up to the age of 40.

Why do older people fall?

The Clinical Guideline 21 on the assessment and prevention of falls in older people (NICE, 2004) has reviewed all the best available evidence to guide clinicians working with older people who fall. The National Institute for Health and Clinical Excellence Guideline 21 reports strong evidence to predict the risk of falling in the older person if there is the presence of one or more factors from the list in Fig. 8.1.

NICE has recommend that *'older people who present for medical attention because of a fall, or report recurrent falls in the past year, or demonstrate abnormalities of gait and/or balance should be offered a multifactorial falls risk assessment'* (NICE, 2004 p. 60). Therefore, Samuel required a full multifactorial risk assessment which included an occupational therapy home hazard assessment to identify possible causes of his fall, with the aim of implementing appropriate interventions which will reduce his risk of falling in the future.

Where do older people fall?

Clinical reasoning and evidence-based practice must be informed by the best evidence available to the occupational therapist (Sackett *et al.*, 1996). In the field of falls prevention, understanding where and why falls occur underpins all of the assessment and intervention strategies. We need to know what the most likely risks are and how to reduce them, and apply this knowledge to individualised assessment and interventions.

In Samuel's situation, he fell on the stairs whilst rushing down to answer the phone one early winter evening. The staircase in his house is narrow and receives no natural light. When Samuel was found by his neighbour, there were no lights on in the hall way or first floor landing. The carpet on the stairs has a floral pattern and from the top of the stairs it is difficult to differentiate between the different

---

- Falls history
- Balance deficit
- Fear of falling
- Cognitive impairment
- Home hazards
- Psychotropic and cardiovascular medications
- Number of medications
- Gait deficit
- Mobility impairment
- Visual impairment
- Urinary incontinence
- Muscle weakness

Figure 8.1 List of factors which may contribute to a fall.

steps. The carpet was also slightly worn and shiny on the edges (nosing) of the steps. When Samuel was found the slippers he had been wearing had come off and were close to the bottom of the staircase.

The Department of Trade and Industry's Home Accidents Surveillance System and Dowswell *et al.* (1999) report where fatal falls occur for the over 65 age group in the UK (1995–1997):

- On/off stairs or step ladders – 62%.
- In between two levels – 15%.
- On the same level – 13%.
- From a ladder – 6%.
- From a building – 4%.

This equates to two or three people dying as a result of a fall on the stairs each day. This may be explained by nature of the trauma experienced on the stairs and complications resulting from those injuries such as a fractured neck of femur. Falling between two levels, such as a bed, chair or WC, is significantly less likely to result in death, as too are falls on the same level, for example tripping and falling on a rug or trailing wire. There is also a seasonal pattern that shows that more fatal falls on stairs occur during the winter months (Department of Trade and Industry, 1999). A long lie following the fall in a cold home will increase the risk of hypothermia, but also joint mobility and strength become impaired in the cold, restricting movement and the ability to react to a loss of balance.

The location of non-fatal falls on stairs and steps in UK homes (1996–1998) is reported as follows (Department of Trade and Industry, 1999):

- Stairs – 62%.
- Interior steps – 17%.
- Exterior steps – 13%.
- Doorstep – 7%.
- Stepladder – 1%.

These figures give a clear indication that stairs present a significant risk to the older person and the consequence of falling on the stairs has a very high risk of resulting in death.

Why do older people fall on stairs?

Fig. 8.2 identifies factors which may contribute to a fall on the stairs. Research commissioned by the Department of Trade and Industry investigated how older people's behaviour contributed to their safety on the stairs. Hill *et al.* (2000) conducted focus groups and then interviewed 157 older people in their own homes to investigate how these older people used their stairs and identified what factors increased the risk of falling on stairs. Different types of behaviour were identified:

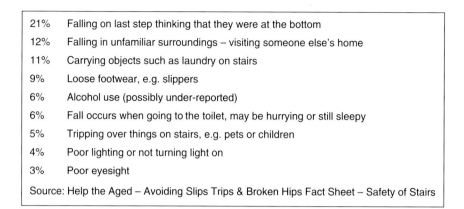

21%	Falling on last step thinking that they were at the bottom
12%	Falling in unfamiliar surroundings – visiting someone else's home
11%	Carrying objects such as laundry on stairs
9%	Loose footwear, e.g. slippers
6%	Alcohol use (possibly under-reported)
6%	Fall occurs when going to the toilet, may be hurrying or still sleepy
5%	Tripping over things on stairs, e.g. pets or children
4%	Poor lighting or not turning light on
3%	Poor eyesight
	Source: Help the Aged – Avoiding Slips Trips & Broken Hips Fact Sheet – Safety of Stairs

Figure 8.2 Factors contributing to non-fatal falls on stairs.

- Behaviour involved in direct use of the stairs. This identified that how people use the stairs increases their risk of falling, for example hurrying, carrying objects, cleaning on the stairs, not turning the light on and not using the handrail.
- Behaviour affecting the stair environment. This included leaving clutter on the stairs or using the stairs as storage, choice of stair covering which may increase the slipperiness of the stairs or the choice of pattern and maintenance of the carpet, types of lighting, if any, and types of lamp shades, which can improve or restrict illumination on the staircase.
- Behaviour affecting the individual's capability to use the stairs safely, for example prescribed medications, alcohol use.

This study makes a useful contribution to the occupational therapist's home hazard assessment in identifying specific environmental hazards (types of lamp shades, patterned carpet) but also in increasing our understanding of the person's behaviour within their home environment. In Samuel's case, it is important, during the occupational therapist's assessment, to identify his behaviour using the stairs as well as a visual check of trip hazards or lack of stair rail. Also, in making recommendations for environmental modifications, the occupational therapist's clinical reasoning must be informed by sound ergonomic principles of fitting the environment to the person and task.

Governmental policy and legislation

Over the past 35 years, successive governments in the United Kingdom have passed legislation and White Papers, setting different policies which have promoted services to support the elderly and disabled people to continue living in their own homes. These policies have shifted the focus of long-term care of vulnerable members of society from institutions to living out their lives in their own homes (Heywood *et al.*, 2002). Key drivers include:

- Chronically Sick and Disabled Persons Act 1970. Between the 1970s and the 1990s the growing numbers of older people with chronic illnesses and disabilities were still spending many weeks and months in hospital beds on long-stay geriatric wards. Many of these people were prevented from being discharged home because their homes presented a potentially hazardous environment and there was a delay in the provision of appropriate equipment and adaptations (Heywood *et al.*, 2002).
- *Caring for People: Community Care in the Next Decade and Beyond* (Department of Health, 1989). This White Paper led the way for what is now known as 'Care in the Community' and the passing of the NHS and Community Care Act 1990 (Griffiths, 1998).
- NHS and Community Care Act 1990. Care managers emerged to assess individual needs and organise either residential care from smaller providers in the private/voluntary sector, or the provision of comprehensive care packages including equipment and adaptations from occupational therapists to support people in their own home.

A change in government in 1997 led to a series of White Papers addressing the modernisation of the National Health Service and Social Services to improve standards and quality:

- *The New NHS: Modern and Dependable* (Department of Health, 1997).
- *A First Class Service* (Department of Health, 1998).
- *Saving Lives: our healthier nation* (Department of Health, 1999).
- *NHS Plan* (Department of Health, 2000).

For the first time, National Service Frameworks were published for different clinical areas, which set milestones for improvement and prioritised where new investment should be targeted. In 2001, the National Service Framework for Older People (Department of Health, 2001a) was published, setting out eight areas of service improvement for older people. Standards which are relevant to Samuel's care during this episode have been summarised in Fig. 8.3.

Both the National Service Framework for Older People (Department of Health, 2001a) and the Clinical Guideline 21 – Falls: The Assessment and Prevention of Falls in Older People (NICE, 2004) provide evidence and information to guide clinical practice in preventing falls for older people. The National Institute for Health and Clinical Excellence (NICE) states:

> *This guidance represents the view of the Institute, which was arrived at after careful consideration of the available evidence. Health professionals are expected to take it fully into account when exercising their clinical judgment. This guidance does not, however, override the individual responsibility of health professionals to make appropriate decisions in the circumstances of the individual patient, in consultation with the patient and/or guardian or carer.*

The evidence referred to in this chapter should only be considered as the best available at the time of writing; as evidence-based clinicians we must

> **National Service Framework for Older People – and Samuel**
>
> **Standard 1 – Rooting out age discrimination**
>
> Eligibility criteria relating to the provision of services including housing adaptations and assistive devices should not discriminate on grounds of Samuel's age.
>
> **Standard 2 – Person-centred care**
>
> Implementation of the single assessment process – *EASY CARE* (Sheffield University, 2004) was used by the intermediate care team and social care services.
>
> **Standard 3 – Intermediate care**
>
> Once Samuel was medically fit, he was referred to the community-based intermediate care team for further assessment and preparation for discharge home.
>
> **Standard 6 – Falls**
>
> Following Samuel's fall and admission into hospital, a *falls care* pathway was followed in which he received specialist assessment and interventions from the multidisciplinary team.

Figure 8.3 Summarised standards from the National Service Framework for Older People (Department of Health, 2001a).

continually strive to update our knowledge and seek out any new research or guidance.

Investment in creating new specialist falls services has been justified compared with the estimated costs of looking after older people who have fallen on the NHS and social care providers. Scuffham reported that the overall cost of falls for people 75 years and over was £647 million (Scuffham *et al.*, 2003), of which hospital admission followed by long-term care is the most costly. Scuffham found that there was significantly less cost associated with people who just attended the accident and emergency department or their GP but did not require hospital admission. In terms of financial burden on the welfare state and the personal consequences on the older person, preventing falls and, therefore, the risk of serious injury in older people is an important health priority.

Overview of Samuel's fall and hospital admission

Samuel had a serious fall on his stairs whilst rushing to answer the telephone. Although he survived the fall without breaking any bones, he was unable to get up to call for help. After lying on the floor for several hours, Samuel was eventually found by his neighbours who had noticed that there were no lights on in the house. An ambulance was called to take him to the local accident and emergency department. Samuel was admitted for investigation and received treatment for a chest infection and dehydration. Samuel was then referred to the local multidisciplinary intermediate care team to investigate the nature of his fall and provide the appropriate interventions to prevent a fall from occurring in the future and prepare him for discharge home.

Models and approaches adopted

Community occupational therapists are trained to carry out home assessments and identify appropriate interventions to ensure safety and enable the client to achieve the level of independence they wish in activities of daily living. The underlying theory which supports the practice of home assessment and modifications relates to an understanding of the dynamic relationship between the home environment and a person's occupational performance. The role of the occupational therapist is to identify incongruence between the person and their environment and to consider a range of interventions which will remove or overcome any environmental barriers which hinder occupational performance. This is often narrowly and incorrectly interpreted solely as an issue of accessibility, for example door widths, stairs or seat heights, but occupational therapists working in the specialist field of falls prevention, must consider the impact of all intrinsic and extrinsic factors on occupational performance.

The chosen model for this case study is the Person–Environment–Occupation Model (Law *et al.*, 1996) (Fig. 8.4). Developed from the work on client-centred practice by the Canadian Association of Occupational Therapists (1997), it offers

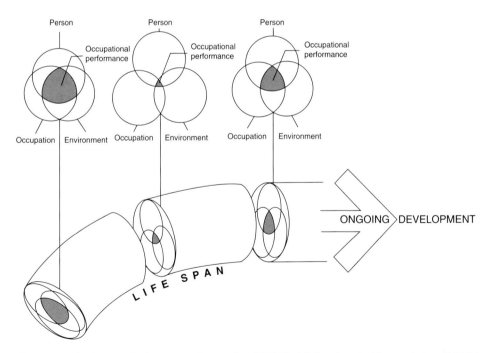

Figure 8.4 The Person–Environment–Occupation (PEO) Model. Reprinted with permission of CAOT Publications ACE, from Law, M., Cooper, B., Strong, S., Stewart, C., Rigby, P. and Letts, L. (1996) The Person–Environment–Occupation Model: a transactive approach to occupational performance. *Canadian Journal of Occupational Therapy*, **63**, 9–23.

a clear explanation of the interdependence between people and their environments (physical, social, economic, cultural and institutional) and their ability to engage in meaningful occupations. This concept is not unique to this model; however the focus of 'person–environmental fit' is specific to this work. Maximising the 'fit' or congruence between the person, their environments and the occupation is central to the role of the occupational therapist's interventions. Traditionally, hospital-based therapists have focused upon rehabilitation of the 'person' to maximise the fit, and community-based occupational therapists have addressed the 'environment' to augment the fit.

The role of the occupational therapist will be to assess Samuel's home environmental hazards, identify what the risks of falling may be and consider appropriate interventions to reduce the risk (Cumming *et al.*, 1999). Samuel, like many clients admitted to hospital following a fall, considers the most important goal is to return home safely, as soon as possible. He is also aware that many of his health conditions, such as his high blood pressure, diabetes and osteoarthritis, can be managed but are not likely to be cured. He seeks a pragmatic solution to him returning home safely and so the occupational therapist will work with him to identify appropriate **compensatory** approaches to enable him to return home. This approach will seek to compensate for any loss of function rather than try to rehabilitate or restore lost abilities. This approach complements the Person–Environment–Occupation Model by seeking ways to 'maximise person–environment fit' through the provision of assistive devices, such as stair rails. The therapist will also work with Samuel to discuss how he carries out his daily tasks and educate him on alternative methods which may be safer. Such advice and re-training utilises both the **adaptive** and **educative** approaches as part of falls and safety advice to Samuel.

Assessment

In line with the falls care pathway, when Samuel was medically fit he was referred to the intermediate care team for a comprehensive multifactorial falls risk assessment. Following Standard 2, Person-Centred Care, of the National Service Framework for Older People (Department of Health, 2001a), the intermediate care team had been trialling the implementation of the single assessment process using the EASY-CARE tool (Sheffield University, 2004) with the local social services department. The electronic version was used to collate and share the assessment data with Samuel's consent. Some of the questions contained in the 'overview' assessment are similar to those explored during the multifactorial falls risk assessment. As Samuel had already been identified as at risk of falling when he was admitted into hospital following his fall, and to avoid unnecessary duplication of assessments, the falls risk screening tool was administered first and the results added to EASY-CARE electronic database. EASY-CARE questions not covered in the falls risk assessment were then asked by members of the nursing team to complete a full picture of how Samuel was coping at home. The EASY-CARE electronic tool was then used to record and monitor the agreed action plan set in place to facilitate Samuel's safe discharge home across health and social care agencies.

Multifactorial risk assessment

The Clinical Guideline 21 (NICE, 2004) concludes that there is currently strong evidence for individualised multifactorial risk assessments being more effective in identifying accurate levels of risk than non-individualised assessments. The multidisciplinary intermediate care team carried out a full falls risk assessment covering the entire known intrinsic risk factors (Fig. 8.1). Samuel's medical conditions linked to his risk of falling are summarised in Fig. 8.5.

In addition, Samuel discussed that he had lost his confidence in going home on his own and having to climb the stairs again. Since his hospital admission he has lost some strength and motivation. He scored 16 seconds in the timed 'Up and Go' test and was then referred to the physiotherapist for further strength and balance training.

Home hazard assessment

NICE (2004) recommends that *'when an older person at increased risk of falling is discharged from hospital, a facilitated home hazard assess should be considered'*. However, the Clinical Guideline goes on to state that there is currently little evidence to support the use of home hazard assessment in isolation, but that assessment and environmental modifications are most effective when delivered as part of a range of targeted fall prevention strategies. A multidisciplinary service was provided for Samuel by the intermediate care team. The multifactorial falls risk screen identified that Samuel had reported problems getting to the WC at night as it is situated on the ground floor in the only bathroom in the house. Samuel's fall occurred on the stairs whilst rushing to answer the phone, but his regular routine of emptying the bucket requires him to carry it downstairs each morning and will also need to be considered as potentially dangerous.

- Non-insulin dependent diabetes mellitus (type II), with some impaired sensation in his feet (diabetic neuropathy). Blood glucose controlled through diet and regular checks with specialist nurse

- Hypertension – uses diuretics and needs to pass urine during night time, uses bucket under bed as WC located on ground floor

- Osteoarthritis in both knees and hips – takes non-steroidal anti-inflammatory medication

- Overweight

- History of tripping and minor falls around the house

Figure 8.5 Summary of Samuel's associated risk factors for falling.

Samuel was referred to the occupational therapist in the team to carry out a home hazard assessment. The significance of the environment hazard has been found to vary in different age groups. Dowswell *et al.* (1999) found that environmental factors are more significant in the cause of falls for the 65–74 age group compared with those aged 85 years or over, for whom personal (intrinsic) factors are considered to outweigh environmental hazards. Environmental hazards may be significant for Samuel, who is 71 years old.

Standardised assessment tools/outcome measures

Occupational therapists are appropriately trained for this role and have a unique understanding of maximising the 'fit' between the person, their environment and occupation. It is common practice for occupational therapists to use non-standardised checklists to record assessments carried out in the home environments. These are frequently concerned with accessibility rather than the identification of risk of falling. The reliability and validity of using such checklists cannot be supported, particularly when they been modified or adapted from existing standardised assessment tools. There is also a need for occupational therapists to use appropriate outcome measures to demonstrate effectiveness of occupational therapy interventions rather than these services being evaluated upon output performance measures, such as waiting lists and numbers of assessments (Eakin and Baird, 1995).

A selection of assessment tools will be considered for their appropriateness for assessing home hazards for Samuel. The assessments chosen for consideration have aspects which have either been designed with falls prevention in mind or have components which assess environmental risk in the home, such as stair climbing, transfers and functional mobility. It is important that clinicians make an informed choice regarding the assessment tools they use and they need to familiarise themselves with the evidence base that supports the use with a specific client group and environment. The tools considered are as follows:

- Safety, Assessment of Function and the Environment for Rehabilitation (SAFER tool) (Community Occupational Therapists and Associates, 1991).
- Community Dependency Index (Eakin and Baird, 1995).
- Falls Efficacy Scale (Tinnetti *et al.*, 1990).
- Westmead Home Safety Assessment (Clemson, 1997).
- Home Falls and Accidents Screening Tool (HOME FAST) (Mackenzie *et al.*, 2000).

Safety, Assessment of Function and the Environment for Rehabilitation (SAFER TOOL)

Developed in Canada by the Community Occupational Therapists and Associates, SAFER is a checklist to be used to record the assessment of a person carrying out their functional activities in the home environment (Oliver *et al.*, 1993). The tool identifies 97 different components of environmental risks and behaviours which allow the therapist to record whether a problem has been identified, addressed or not applicable. The authors suggest that a summary score, which provides a percentage of the problems out of the total components assessed, can be used as an outcome measure. It is suggested that the tool could be re-used to measure change post interventions by comparing the summary score.

Letts *et al.* (1998) tested the tool on 38 subjects and concluded test–retest, and inter-rater reliability, was acceptable. This tool was designed to be used by community occupational therapists and does resemble many bespoke home visit checklists. The 'summary score' is not a precise measure of functional safety and overall the development of this tool lacks rigour. There is no evidence that this tool can be used to predict the risk of falling as required for this case study.

Community Dependency Index

Originally developed from the Barthel Index (Mahoney and Barthel, 1965), this is another community occupational therapy standardised assessment, originally designed to be used within the framework of new community care legislation (National Health Service and Community Care Act 1990) policy in the United Kingdom. Eakin and Baird (1995) explain that the Community Dependency Index has been developed as an outcome measure of the person's dependency within the home environment and is not a measure of their disability or impairment. In measuring dependency not disability, this tool can enable community care managers to identify a person's needs for community care services based upon actual need (dependency), rather than prioritise resources based upon diagnosis. The underlying principle for the role of the community occupational therapist is maximising person–environment fit once again.

This assessment measures performance in ten self-care occupations and mobility-related activities, including stair climbing. The chosen categories for assessment have been selected from custom and practice of occupational therapy home assessments and community care policy. A scoring system is used to identify levels of dependency for each activity at initial assessment and follow-up. The scoring of dependency in the different activities attracts different weighting which reflects the significance of the activity being performed, with independence in outside mobility and transferring on and off chairs and getting into bed being scored more highly than being independent washing face and hands or bathing. The lower the score, the more dependent the client is assessed as being and, therefore, the more in need of services. Eakin and Baird (1995) report high inter-rater and intra-rater reliability on 38 subjects using Kendall's coefficient of concordance.

This assessment tool will identify the person's independence carrying out daily activities in their own home, but it is not able to predict the relative risk of falling specifically, even though mobility and transfers are assessed. Levels of dependency identified in this assessment tool (i.e. low scores) cannot be mistaken for levels of risk.

Falls Efficacy Scale

Developed to be used as part of a multidisciplinary falls prevention programme, the Falls Efficacy Scale measures a person's confidence in carrying out daily activities without falling. Many high-quality studies have identified the fear of falling is significantly predictive of the occurrence of future falls in the older population (Cumming *et al.*, 2000; Tromp *et al.*, 2001; Friedman *et al.*, 2002). This assessment uses a ten-point scale ranging from 0 (not confident at all) to 10 (completely confident). The older person is asked to rate their confidence on ten different activities, e.g. getting out of bed, taking a bath or shower, light housekeeping. It has good test–retest reliability (Cumming *et al.*, 2001).

This assessment can be used with Samuel as he has a history of falling, and a fear of falling carrying out his daily activities is predictive and a significant risk factor of him falling again. The Falls Efficacy Scale does not assess environmental hazards and therefore another suitable standardised assessment must be chosen for the occupational therapist on the home assessment.

Westmead Home Safety Assessment

A strength of the Westmead Home Safety assessment is that it has been specifically developed to identify home fall hazards rather than being a generic occupational therapy home visit assessment. This tool has undergone thorough development, including expert review. The tool has achieved a high level of content validity and Clemson *et al.* (1999b) suggest that this tool could offer a gold standard for occupational therapists in identifying home falls hazards. Seventy-two hazards have been organised under categories, including external/internal traffic ways, seating, bedroom, footwear and medication management (Clemson *et al.*, 1999b). The detailed nature of this tool takes a long time to administer which impacted upon its clinical utility. In response a shorter version has been created. A manual supports the assessment, and reliability has been found amongst therapists who have used the manual.

Home Falls and Accidents Screening Tool (HOME FAST)

HOME FAST has been developed in Australia to be used as a screening tool of older people living in the community, to identify home environmental hazards which increase the person's risk of falling (Mackenzie *et al.*, 2000). Unlike the Westmead Home Safety Assessment, this tool was specifically designed to be a simple-to-use screening tool. It has 25 questions relating to known environmental hazards, which have been developed through field testing, literature review and expert opinion. Currently responses are marked as 'yes', 'no' or 'not applicable', but further work on developing a scoring system is being carried out. Reliability studies have been conducted in Australia and the UK. The overall inter-rater reliability of this tool was found to be fair to good with a Kappa score of 0.62 (Mackenzie *et al.*, 2002). On four specific criterions, excellent reliability (Kappa

≤0.75) between the raters was found, these being the proximity of the toilet to the bedroom, safety using the bath and shower, and absence of rails in bathroom. It has good clinical utility and is used in many falls services in the UK, Australia and Canada.

Samuel was assessed in his home environment by the physiotherapist and the occupational therapist; he also invited his daughter to be present on the visit. The occupational therapist assessed his environmental hazards of falling using the HOME FAST assessment tool and information from the overview and this specialist assessment was collated using EASY CARE (Single Assessment Process). HOME FAST was used before and after occupational therapist's interventions as an outcome measure (Chartered Society of Physiotherapy, 2002). Fig. 8.6 summarises Samuel's initial HOME FAST assessment record.

This assessment showed that, from the 25 questions identifying risk in the HOME FAST tool, the occupational therapist had identified 16 different risk environmental risk factors which were either associated with Samuel's fall or pose a potential risk of falling in the future.

Goals

Long-term goals

The nature of setting long-term goals is for the team and Samuel to have an agreed direction and long-term outcome of any interventions he is to receive. Long-term goals, which indicate an outcome which may span over several months or years, need to be broken down into more specific medium- and short-term goals, which, when achieved, enable the long-term goal to be realised.

The generic long-term goals set by Samuel and the intermediate care team were:

▨ To facilitate a safe home discharge for Samuel.
▨ For Samuel to continue to live in his home for as long as possible without falling.

The multifactorial assessment carried out by the team has identified the following areas that will need addressing in order for Samuel to realise his long-term goal.

Medium-term goals

▨ Review and monitor medication and management of Samuel's medical conditions: diabetes, hypertension, osteoarthritis (specialist nurse and doctor).
▨ To improve his overall mobility, strength and balance to enable safe transfers and stair climbing (physiotherapist).

1. **Walkways** – upstairs – bedroom and hallway generally clear from clutter however there was a trailing wire for an additional electric heater he used in his bedroom and there was the bucket he used during the night on the floor beside his bed. All doorways were free from obstruction and could be properly closed. Downstairs there was a sideboard positioned at the bottom of the stairs and some washing on the bottom step waiting to be carried up stairs.
2. **Floor coverings** – overall the carpet throughout the house was old and worn but not lifting anywhere. The carpet on the stairs was particularly worn out on several of the nosings on the stairs.
3. **Non-slip floor surfaces** – kitchen and bathroom had lino tiles which were non-slip and old.
4. **Loose mats securely fixed to floor** – Samuel did not use mats or rugs in the house.
5. **In and out of bed safely** – Samuel had a very old low bed (37 cm (15 inches) from floor) with a mattress which was worn and sunken in the middle. Samuel had difficulty standing from sitting at the edge of this low bed and would sometimes lean on the bedside cabinet and push up to help him stand.
6. **Get up from lounge chair** – Samuel had a three piece suite and he mainly sat in the arm chair but this was soft and low (37 cm (15 inches) seat height) and he struggled to rise to stand from sitting position. Relied heavily upon his upper arm strength to push himself up as his knees were generally stiff and sore from his osteoarthritis.
7. **Lighting** – downstairs hallway had very dark solid plastic lampshade with only a 40 Watt light bulb, which cast shadows at the bottom of the stairs. There was no light directly above the stairs just one on the top landing. This had the effect of a very dark area in the middle of the stairs. Generally Samuel used 40 Watt light bulbs around the house and a fluorescent tube lighting in the kitchen and bathroom.
8. **Turning on light easily from bed** – he had a bedside lamp which he found fiddly to turn on during the night when it is dark.
9. **Lighting to outside paths, steps and entrances** – Samuel had no external lights for either entrance to his house.
10. **On and off toilet safely** – WC seat height was 40 cm (16 inches) and as Samuel is approximately 6? tall he finds this difficult to stand up from, pulls himself up on pedestal hand basin. No rails in situ.
11. **In and out bath easily and safely** – Samuel had stopped using the bath as he has experienced difficulty standing up from the bottom of the bath. He has strip washed for the past 6 months but expressed a wish to be able to bath again in the future as he found the warm water helped alleviate his stiffness in his legs.
12. **Shower** – N/A no shower in situ.
13. **Accessible grab rail beside bath** – no rail in situ.
14. **Slip-resistant mats** – none present or have been used previously.
15. **Proximity of WC to bedroom** – WC situated on ground floor and bedroom upstairs.
16. **Reaching items to use in kitchen** – only cooked for himself and tended to use the grill or microwave. Cooking utensils and foods well organised and no need to climb or bend except to get milk from bottom of fridge door.
17. **Carrying meals safely** – Samuel tended to eat meals in kitchen and only carried light snacks and hot drinks into his living room on a tray with no problems.
18. **Indoor steps and stairs** – staircase was narrow enclosed by two walls – no stair rail present on either wall. No other internal steps present.
19. **Outdoor steps** – just one step up to front door porch and a threshold step at front door. No rails present and no problems with Samuel managing these two steps.
20. **Easily and safely go up and down stairs** – Samuel reported that depending upon his high blood pressure, he could at times get breathless climbing the stairs and tired easily. Diabetic neuropathy had impaired sensation in his feet although Samuel was unaware that this might affect his safety climbing the stairs. His knees and hips can become stiff and painful at the end of an active day which made stair climbing more difficult.
21. **Edges of steps/stairs** – standing at the top of the stairs, Samuel found it hard to differentiate between the different steps due to poor lighting and a continuous patterned carpet.
22. **Entrance door** – Samuel reported no history of problems with front entrance nor were there any problems observed.
23. **Paths around house** – paths were free from clutter and no hazards observed.
24. **Shoes & slippers** – Samuel was wearing open-backed slippers when he fell on the stairs.
25. **Pets** – Samuel had no pets to care for.

Figure 8.6 Summary of Samuel's HOME FAST assessment.

▦ To make appropriate modifications to his home to reduce environmental risks (occupational therapist).
▦ To educate and advise Samuel about potential risks of falling and offer education on how to prevent a long lie if he were to fall again (falls prevention group).
▦ To improve confidence to return home and reduce his fear of falling (falls prevention group and multidisciplinary team).

Short-term goals

Each profession will work towards their own specific short-term goals which may be set for a specific session or as goals for the week. Together, achieving the sessional or weekly goals, the medium-term goals are achieved. These short-term goals should be 'SMART' and are generally graded to increase independence or performance.

Occupational therapy interventions for Samuel

Gillespie's systematic review of studies which investigated the effectiveness of interventions which prevent falls in elderly people (Gillespie *et al.*, 2005) concluded that home hazard assessment and home modifications carried out by occupational therapists are only effective with elderly people who have a history of falling. Samuel who has a history of falls is therefore a suitable candidate to benefit from home modifications to reduce his environmental risks.

The main areas identified from the Home Falls and Accidents Screening Tool (HOME FAST) were:

▦ Stairs – no rails, carpet, poor lighting, hurrying and carrying things whilst climbing stairs.
▦ Transfers on WC, armchair, bed and bath.

The occupational therapist spent a long time discussing the home hazards identified on the previous home visit with Samuel and his family and actively engaged him in the process of identifying solutions so that Samuel was happy to accept the changes to his home and routines. There is rarely one solution to a reducing an environmental hazard and time is required to work with the client to choose the appropriate solution they are likely to adhere to long term. The long-term effectiveness of home modifications prescribed by occupational therapists was studied by Cumming *et al.* (2001) who considered whether home modifications were still being used 12 months after delivery. At 12 months, only 52% of occupational therapist recommended modifications were still being used fully or partially. The authors concluded that the major barrier to older people adhering to the occupational therapist's recommendation was their belief that the modification will not reduce their risk of falling.

Adherence of the advice and ongoing use of the modifications given by occupational therapists is significant to the successful outcome of falls prevention
(Lyons *et al.*, 2003). Gosselin *et al.* (1993) studied 255 older people in Canada to
examine factors which determine adherence to home modifications recommended
by occupational therapists. They found that the most significant predictor for
adherence was the perceived need by the older person for the recommended
modification, followed by the cost of the work and the ability to fund such work.
A much smaller study by Clemson *et al.* (1999a) concluded that adherence was
more likely if the older person was part of the decision-making process and that
they felt in control over changes to their home. Heywood (2001), in the UK-based
study evaluating the effectiveness of housing adaptations, concluded that inadequate assessment and recommendation of the person's needs resulting in modifications which were inadequate, was the major cause for ineffective interventions.
Poor consultation and lack of inclusion of the client in the assessment and design
process all contributed to dissatisfaction and wasted expenditure.

With all this in mind the following solutions and modifications were agreed
with Samuel.

Stairs

Samuel was of the firm opinion that the main cause of his fall was that he was
rushing to answer the phone in the dark with no rails to hang on to.

Aim

The aim of the intervention was to improve Samuel's safety when using the
stairs.

Action

- Update telephone system to a wireless handset with base units upstairs and
  downstairs, so that Samuel can answer the phone anywhere in the house
  without rushing downstairs.
- Change light bulbs to 100 Watt long-life options to avoid need to replace bulbs
  frequently. Replace existing dark light shade to plain white colour to reflect
  more light.
- Install handrail the total length of the stair case at a height 950 mm and design
  which complies with Part M of Building Regulations (Office of the Deputy
  Prime Minister, 2004). The stair case is very narrow and the physiotherapist
  agreed that the provision of a single stair rail should be sufficient at this stage
  to provide adequate support and stability for Samuel when climbing stairs and
  carrying light loads.
- Samuel was advised to avoid leaving his washing on the bottom step as this
  was a potential trip hazard, and when carrying the washing upstairs, to take

small loads rather than one large bundle which might obscure his vision on the stairs.
- Carpet. Samuel was advised that the patterned carpet was contributing to his difficulty seeing the edge of each step. As a short-term measure, white heavy duty tape was stuck down on the edges of each step and advice given that when replacing the worn carpet he should try a non-patterned, light-coloured carpet.
- Intercom. Samuel does not receive many visitors and so there was no need to consider an intercom for use upstairs at this stage but he was given an information leaflet of the local social services occupational therapy department and 'Care and Repair' service for future advice.
- Samuel was advised to change his slippers to a more secure design which are less likely to fall off his feet.

Transfers

Aim

- To enable Samuel to move from a sitting to standing position safely.
- To enable Samuel to safely resume taking a bath.

Samuel, who is quite tall, has been having difficulty standing up from his armchair, WC and bed, and had given up trying to get into the bath for fear of getting stuck. Generally the furniture was too low and too soft for Samuel to stand up from.

Action

- The bed was raised with bed blocks and a board placed under the mattress to provide more firm base to stand up from. These modifications worked sufficiently for Samuel at that time but advice was given about the type of bed that would suit his needs if he were to buy a new one in the future and that specialist rails are available to assist with bed transfers if he has difficulty in the future.
- The WC was fitted with a 10 cm (4 inch) raised toilet seat and a short grab rail fitted to the adjacent wall at a height individually assessed for Samuel.
- The armchair was also too low but fitted him well and had two arm rests. The chair was raised using chair raisers and again advice given to Samuel about good features of a chair if buying a new one.
- The bath. Samuel was assessed with a bath board, seat and rubber mat. He was able to lift his legs over the side of the bath whilst sitting on the bath board but experienced a lot of pain in his knees when they were bent going down on to the bath seat. There was very little space for his long legs when down on the bath seat. These problems combined with his existing fear of getting stuck in the bath again suggested that the bath board and seat would not meet his needs

safely and so a battery operated bath seat was recommended. This only required Samuel to sit on the seat and swivel his legs around into the bath which he was able to do. In addition a grab rail was fitted to the bath wall to aid lifting his legs over the side of the bath whilst sitting.

Lighting

- General advice was given regarding the types of light bulbs used around the house. Use of bulbs of minimum 75 Watts and long-life bulbs are recommended.
- The bedside lamp could be replaced with a light that comes on by touching the shade rather than fiddling around to find the switch.

An external light with passive infrared heat sensors to automatically turn on and off when Samuel approaches the front door was also recommended.

Fear of falling

The falls prevention groups discussed strategies on what to do if you fall. Whilst on a home visit, the occupational therapist discussed individualised strategies of how Samuel might cope if he were to fall again. Training and advice were given on how to get up from the floor using the 'backward chaining' method (Reece and Simpson, 1996). Samuel had lost a lot of confidence following his fall and was worried about returning home alone whilst he was still physically frail. He agreed to be referred for the community alarm system which included a pendant alarm and fall detector.

Evaluation

Samuel was discharged home after 6 weeks' rehabilitation with the intermediate care team. He felt that he had regained his strength and mobility to the levels prior to his fall. All equipment and rails had been installed prior to his discharge home in cooperation with the integrated community equipment store and social services department. A follow-up home visit was carried out by the occupational therapist to check how Samuel was managing. A review of the Home Falls and Accident Screening Tool identified that Samuel's home hazards had been significantly reduced and that he was managing the stairs with more confidence. The family had changed the lighting as advised in the hallways and bedroom and they were saving up to buy him a new bed. Samuel was managing well with the bath lift and all his transfers were significantly easier for him to manage. He had not had a fall or had needed to use the alarm cord, but was reassured that it was there in case of an emergency.

Reflection and comment

The evidence-based practice discussed in this chapter has been based upon the NICE Clinical Guideline 21 (2004). Readers are advised to refer to the full text version of that document for specific guidance and references. This is a dynamic area of practice and new research and systematic reviews are being published all the time. Readers need to ensure that they check for the most recent evidence base if it is to be used to change practice.

The author has used her clinical and teaching experience to discuss a case study which reflects current best practice in light of current government guidance on falls services and the single assessment process. The author has avoided procedural detail with regards to the procurement of equipment and eligibility criteria as this can vary from trust to trust.

Challenges to the reader

- How can the single assessment process be used in your locality to improve the effective management of risk for the older person who has a history of falling?
- How can assistive technologies (including Telecare) be used to help maintain and manage the independence of the older person who falls?
- In your locality, is there a specialist falls service and, if so, how often do you refer to it?
- What alternative strategies could have been adopted in helping Samuel and why might they have been used?

Resources

College of Occupational Therapy Specialist Section of Occupational Therapy for Older People (OTOP)

National Occupational Therapy Falls Clinical Forum (affiliated to OTOP)

Department of Trade and Industry – Home Safety Network www.dti.gov.uk/homesafetynetwork. htm Help the Aged Preventing Falls Campaign 'Slips Trips and Broken Hips' www.helptheaged. org.uk/adviceinfo/slips+trips.htm

References

Canadian Association of Occupational Therapists (1997) *Enabling Occupation: an Occupational Therapy Perspective.* CAOT Publications ACE, Ottawa

Chang, J.T., Morton, S.C., Rubenstein, L.Z., Mojica, W.A., Maglione, M., Suttorp, M.J., Roth, E.A. and Shekelle, P.G. (2004) Interventions for the prevention of falls in older adults: systematic review and meta-analysis of randomised clinical trials. *British Medical Journal*, **328(7441)**, 680

Chartered Society of Physiotherapy and College of Occupational Therapy (2002) *Falls Audit Pack – Guideline for the Collaborative, Rehabilitative Management of Elderly People who have Fallen.* www. csp.org.uk (accessed 15 December 2005)

Clemson, L. (1997) *Home Fall Hazards and the Westmead Home Safety Assessment.* Coordinates Publications, West Brunswick

Clemson, L., Cusick, A. and Fozzard, C. (1999a) Managing risk and exerting control: determining follow through with falls prevention. *Disability and Rehabilitation*, **13**, 531–541

Clemson, L., Fitzgerald, M. and Heard, R. (1999b) Content validity of an assessment tool to identify home fall hazards: the Westmead Home Safety Assessment. *British Journal of Occupational Therapy*, **62(4)**, 171–179

Community Occupational Therapists and Associates (1991) *Safety Assessment of Function and the Environment for Rehabilitation (SAFER Tool).* COTA, Toronto

Cryer, C. (2001) *What Works to Prevent Accidental Injury Amongst Older People? Report to the Health Development Agency.* HDA, London

Cumming, R., Salkeld, G., Thomas, M. and Szonyi, G. (2000) Prospective study of the impact of fear of falling on activities of daily living, SF-36 scores, and nursing home admission. *Journals of Gerontology, Series A Biological Sciences and Medical Sciences*, **55(5)**, M299–M305

Cumming, R., Thomas, M., Szonyi, G., Frampton, G., Salkeld, G. and Clemson, L. (2001) Adherence to occupational therapist recommendations for home modifications for falls prevention. *American Journal for Occupational Therapy*, **55**, 641–648

Cumming, R., Thomas, M., Szonyi, G., Salkeld, G., O'Neill, E., Westbury, C. and Frampton, G. (1999) Home visits by an occupational therapist for assessment and modification of environmental hazards: a randomized trial of falls prevention. *Journal of American Geriatrics Society*, **47**, 1397–1402

Day, L., Fildes, B., Gordon, I., Fitzharris, M., Flamer, H. and Lord, S. (2002) Randomised factorial trial of falls prevention among older people living in their own homes. *British Medical Journal*, **325(7356)**, 128

Department of Health (1989) *Caring for People: Community Care in the Next Decade and Beyond.* The Stationery Office, London

Department of Health (1997) *The new NHS: Modern and Dependable.* HMSO, London

Department of Health (1998) *A First Class Service.* HMSO, London

Department of Health (1999) *Saving Lives: Our Healthier Nation.* HMSO, London

Department of Health (2000) *NHS Plan.* HMSO, London

Department of Health (2001a) *National Service Framework for Older People.* The Stationery Office, London

Department of Health (2001b) *Saving Lives: Our Healthier Nation.* The Stationery Office, London

Department of Trade and Industry (1999) *Accidental Falls in the Home – Regional Distribution of Cases Involving People Aged 65 in the UK.* www.helptheaged.org.uk/adviceinfo/slips+trips.htm (accessed 15 December 2005)

Dowswell, T., Towner, E., Cryer, C., Jarvis, S., Edwards, P. and Lowe, P. (1999) *Accidental Falls: Fatalities and Injuries. An examination of the data sources and review of the literature on preventative strategies. A report for the Department of Trade and Industry ref: URN99/805* www.dti.gov.uk/homesafetynetwork/fl_rsrch.htm (accessed 15 December 2005)

Eakin, P. and Baird, H. (1995) The Community Dependency Index: a standardized assessment of need and measure of outcome for community occupational therapy. *British Journal of Occupational Therapy*, **58**(1), 17–20

Friedman, S., Munoz, B., West, S., Rubin, G. and Fried, L. (2002) Falls and fear of falling: which comes first? A longitudinal prediction model suggests strategies fro primary and secondary prevention. *Journal of American Geriatric Society*, **50**(8), 1329–1335

Gibson, M., Andres, R., Isaacs, B., Radebaugh, T. and Worm-Petersen, J. (1987) The prevention of falls in later life. A report of the Kellogg International Working Group on the prevention of falls by the elderly. *Danish Medical Bulletin*, **34**(4), 1–24

Gillespie, L., Gillespie, W., Robertson, M., Lamb, S., Cumming, R. and Rowe, B. (2005) Interventions for preventing falls in elderly people. *The Cochrane Database of Systematic Reviews*. Issue 4 Art No CD000340

Gosselin, C., Robitaille, Y., Trickey, F. and Maltais, D. (1993) Factors predicting the implementation of home modification among elderly people with loss of independence. *Physical and Occupational Therapy in Geriatrics*, **12**(1), 15–23

Griffiths, R. (1998) Community Care: an Agenda for Action. The Stationery Office, London

Health Education Authority (1999) *Older People and Accidents. Fact Sheet 2.* www.helptheaged.org.uk/HealthyAging/Falls/_practitioners.htm#factsheets

Health Promotion England (2001) *Older People in the Population. Avoiding Slips Trips and Broken Hips – Fact sheet 1.* www.helptheaged.org.uk/Health/HealthyAgeing/Falls/_practitioners.htm#factsheets (accessed 15 December 2005)

Heywood, F. (2001) *Money Well Spent: the Effectiveness and Value of Housing Adaptations.* The Policy Press, Bristol

Heywood, F., Oldman, C. and Means, R. (2002) *Housing and Home in Later Life.* Open University Press, Buckingham

Hill, L., Haslam, R., Howarth, P., Brooke-Wavell, K. and Sloane, J. (2000) *Safety of Older People on Stairs Behavioural Factors.* www.dti.gov.uk/homesafetynetwork/fl_rsrch.htm (accessed 15 December 2005)

Jørstad, E.C., Hauer, K., Becker, C. and Lamb, S.E. (2005) Measuring the psychological outcomes of falling: a systematic review. *Journal of the American Geriatrics Society*, **53**(3), 501–510

Law, M., Cooper, B., Strong, S., Stewart, D., Rigby, P. and Letts, L. (1996) The Person-Environment-Occupation Model: a transactive approach to occupational performance. *Canadian Journal of Occupational Therapy*, **63**(1), 9–23

Letts, L., Law, M., Rigby, P., Cooper, B., Stewart, D. and Strong, S. (1994) Person–environment assessments in occupational therapy. *American Journal of Occupational Therapy*, **48**(7), 608–618

Letts, L., Scott, S., Burtney, J., Marshall, L. and McKean, M. (1998) The reliability and validity of the Safety Assessment of Function and the Environment for Rehabilitation (SAFER TOOL). *British Journal of Occupational Therapy*, **61**(3), 127–132

Lord, S. (2001) *Falls in Older People: Risk Factors and Strategies for Prevention.* Cambridge University Press, Cambridge

Lyons, R., Sander, L., Weightman, A., Patterson, J., Jones, S., Rolfe, B., Kemp, A. and Johansen, A. (2003) Modification of the home environments for the reduction of injuries. *The Cochrane Database of Systematic Reviews.* Issue 4 Art no CD003600

Mackenzie, L., Byles, J. and Higginbotham, N. (2000) Designing the Home Falls and Accidents Screening Tool (HOME FAST): Selecting the items. *British Journal of Occupational Therapy,* **63(6)**, 260–269

Mackenzie, L., Byles, J. and Higginbotham, N. (2002) Reliability of the Home Falls and Accidents Screening Tool (HOME FAST) for identifying older people at increased risk of falls. *Disability and Rehabilitation,* **24(5)**, 266–274

Mahoney, F. and Barthel, D. (1965) Functional evaluation: the Barthel Index. *Mid-State Medical Journal,* **14**, 61–65

McClure, R., Turner, C., Peel, N., Spinks, A., Eakin, E. and Hughes, K. (2005) Population-based interventions for the prevention of fall-related injuries in older people. *The Cochrane Database of Systematic Reviews.* Issue 1 No. CD004441.pub2

Millward, L., Morgan, A. and Kelly, M. (2003) *Prevention and Reduction of Accidental Injury in Children and Older People. Evidence Briefing.* London: Health Development Agency. Internet: www.publichealth.nice.org.uk/page.aspx?0=502599 (accessed 15 December 2005)

National Institute for Health and Clinical Excellence(NICE) (2004) *Clinical Guideline 21 – Falls: The assessment and prevention of falls in older people.* http://www.nice.org.uk/pdf/CG021fullguideline.pdf (accessed 15 December 2005)

Office for National Statistics (2000a) *People Aged 65 and Over: Results of a study carried out on behalf of the Department of Health as part of the 1998 General Household Survey.* The Stationery Office, London

Office for National Statistics (2000b) *Living in Britain: Results from the 1998 General Household Survey.* The Stationery Office, London

Office for National Statistics (2002). *Living in Britain. General Household Survey.* The Stationery Office, London

Office for National Statistics (2005) 16% of United Kingdom's population is aged 65 or over. www.statistics.gov.uk/cci/nugget.asp?ID=949 (accessed 15 December 2005)

Office of the Deputy Prime Minister (2004) Building Regulations 2000. Access to and use of buildings, approved document M – 2004. The Stationery Office, London

Oliver, R., Blathwayt, J., Brackley, C. and Tamaki, T. (1993) Development of the Safety Assessment of Function and the Environment for Rehabilitation (SAFER TOOL). *Canadian Journal of Occupational Therapy,* **60(2)**, 78–82

Reece, A. and Simpson, J. (1996) Teaching elderly people how to cope after a fall. *Physiotherapy,* **82**, 227–235

Sackett, D., Richardson, W., Rosenberg, W. and Haynes, R. (1996) *Evidence-based Medicine.* Churchill Livingstone, Edinburgh

Scuffham, P., Chaplin, S. and Legood, R. (2003) Incidence and costs of unintentional falls in older people in the United Kingdom. *Journal of Epidemiology and Community Health,* **57**, 740–744

Sheffield University (2004) EASY CARE 2004. www.shef.ac.uk/sissa/easycare (accessed 15 December 2005)

Sherrington, C., Lord, S.R. and Finch, C.F. (2004) Physical activity interventions to prevent falls among older people: update of the evidence, *Journal of Science and Medicine in Sport*, **7(1)**, 43–51

Tinnetti, M. (2001) Where is the vision for falls prevention? *Journal of the American Geriatrics Society*, **49**, 676–677

Tinnetti, M., Richman, D. and Powell, L. (1990) Falls efficacy as a measure of falling. *Journal of Gerontology*, **45(6)**, 239–243

Tromp, A., Pluijm, S., Smit, J., Deeg, D., Bouter, L. and Lips, P. (2001) Fall-risk screening test: a prospective study on predictors for falls in community-dwelling elderly. *Journal of Clinical Epidemiology*, **54(8)**, 837–844

Tse, T. (2005) The environment and falls prevention: do environmental modifications make a difference? *Australian Occupational Therapy Journal*, **52(4)**, 271–281

9: Enabling participation in occupations post stroke

Janet Golledge

Introduction

The variations in functional presentation associated with stroke are a direct consequence of the disruption of the blood supply to a location within the brain (Bartels, 2004). The range of potential motor, cognitive–perceptual, psychological and emotional variables means that programmes of intervention must be tailored to the individual. In this chapter, two approaches are justified using established theory and best available evidence:

- The Bobath Concept (International Bobath Instructors Training Association, 2005) is applied to enhance motor control. This approach may be contentious in that it is justified according to its theoretical and philosophical foundations rather than evidence advocating its efficacy (Luke *et al.*, 2004).
- The multicontext approach (Toglia, 1998; 2003) is also critically evaluated in relation to improving cognitive and perceptual processing following stroke. This approach is based on a dynamic interaction model of cognition, analysing interaction between the individual, environment(s) and task(s). Much of the evidence for this approach is based on qualitative data in order to reflect the client's experience.

A stroke is often associated with older individuals but younger adults are also diagnosed with this disabling condition. Each year, over 130 000 people in England and Wales have a stroke, and 10 000 of these are under retirement age (Stroke Association, 2004). Approximately 30% of individuals die following their stroke and, of those who survive, about 35% require considerable help with daily occupations (Stephen and Rafferty, 1994; Department of Health, 2001b). As a result, a significant proportion of health and social care resources are needed for immediate and continuing care (Wolfe *et al.*, 1996). The cost of stroke care to the NHS is estimated to be over £2.3 billion per year, or approximately 4–5% of the NHS budget (Department of Health, 1996).

From this statistical information, it is evident that many individuals will have significant difficulties completing occupations and consequent problems engaging in their roles to support their lifestyles. Occupational therapists enable individuals to participate in their daily occupations and assist them on their journeys towards recovery. Occupational therapy for individuals who have had a stroke *'focuses on the nature, balance, pattern and context of occupations and activities in the lives of individuals, family groups and communities'* (Creek, 2003) with relevant interventions being selected according to individual need.

The National Service Framework for Older People (Department of Health, 2001b) outlines the needs and interventions for people post stroke in Standard 5. The key aim is to *'reduce the incidence of stroke in the population and ensure that those who have had a stroke have prompt access to integrated stroke care services'* (Department of Health, 2001b, p. 62). This chapter will present the occupational therapy intervention for a 70-year-old lady named Sally, during the first 4 weeks post stroke. Aetiology, prevalence and incidence statistics will be presented in addition to strategies for intervention. A structure will be provided using the occupational therapy process, beginning with assessments used and the plan, incorporating goal planning, selection of therapy approaches and a model of practice. An example of a therapy session will be presented, followed by the evaluation, which will conclude the intervention.

Explanation of stroke

Stroke was originally explained by the World Health Organization in 1978 and remains defined as *'a clinical syndrome typified by rapidly developing signs of focal or global disturbance of cerebral functions, lasting more than 24 hours or leading to death, with no apparent cause other than of vascular origin'* (Intercollegiate Stroke Working Party, 2004, p. 3).

A stroke is also known as a cerebrovascular accident (CVA) but stroke is the currently accepted term. A stroke occurs in one side of the brain (usually a cerebral hemisphere) or in the brain stem. It involves interruption of the blood supply to a part of the brain, with subsequent inadequate supply of oxygen. This results in a range of functional problems, depending on the location of this interruption (Bartels, 2004). It is important to understand the anatomy and physiology of the central nervous system (CNS) to appreciate these consequences. Damage to the posterior part of the frontal lobe will have a different impact on function than damage to the posterior parietal lobe. Most strokes occur as a consequence of a cerebral infarction (69%). Haemorrhages account for 19% whilst 12% result from uncertain origin (Wolfe *et al.*, 2002). Between 30 and 43% of individuals have a further stroke within 5 years (Mant *et al.*, 2004). Closely related to strokes are transient ischaemic attacks (TIA). This is a *'clinical syndrome characterised by an acute loss of focal cerebral function with symptoms lasting less than 24 hours'* (Intercollegiate Stroke Working Party, 2004, p. 3). Individuals recover from a transient ischaemic attack more effectively than after stroke but a transient ischaemic attack is associated with a high risk of stroke in the next month and up to 1 year later (Coull *et al.*, 2004).

Consequences of stroke

The effects of the stroke may be influenced by the individual's general health and the extent of damage to the brain (Department of Health, 2001b). Texts will typically describe these consequences in terms of *impairments* or *components* of dysfunction:

▢ **Motor**, which may include hypertonia, hypotonia, spasticity, impaired dexterity, weakness.
▢ **Cognitive–perceptual**, which includes visual processing deficits, executive problems, neglect, impaired memory or insight, apraxia, hemianopia.
▢ **Emotional and psychological** effects, may include depression, anxiety, emotional lability and low motivation.
▢ **Social** interaction may be affected due to receptive or expressive dysphasia, dysarthria or difficulties with facial expression, limiting an individual's opportunities for satisfying interactions with others.

Although these terms are valid, help to clarify impairments and provide a consistent terminology for the different health team members, they reflect a biomedical focus, rather than a lifestyle focus. A stroke is a revolutionary event that interrupts the continuity of the individual's journey through life (Golledge, 2004). Focusing on impairments does not sufficiently reflect the enormity of the consequences for individuals. Occupational therapists look beyond these impairments and analyse the impact at an **occupational level**. For example:

▢ **Hypertonia** in elbow flexors of the affected upper limb would impact on occupations requiring reaching, due to difficulty lengthening these muscles, e.g. to select items from a kitchen cupboard, reach for the telephone or put on shoes.
▢ **Impaired dexterity** in the affected hand will influence most occupations, including the ability to use cutlery to eat, select coins from a purse or fasten clothing.
▢ **Visual processing** deficits may result in difficulties visually locating items in a fridge or a room, putting the lid on a jar, pouring a drink.
▢ **Anxiety** compromises engagement and problem solving in occupations, impacting on the ability to attend and learn, which are key influences on successful therapy.
▢ **Dysphasia** impacts on the ability to participate in conversation with others, listen to the television, answer the telephone, and access e-mails and the internet.

The above examples represent a fraction of the potential occupations influenced by just a few selected impairments (Golledge, 2004). Two significant but sometimes misunderstood consequences will now be clarified: motor and cognitive–perceptual.

Motor consequences

Difficulties with movement are observed post stroke with a **hemiplegia** (paralysis) or **hemiparesis** (weakness) on the side of the body contralateral to the side of the stroke. If the stroke occurs in the left cerebral hemisphere, this will result in a right hemiplegia or hemiparesis. Although most difficulty with movement occurs on the affected side, individuals often struggle to move the whole body, so therapy attends to the whole body moving functionally. Motor control is not the sole contributor to moving; general mood and cognitive–perceptual problems adversely affect movement.

A stroke often damages neurones on motor control areas of the cerebral cortex on the frontal lobe or axons of descending **upper motor neurones** (UMNs, linking the cortex and other CNS structures to the spinal cord) from the corticospinal and dorsal reticulospinal pathways. These motor pathways, along with others, contribute to the regulation and control of movement for different parts of the body. When these pathways are damaged, there is an imbalance of descending motor impulses synapsing on the **lower motor neurones** (LMNs) at all levels of the spinal cord. The lower motor neurones link the spinal cord to the muscles and innervate these muscles via peripheral nerves. If the lower motor neurones do not receive the normal range of influences from all the upper motor neurone pathways, alterations in muscle tone are evident.

Hypotonia

Initially after a stroke, **hypotonia** (lower than normal muscle tone) is present, influenced by neuronal shock. Hypotonia impacts on normal concentric and eccentric muscle action. Additionally, there are problems with reciprocal inhibition – the graded interaction between prime movers and antagonists. Muscles need to be able to lengthen and shorten for function; individuals who cannot actively alter the length of their muscles cannot interact effectively with a base of support, e.g. in sitting, standing or to complete occupations. After stroke, electromyographic studies have shown that there is inadequate recruitment of motor units in muscles for movement, resulting in weakness, impaired dexterity, slowness of movement, increased sense of effort and difficulty generating force. These problems are also influenced by non-synchronous timing of activity in both prime movers and antagonists. When the individual tries to move his/her limbs, it is often in an abnormal way, using **mass movement synergies** where coordinated and selective movements at individual joints are not apparent. Given the reduced activity in the muscles, this is the best he/she can do, presenting as inefficient, awkward movements.

Hypertonia

Over the next few weeks, some muscles may develop **hypertonia**, an increased resistance to passive movement (Carr and Shepherd, 2003) and potentially, active movement, as a result of:

▨ **Biomechanical changes** occurring in muscle tissue (loss of sarcomeres, changes in muscle fibre types, shortening, atrophy from disuse, increases in collagen around muscle fibres with resultant stiffness), as a consequence of difficulties moving and immobility.

▨ Altered synaptic connections at the spinal cord level, occurring as a result of **neuroplasticity** (the capacity of the CNS to modify its structural organisation and functioning in response to damage). The alterations in synapses around the lower motor neurones occur because of the reduction in descending motor influences from the damaged cerebral hemisphere. These neuroplastic changes result in a phenomenon known as **spasticity**, which contributes to hypertonia.

Spasticity and the stretch reflex

Spasticity is a motor disorder characterised by a velocity dependent increase in tonic stretch reflexes (muscle tone) with exaggerated tendon jerks, resulting from a hyperexcitability of the stretch reflex, as one component of the upper motor neurone syndrome (Lance, 1980, p. 486).

This acknowledged and current definition contains some important terminology. Although spasticity contributes to eventual hypertonia, its influence on movement difficulties is overstated (O'Dwyer *et al.*, 1996; Carr and Shepherd, 2003).

The **stretch reflex** (one of the spinal network of reflexes that support inter-limb coordination and upright posture), influences the length and stretch in a muscle but is dependent for normal function on modulation, or fine tuning, from all descending upper motor neurones. This allows variation in muscle length and tone relevant for different tasks. It is a bit like mixing all the ingredients for a cake. If one or two ingredients have been omitted, this affects the quality of the cake. Balance reactions and smooth movements are dependent on the ability to alter muscle tone and length, selectively moving those parts of the body required for the task and inhibiting activity of other parts, e.g. to drive a car or brush the teeth. This modulation is impaired after stroke, due to damage to some upper motor neurones. The stretch reflex does not work as it should: it is not receiving all the ingredients.

Upper motor neurone syndrome

The motor consequences of stroke may be presented as positive and negative features, known as the **upper motor neurone syndrome** (Sheean, 1998; Carr and Shepherd, 1998):

▨ **Positive**: spasticity, hyperreflexia (e.g. stretch reflex), parapyramidal dysfunction (including the reticulospinal, vestibulospinal and rubrospinal pathways).

▨ **Negative**: weakness, slowness of movement, loss of dexterity, fatiguability, pyramidal deficits (predominantly corticospinal pathway).

The positive features of the upper motor neurone syndrome have often been stressed as the key focus for intervention, but investigations suggest that the negative consequences are the principal influences on movement problems. These are apparent initially when hypotonia is present, but remain an issue when hypertonia develops and the biomechanical changes take place. This has implications for the structure of therapy.

Spasticity is not the most significant influence on individuals' difficulties with movement; the biomechanical changes are more important (O'Dwyer et al., 1996; Sheean, 1998; Carr and Shepherd, 1998, 2003). Inhibiting spasticity does not generally result in improved motor performance. This contrasts with the sometimes overt emphasis in some services that spasticity is the key aspect to which therapists should attend. The apparent spasticity, felt by some therapists, is primarily due to the biomechanical changes contributing to hypertonia or the individual's efforts to move, recruiting those muscles that have most activity and, because moving is difficult, co-contraction of muscle groups. To the uninformed, this may be interpreted as spasticity. There is inconsistent use of the terms spasticity and hypertonia in the literature, particularly in the dissemination of research. This creates uncertainty for the reader: what is being investigated and reported? It would be helpful if authors could present accurate use of the terms, to enable therapists to understand the distinction.

The focus in occupational therapy will be to assist Sally to move and act in everyday contexts. Active attempts at movement will not be prevented under the mistaken perception that spasticity is being inhibited. There is no evidence that providing resistance in tasks, exercise or occupations increases spasticity, so handling techniques will be used to facilitate Sally's active movements. This will enable the occupational therapist to analyse the initial presence of hypotonia and potential development of hypertonia, which, in turn, will influence the selection of therapeutic techniques.

Cognitive–perceptual consequences

The incidence of cognitive–perceptual problems amongst individuals who have had a stroke is varyingly reported in the literature. Tatemichi et al. (1994) noted that significant cognitive deficits were found in 35% of individuals but Dreissen et al. (1997) noted that 63% had deficits influencing their function. Individuals with cognitive impairments in addition to motor difficulties have less functional recovery (Paolucci et al., 1996; Katz et al., 2000; Stephens et al., 2005). The Intercollegiate Stroke Working Party (2004) stresses the significance of and assessment for cognitive–perceptual problems, and notes that '25% of long-term survivors have such severe generalised impairment that they may be diagnosed with dementia'. Cognitive impairment remains significant 3 years post stroke and may show minimal changes without therapy (Patel et al., 2003).

It is essential, therefore, that cognitive–perceptual problems are assessed and effective therapy employed, although the National Service Framework for Older

People (Department of Health, 2001b) does not specify therapy for cognitive–perceptual problems. Occupational therapists have particular expertise regarding this issue (Intercollegiate Stroke Working Party, 2000) and share their knowledge and expertise with other team members, since these problems impact on the effectiveness of all interventions (Golledge, 2005a). Cognitive and perceptual deficits may be listed separately in texts but they both work in tandem to support function. A visual perceptual deficit in spatial relations will influence learning, judgement and memory (i.e. cognitive components), so it is better to appreciate them as linked. In the literature, they are increasingly presented as *cognitive problems,* categorised as difficulties in (Golisz and Toglia, 2003):

- Orientation.
- Insight and awareness.
- Attention (detect/react, select, sustain, shift, mental tracking).
- Visual processing – visual discrimination and visual motor.
- Neglect.
- Motor planning.
- Memory.
- Executive functions, organisation, problem solving.

The functional consequences of these are varied, from difficulties selecting items on supermarket shelves to orientating clothes to the body for dressing. Individuals who have cognitive–perceptual problems may have damage to any of the lobes of the brain. The right parietal lobe helps support spatial processing, for example, so if this is damaged, function will be impaired (Golledge, 2005a). Individuals struggle to analyse the interaction between the demands of the occupation, the environment and the strategies required for completion. There is a breakdown in the information processing system, with difficulty comprehending why they are unable to do an occupation that was quite automatic prior to the stroke. This requires careful explanation. Some people may think that Sally is being difficult or not trying because they may not understand why Sally is unable to cooperate. Cognitive–perceptual dysfunction can occur with little or no muscle tone changes influencing movement but can create considerable occupational difficulties. It is important that all team members understand the implications of these distressing consequences (Zinn *et al.,* 2005).

Key legislation and professional documentation

Health care professionals use legislation and clinical guidelines to inform their practice. This documentation aims to ensure that all occupational therapists understand care pathways and the overall aims of fair, high-quality and integrated intervention. The aims reflect government programmes of health reform, disseminating results of research to support evidence-based practice.

Key documentation influencing intervention with people following stroke includes:

- *NHS Plan: A Plan for Investment. A plan for Reform* (Department of Health, 2001a).
- National Service Framework for Older People (Department of Health, 2001b).
- *National Clinical Guidelines for Stroke*, 2nd edn (Intercollegiate Stroke Working Party, 2004).

Guidelines for intervention

Currently, evidence is not unequivocal in stroke rehabilitation. Whilst there is considerable emphasis on evidence-based practice in health care, it is acknowledged that stroke is a very heterogeneous condition, so there is unlikely to be a single, definitive approach for therapy. The quest for best practice also requires reflective practice, using sound clinical reasoning, interpretation of results and professional judgement (Blair and Robertson, 2005). Research studies regularly do not demonstrate the benefits of one therapy approach or intervention over another and may present with conflicting results, often due to methodological flaws (Foley *et al.*, 2003; Jutai and Teasell, 2003; Steultjens *et al.*, 2003; Teasell *et al.*, 2003). The *National Clinical Guidelines for Stroke* (Intercollegiate Stroke Working Party, 2004) and the National Service Framework for Older People (Department of Health, 2001b) both note that there should not be adherence to only one approach. Positive outcomes are likely to occur with individualised therapy programmes that respond to individual needs and circumstances, fitting with the philosophy of occupational therapy.

Studies and systematic reviews reflect the importance and influence of neuroplasticity and learning theories from neuropsychology for informing effective therapy (Bergquist *et al.*, 1994; Cicerone *et al.*, 2000; Heddings *et al.*, 2000; Johannsson, 2000; Selzer, 2000; Bach-y-Rita, 2001; Fisher and Sullivan, 2001; Unsworth and Cunningham, 2002; Steultjens *et al.*, 2003; Teasell *et al.*, 2003). The Cochrane Database for Systematic Reviews (Stroke Group) (2004) presents four reviews investigating the evidence for interventions for attention deficits (2000), cognitive impairment (2002), memory deficits (2000) and spatial neglect (2002). They report inconclusive evidence to support any specific therapy approach and stress that there should be a serious attempt to investigate the interventions for cognitive problems, learning from cognitive neuroscience and neuropsychology literature. Efforts to establish sound practice are stressing the importance of these points, for example in the multicontext therapy approach (Toglia, 2003). The very nature of cognitive deficits, combined with the other consequences of stroke, makes it unlikely that a definitive approach will be established to meet the strict criteria acceptable to the Cochrane group. The components of reflective practice, a fundamental aspect of occupational therapy, are particularly relevant for establishing effective therapy, in contrast to the more reductionist evidence-based practice rationale. The range of potential consequences for motor, cognitive–perceptual, psychological and emotional variables means that programmes of intervention must be tailored to the individual. This is evident in goal planning for Sally.

Assessment

The World Health Organization *International Classification of Functioning, Disability and Health* (ICF) is an international standard developed to describe and measure health and functioning (World Health Organization, 2001). The emphasis on occupational functioning and contextual factors is compatible with the application of occupational therapy (College of Occupational Therapists, 2004). The ICF exhorts professionals to work with clients at the activity and participation levels, rather than the impairment level. Assessment details may include some results at this level, but, to reflect the philosophy of occupational therapy, most assessments used as outcome measures with Sally reflect activity and participation. This issue is also stressed by the Intercollegiate Stroke Working Party (2004) and the National Service Framework for Older People (Department of Health, 2001b). An outcome measure used at the end of Sally's inpatient stay, the Stroke Impact Scale, is a participation measure. No single measure will collect data that illustrates the wide range of outcomes after stroke (Mayo *et al.*, 2002). Consequently, a variety of assessments are used by the occupational therapist to provide an accurate picture of Sally's outcomes. All data collected reflect the Single Assessment Process outlined in Standard 2 of the National Service Framework for Older People (Department of Health, 2001b). Details of the Single Assessment Process can be found at www.dh.gov.uk.

Standardised assessments can be divided into three categories: discriminative, predictive and evaluative. Some assessments may include elements of all three. Discriminative assessments aim to distinguish between individuals and describe their particular level of functioning on the measure. Predictive assessments aim to try to predict outcome, based on initial assessment scores, or to make a prognosis. Evaluative instruments are used to measure change over time (Bowling, 2001). Relevant categories will be noted in the assessments used with Sally.

Initial interview

The initial interview is the first opportunity for interaction between the occupational therapist and Sally. Information is first gathered from the case notes and used during the interview to explore Sally's perspective of the stroke, her concerns and her hopes for the future. Clinical reasoning is used to formulate ideas about Sally's occupational performance difficulties, based on an understanding of the consequences of stroke; for intervention to be meaningful, however, the occupational therapist needs to know the particulars of Sally's situation (Henry, 2003). The following information has been gathered in the initial interview, lasting approximately 30 minutes, through discussion and observations.

Sally Hunter is 70 years old and lives with her husband, Tom, who is 75 years old. He is relatively well but has high blood pressure and late-onset diabetes. They own and live in a semi-detached bungalow on a suburban housing estate with their small dog, Lulu. They have a son and daughter, who each have two teenage children. They all live locally and see each other regularly. Sally and Tom used to work for the local bus service for many years. Tom was a driver and Sally was a secretary. Tom still drives a car, which they use to maintain their lifestyle, e.g. shopping, visiting the library and family and friends, and to attend social events, such as dances, theatre and musicals. Sally's spirituality was evident in her values, beliefs and goals. Her drive, determination and motivation to resume and take control of her life, were evident. Sally is keen to return home and expresses her desire to use her left side effectively, rather than compensating with her right side. This is beginning to inform the occupational therapist's selection of therapy approaches.

Diagnosis

Sally has had an ischaemic stroke (subcortical) in the right cerebral hemisphere. She had a myocardial infarction 8 months ago and it is thought that her stroke is the result of a cardiac embolus. This has caused an interruption of cerebral blood flow in the upper division of her right middle cerebral artery. This anatomical information will explain some of Sally's functional difficulties. Prior to her myocardial infarction, Sally felt that she enjoyed good health. She is right handed.

Roles and occupations

Sally was independent in all personal care occupations prior to her stroke – toileting, showering, grooming, dressing and eating.

- Home maintainer: Sally and Tom shared many domestic tasks, including cooking and meal preparation, shopping and cleaning. Sally does laundry and ironing. Their small garden, where they enjoy sitting, is structured for easy maintenance.
- Parent and grandparent: Sally and Tom see their children most weeks and regularly see their grandchildren. They all have Sunday lunch at one of their homes once a month. Sally likes to see all the family together and the monthly lunches are important to her.
- Friend: Sally has a few close friends from the local embroiderer's guild, which she attends monthly. She and Tom meet another couple monthly, for dinner.
- Hobbyist: Sally enjoys embroidery, alone at home and in the local group. She likes reading crime novels and watching similar programmes on television. Sally and Tom go ballroom dancing, where they meet friends.
- Pet owner: Sally and Tom jointly care for Lulu and enjoy taking her for walks.

Motor skills

Sally has difficulty moving her left arm and leg, saying that they feel weak. She is able to stand and transfer with some assistance but is anxious that she will fall.

Coordination and manipulation of objects is difficult; she is unable to generate enough activity in relevant muscles. This is presenting as hypotonia at this early stage, making it difficult for her to reach and move her left arm against gravity.

Processing skills

Sally is experiencing problems with visual processing and organising space around her and the objects she needs for occupations. She reports feeling confused about her difficulties and may have some attention deficits.

Communication/interaction skills

Sally does not have receptive or expressive dysphasia or dysarthria. She finds speaking tiring but interacts with others, orientating herself and engaging in conversation. She uses appropriate affect, demonstrating concern, respect, patience and interest in events around her. She tries to watch television and read.

Standardised assessments

Subsequent to the initial interview, the occupational therapist selects standardised assessments to investigate Sally's abilities and difficulties in more depth. Accurate assessment results are required to construct a therapy programme that will meet Sally's needs and hopes for future function.

Behavioural Inattention Test (BIT)

This standardised assessment (discriminative) is an instrument for measuring unilateral visual neglect (Wilson *et al.*, 1987). Neglect manifests as a range of difficulties with personal, peripersonal and distant space. Neglect has a significant negative effect on rehabilitation outcomes (Katz *et al.*, 2000; Buxbaum *et al.*, 2004) and should not be confused with hemianopia or attention problems. It is noted to be most prevalent after right cerebral hemisphere damage (Buxbaum *et al.*, 2004). As this reflects Sally's situation, it is important to confirm or not the presence of neglect since this would have significant impact on her therapy and outcomes (Katz *et al.*, 2000; Gillen *et al.*, 2005). There is inconsistent reporting of spontaneous recovery from neglect in the first few weeks after stroke, with suggestions for delayed assessment. Appelros *et al.* (2004) note that many individuals retain some element of neglect 6 months post stroke, whilst Gillen *et al.* (2005) stress the negative impact on rehabilitation outcomes. Neglect is known to promote longer in-patient stays and slower progress. With these points in mind, it was relevant to assess Sally for neglect. The BIT has good reliability and validity, discriminating between individuals with and without neglect. The results of this assessment concluded that Sally does not have neglect.

Functional Independence Measure (FIM)

This is a commonly used instrument (Sangha *et al.*, 2005) for assessment of activities of daily living, measuring progress in rehabilitation and designed as an outcome measure to predict effectiveness of rehabilitation and required level of care (Guide for Uniform Dataset for Medical Rehabilitation, 1997). It does not measure level of competence or quality of task performance. It measures function at the activity level of the ICF. As a standardised assessment, it is discriminatory, evaluative, predictive and sensitive to changes in disability following stroke (Dromerick *et al.*, 2003). Many studies have confirmed its reliability and validity (Hamilton *et al.*, 1994; Hsueh *et al.*, 2002; Lundgren-Nilsson *et al.*, 2005).

Sally is observed completing basic self-care tasks and rated on a seven-point score range for 13 items on a physical scale and five items on a social cognition scale. Scoring reflects the level of dependence and assistance required, with a score of 7 indicating a higher level of independence than 1. The data is ordinal and, as such, should not be added as a summed score but as an outcome measure; this is often done with FIM. A detailed critique of this issue is beyond the scope of this section. Sally's scores are presented below. Timbeck and Spaulding (2004) and Lutz (2004) note that admission total FIM score is a strong predictor of discharge score, outcome disability and discharge destination. Individuals with admission FIM scores of less than 50 remain dependent with self-care activities at discharge whereas those with scores higher than 90 are more likely to be discharged home and have greater independence. Sally's total score of 78 implies that she is in a good initial position to make progress towards further recovery.

Scoring levels are as follows:

- 7 = complete independence, timely, safe, no helper.
- 6 = modified independence, use of device, no helper.
- 5 = modified independence, supervision needed, person does 100%.
- 4 = minimal assistance, person does 75%+.
- 3 = moderate assistance, person does 50%+.
- 2 = complete dependence, person does 25%+.
- 1 = total assistance, person does less than 25%.

Results

Each score is out of 7.

- Self care:
  - Eating 5.
  - Grooming 3.
  - Bathing 3.
  - Dressing – upper body 3; lower body 3.
  - Toileting 3.
- Sphincter control:
  - Bladder management 7.
  - Bowel management 7.

- Transfers:
  - Bed, chair, wheelchair 3.
  - Toilet 3.
  - Shower 3.
- Locomotion:
  - Walking 2.
  - Stairs 2.
- **Motor subtotal score 47/91.**
- Communication:
  - Comprehension (auditory and visual) 7.
  - Expression (vocal and non-vocal) 7.
- Social cognition:
  - Social interaction 7.
  - Problem solving 3.
  - Memory 7.
- **Cognitive subtotal score 31/35.**
- **Total FIM score = 78/126.**

The motor scores are influenced by hypotonia on Sally's left side. This makes it difficult for her to move, but she has some slow, effortful, active movements in her left upper and lower limb, reflected in the level of scores. Her trunk control is good, resulting in stability in static sitting and standing. Reaching for items and moving in these postures results in some instability. At this early stage, she walks for short distances with assistance and the use of a walking frame.

Lowenstein Occupational Therapy Cognitive Assessment (LOTCA)

The LOTCA is a basic cognitive assessment for evaluating clients with neurological dysfunction (Itzkovich *et al.*, 1990). It includes 20 subtests covering four areas: orientation, perception (including praxis), visuomotor organisation and thinking operations. It is a performance measure, requiring few verbal responses and takes approximately 45 minutes to complete. Results will clarify Sally's abilities and difficulties with cognitive–perceptual processing at an impairment level (ICF) and how these may influence her completion of occupations. This assessment is discriminatory and evaluative and two studies have confirmed its predictive qualities (Katz *et al.*, 2000; Zwecker *et al.*, 2002). Investigations have confirmed its validity and reliability. Cognition is essential for effective completion of occupations, so any deficits that Sally may have will influence her progress and inform selection of relevant therapy approaches. Katz *et al.* (2000) stress that the more complex visuomotor and thinking skills are significantly related to functional outcomes for individuals with cognitive problems and no neglect, reflecting Sally's situation.

The LOTCA is scored on a scale of 1–4 for 17 subtests and 1–5 for three subtests. A score of 1–2 is low, and 3–5 are high scores, indicating greater skill.

Results

▪ Orientation for time and place had maximum scores of 4 each.
▪ Perception for object identification and praxis both scored 4; shapes identification, overlapping figures, object constancy and spatial perception all scored 3.
▪ Visuomotor organisation resulted in five subtests scoring 3 each, two subtests scoring 2. Some constructional aspects presented challenges.
▪ Thinking operations has six subtests – Sally's scores ranged from 3–5. Sequencing was a problem.

It is anticipated that these difficulties will be more evident during the AMPS assessment, since Sally will be completing more complex domestic occupations.

Assessment of Motor and Process Skills (AMPS)

This is an observational, standardised assessment that enables the occupational therapist to measure Sally's ability to complete mostly domestic occupations (Fisher, 2003). It is discriminative and evaluative, assessing at the activity level. Sally completed three familiar occupations in context to score the assessment and identify the aspects that impede or support her function. The quality of Sally's performance is assessed by rating 16 motor and 20 process skills, reflecting her degree of effort, efficiency and safety. Motor skills include actions Sally did to move her body or objects used during an occupation, e.g. aligning her body to work surfaces in the kitchen or reaching for the tap. Process skills were evident as Sally organised herself, sequenced events or adapted what she did for successful completion (Robinson and Fisher, 1996).

Each skill receives a score of 4, 3, 2 or 1 (Fisher, 2003):

▪ 4 = competent, good outcome, no evidence of problem.
▪ 3 = questionable, uncertainty, possible problem.
▪ 2 = ineffective, undesirable use of time or amount of effort, potential for unsafe performance.
▪ 1 = markedly deficient, unacceptable use of time or amount of effort, task breakdown, imminent safety risk or need for assistance.

This assessment measures Sally's occupational performance and goal-directed behaviour (Fisher, 2003). Sally has difficulty completing occupations that are important to her, so this is a relevant assessment. It will not only outline her motor difficulties but provide essential information to clarify her processing difficulties and abilities. It will be used to evaluate changes in her abilities but does not aim to quantify the amount of assistance required. This contrasts effectively with another assessment used with Sally, the Functional Independence Measure (FIM), which does look at this issue. Congruent validity is demonstrated between AMPS and FIM (Robinson and Fisher, 1996). The reliability and validity of AMPS is very good and has been extensively studied (see Fisher, 2003 for a summary of studies).

Sally was observed completing:

▦ Upper body grooming/bathing.
▦ Hand washing dishes.
▦ Making a ham sandwich with pre-sliced meat.

These occupations were selected for level of difficulty at this early stage. Sally walks for short distances with a frame but is unsteady and needs some guidance.

The skills assessed are as follows, with the skills items assessed by observation listed for each skill:

▦ Motor skills:
  Posture: stabilises, aligns, positions.
  Mobility: walks, reaches, bends.
  Co-ordination: co-ordinates, manipulates, flows.
  Strength and effort: moves, transports, lifts, calibrates, grips.
  Energy: endures, paces.
▦ Process skills:
  Energy: paces, attends.
  Using knowledge: chooses, uses, handles, heeds, inquires.
  Temporal organisation: initiates, continues, sequences, terminates.
  Space and objects: searches/locates, gathers, organises, restores, navigates.
  Adaptation: notices/responds, accommodates, adjusts, benefits.

Scoring is very structured with detailed operationalising of skills terms to ensure consistency of scoring. Occupational therapists attend a 5-day training course to use AMPS accurately.

Results

Sally has scores of 2 on all the motor skills except flows, manipulates and coordinates, each scoring 1. In the process skills, Sally shows particular difficulty in space and objects and adaptation sections, with scores of mostly 2. In most other process skills, Sally scores 3 or 4. These process skills scores confirm the difficulties Sally displayed during the completion of the LOTCA and establish accurate assessment results. Explanations of these individual skills can be found in the American Occupational Therapy Association's Occupational Therapy Practice Framework (American Occupational Therapy Association, 2002). Park (2004) also provides a helpful overview of the application of this assessment.

Additional Assessments

The Rivermead Assessment of Somatosensory Performance (RASP) (Winward *et al.*, 2000) was used to investigate **somatosensory** function. Deficits in appreciation of sensory stimuli are known to influence outcomes, so it was important to ascertain any problems for Sally. Results confirmed no deficits.

Upon examination by the consultant at her admission, Sally was noted to have a **left hemianopia**, a visual field deficit. She does not fully see details in her left visual field, for which she will need to compensate by developing good scanning techniques. These will be encouraged by all members of the team to ensure she attends to everything in the environment, crucial for completing occupations.

It is important that Sally's mood is regularly evaluated. Low mood, depression and anxiety are significant consequences of stroke and have a detrimental effect on outcomes (Paolucci *et al.*, 1999; Rigler, 1999; King *et al.*, 2002; Turner-Stokes and Hassan, 2002).

Intervention plan

In this stage, decisions are made about how to structure the therapy sessions, the approaches to be used and to construct the anticipated outcomes. Stating the outcomes helps Sally to clarify her desired occupational performance. Clinical reasoning, understanding of relevant theory and knowledge of available evidence are required to justify the plan and subsequent therapy. The plan states overall aims and specific goals (Intercollegiate Stroke Working Party, 2004).

Aims and goals

The results of the assessments are discussed with Sally and Tom. More positive outcomes from therapy are achieved when the individual and carers value and own the plan, improving active collaboration within therapy (Foster, 2002; Randall and McEwen, 2000; Cohn *et al.*, 2003). The aims are statements of what Sally hopes to attain in the long term whilst the goals are more concise, positively written descriptions of specific outcomes to achieve during therapy.

Agreed aims are as follows:

- Sally will return home to live with Tom.
- Sally will cook and prepare a meal for herself and Tom.

To achieve these aims, goals were agreed, reflecting activity and participation (World Health Organization, 2001). They are meaningful and purposeful and positively influence Sally's quality of life.

Long-term goals

In 4 weeks, Sally will:

- Put on and fasten all her day clothes independently in 30 minutes.
- Prepare potatoes, carrots and cabbage for cooking in 45 minutes.
- Shower in 20 minutes, using an over-bath shower, transferring into standing from a bath board. Sally will hold a wall-mounted rail in her left hand to maintain stability and wash with her right hand, with Tom's assistance.
- Prepare a casserole with stock, meat and onion in 1 hour. Tom will put the casserole in the oven.

- Make a pot of tea and serve with milk in mugs, in 15 minutes. Sally will fill the kettle and gather all items required from containers, cupboard and fridge.
- Stabilise her standing embroidery frame with her left hand and stitch with her right hand for 30 minutes.
- Push a trolley around the supermarket for 30 minutes, using both hands, whilst Tom puts items into the trolley.

Short- to medium-term goals

In 2 weeks, Sally will:

- Walk to the bathroom (15 metres) using a stick in her right hand and carrying her toiletries bag in her left hand in 5 minutes, without support from the occupational therapist.
- Sit on a perching stool to wash and dry her face and upper body in 20 minutes using both hands. The occupational therapist will facilitate movements in her left arm. Sally will arrange her toiletries on the sink and shelf using her right hand.
- Stand in front of a mirror in the bathroom and put on her makeup (foundation, lipstick and blusher) in 20 minutes, holding the containers in her left hand, facilitated by the occupational therapist, and applying them with her right hand.
- Put on day clothes using both hands in 45 minutes, with the occupational therapist facilitating her left arm and assisting with buttons, hooks and zips.
- Reach out to open (and close) the fridge with her left hand and bend to select items with her right hand within 5 minutes. Items to be placed on the counter.
- Place 250 ml of water in the kettle using a jug held in her left hand after collecting water from the tap. Sally turns on the tap and switches on the kettle with her right hand; all within 5 minutes.

Model of practice and therapy approaches

To help Sally achieve these goals, restorative therapy approaches are utilised to provide techniques that the occupational therapist will use within therapy. A model of practice is selected to provide a framework to guide overall intervention and limit stereotyped routine therapy. The model of practice reflects the purpose of occupational therapy, integrates theory with practice and explains the complex relationships between concepts. These concepts are the influences on human function and include (Golledge, 2005b and c):

- Context, e.g. the environment, culture, society, political influences.
- Nature of the different occupations.
- Physical, psychosocial components.
- Motivation.
- The individual's personal characteristics.

Sally's skills, deficits, view of the future, her spirituality, understanding of her diagnosis and the occupations and roles she wishes to resume become apparent after the initial interview and the completion of assessments. These points have guided the selection of the Human Subsystems Influencing Occupation Model to provide an overall structure to the intervention with Sally.

Human Subsystems Influencing Occupation Model (HSIO)

The HSIO model has developed from occupational science, the study of the human as an occupational being (Clark *et al.*, 1991; Clark and Larson, 1993). This model uses holism and general systems theory to represent the individual as an open system, interacting with the environment and influenced by historical and socio-cultural contexts. Occupational behaviour is presented as emerging from the interaction of six subsystems arranged hierarchically, with **physical** as the lowest, rising to the **biological**, then **information processing**, **symbolic–evaluative** and, finally, **transcendental** (reflecting spirituality) as the highest subsystem. This model recognises that although occupations (the output) can appear simple and ordinary, they are infinitely complex. The subsystems reflect the influences on Sally's occupational behaviour and using the HSIO model will ensure that the occupational therapist attends to all of these in therapy, rather than becoming reductionist and focusing only on motor difficulties. Figs. 9.1, 9.2 and 9.3 provide an overview of Sally's occupational behaviour, organising the results of assessments and conversations and to guide future intervention.

Clinical reasoning was employed in the decision making for selection of therapy approaches. In discussion, Sally confirmed her wish to try to regain as much of her pre-stroke level of functioning as possible, so remedial/restorative therapy approaches were selected, rather than compensatory, to address her occupational difficulties. The following therapy approaches were selected by the team to meeting Sally's needs:

▨ The Bobath concept, to enhance motor control.
▨ The multicontext approach, to improve Sally's cognitive processing.

The client-centred approach will also influence the delivery of the programme.

Bobath concept

This therapy approach is *'a problem-solving approach to the assessment and treatment of individuals with disturbances of function, movement and postural control due to a lesion of the central nervous system'* (International Bobath Instructors Training Association, 2005, p. 1) and will be helpful for Sally's motor control difficulties. The occupational therapist will utilise facilitation techniques to help Sally actively participate in therapy. Reflecting the physical subsystem of HSIO, this approach requires the occupational therapist to analyse Sally's *'components of movement and underlying impairments'* (International Bobath Instructors Training Association,

Transcendental
▓ Sally previously had a good quality of life and felt in control.
▓ She had participated in a range of meaningful and purposeful occupations that made her feel good about herself, positive and optimistic.
▓ Taking care of her health and Tom's is important so their future years are happy and comfortable.
▓ Sally, Tom and family plan to go on a cruise next year, cementing family relationships – wants to recover from her stroke and is motivated to achieve this future goal. Has a strong drive to 'do'; she feels a sense of purpose.

Symbolic–evaluative
▓ Sally assigns considerable value to her roles of wife, mother, grandmother and the occupations that support these roles.
▓ She wants her family and friends to view her positively, anticipating their support. Emotionally, she feels a strong sense of commitment to her family and wants to do her best for them and herself.
▓ Sally realises her current skill level does not meet her needs but is determined to overcome her difficulties. She wants to be able to go to the theatre, musicals and dancing; they make her 'feel young', joyful, relaxed.

Sociocultural
▓ Sally has strong ideas about the occupations she wants to do that reflect her femininity and her views on maintaining her home.
▓ She feels responsible for doing housework, meeting family/friends' expectations.
▓ Sally is sociable, deriving pleasure from interacting with people and being part of social groups. Sally adopts a nurturing and supportive role and feels valued for this.

Information processing
▓ Sally has problems organising herself and objects to complete occupations.
▓ Difficulties with attention present challenges.
▓ Sally's left hemianopia impacts on her impaired temporal organisation and use of tools/equipment.
▓ Problem solving is OK but some adaptive responses (AMPS) are difficult.
▓ Sally's memory is good; she knows what she wants to be able to do and can make decisions.

Biological
▓ Sally is trying her best to cope, adapting to problems, eg. eating, toileting. She is determined to overcome her difficulties.
▓ Uses exploratory behaviour, increasing her familiarity with the stroke unit.
▓ Using senses collectively; tactile and vision to put clothes on, smell and taste to eat, vision and hearing to interact with others.

Physical
▓ Some muscles on her left side do not have effective eccentric and concentric action to support function. Hypotonia is evident but hypertonia may develop in some muscles in the next few weeks.
▓ Altered tone in hand muscles impedes grip in occupations.
▓ Altered neurotransmitter action in her CNS impacts on her function.
▓ Sally can see (but has a left hemianopia), hear and has intact sensory feedback on her affected and non-affected side.

Figure 9.1 Subsystems.

2005, p. 2) within the context of occupational performance. Although occupational therapists do not work at this impairment level (World Health Organization, 2001), an understanding of movements and influences on muscle tone post stroke is essential for using the Bobath concept. Knowledge of the musculoskeletal system

---

Historical
Sally has experience of completing all the occupations she wishes to do in her therapy, reflected in her goals. Consequently, she has a level of expertise and knowledge of the process and outcomes of her occupations.

Sociocultural
Sally is working with social groups, eg. staff, family, friends, who will support her endeavours to overcome her difficulties. Her husband wants to be actively involved in her therapy and for Sally to return home. The culture of the rehabilitation service is client centred, reflecting Sally's hopes and aspirations.

Environmental challenges
Distances, novelty, layout of rooms and stroke unit routine all present challenges. These will be structured to facilitate Sally's occupational behaviour, rather than impede it.

Figure 9.2 Contextual influences.

The output is Sally's participation in occupations that are meaningful and purposeful. These are facilitated by the occupational therapist, Tom, family, friends and other staff and by the interaction of the different subsystems in supporting her occupational behaviour.

Figure 9.3 Output.

and typical (normal) movements for people without CNS damage helps to ascertain when Sally is or is not using movement patterns that will help her to be more independent. The occupational therapist uses clinical reasoning whilst observing Sally completing occupations during assessment and later in therapy sessions, but therapy is not implemented at this component (impairment) level. Therapy should not focus on trying to facilitate specific movements at particular joints or use protracted periods of time to alter muscle tone when these are divorced from their implicit integration within occupations. Indeed, neuroplasticity research exploring the most effective methods for restoring motor control, stresses that therapy must be completed with 'activities' (occupations) that are meaningful and purposeful and relate to the individual's life situation (Heddings *et al.*, 2000; Johannsson, 2000; Nudo *et al.*, 2000; Bach-y-Rita, 2001; Fisher and Sullivan, 2001; Nudo *et al.*, 2001; Umphred *et al.*, 2001).

There is no evidence that the Bobath concept is superior to other therapy approaches but neither is there evidence that refutes its usefulness. Recent teaching on Bobath courses includes theory from neuroplasticity, motor control, current knowledge on causes of hypertonia beyond spasticity and some motor learning with the importance of task-orientated therapy (Brown, 2005). This reflects current theoretical guidance. Access to current Bobath methods is only available by attending courses, which is professionally questionable and a point for critique.

Multicontext therapy approach

This will be used to help Sally to overcome her cognitive–perceptual difficulties and address issues of generalisation. The ability to generalise and transfer learning is crucial for effective therapy but this is noted to be problematic for individuals post stroke (Neistadt, 1994; Katz, 1998; Cicerone *et al.*, 2000; Toglia, 2001 and 2003; Patel *et al.*, 2003). This approach is based on a dynamic interaction model of cognition analysing interaction between the individual, environment(s) and task(s), linking effectively with the HSIO model and the information processing subsystem.

Cognitive–perceptual difficulties are regarded as deficiencies in processing strategies, used daily to support function. Processing strategies are *'organised approaches, routines or tactics which operate to select and guide the processing of information'* (Toglia, 1998) and are grouped into four categories. Some examples are provided to aid clarification:

▓ Attention:
  React to gross change in environment.
  Initiate exploration of environment.
  Easily disengage focus of attention.
▓ Visual processing:
  Initiate active visual search.
  Detect and compare subtle visual details.
  Look at whole and divide into parts.
▓ Memory:
  Recognise overall context.
  Use rehearsal, visual imagery.
  Spontaneously use aids to assist recall.
▓ Problem solving:
  Recognise when information is incomplete; actively search for missing object.
  Formulate or initiate a plan.
  Spontaneously check progress.

Assessment confirmed that Sally has some attention deficits in shifting attention and mental tracking (Golisz and Toglia, 2003) and visual processing difficulties. Therapy alters the occupations and environments to improve Sally's ability to process, monitor and use information in all occupations and new situations. To promote this transfer of learning, the occupational therapist will ensure:

▓ Use of multiple environments for completing occupations.
▓ Task analysis to aid transfer of learning.
▓ Metacognitive and processing strategies are taught.
▓ Sally understands the relation of new information to knowledge and skills learnt in previous therapy sessions. Overt links will be made so that Sally understands the similarities of the underlying demands between occupations. Transfer of learning must be taught, not presumed to occur.

Metacognitive strategies will be taught throughout therapy, helping to rebuild Sally's sense of self, her understanding of her abilities and difficulties, through systematic feedback and self-monitoring techniques. Sally will learn how to evaluate her own performance. Metacognitive strategies include:

- **Anticipation**.
- Self-prediction.
- Self-checking.
- **Self-questioning**.
- Time monitoring.
- Role reversal.

The metacognitive and processing strategies in **bold** are used with Sally. Sally's self-questions, reflecting her difficulties in occupations, are:

- 'Is my walking stick safe?'
- 'Am I in the right position?'
- 'Am I getting sidetracked?'

Processing strategies are organised tactics or rules that are used consciously or unconsciously to guide behaviour. Some are useful in specific situations whilst others have more general applicability. They include:

- **Visual imagery prior to commencing occupations or prior to searching for items.**
- Rehearsal.
- Rearrangement of items.
- **Looking all over before starting occupations.**
- Pointing to help focus on details.
- Categorisation; grouping.
- **Use of self-instruction procedures.**

The responsibility for cueing the use of the strategies and structuring the occupations will gradually move from the therapist to Sally. This therapy approach capitalises on the compatible elements of remedial and adaptive theories. Sally will be assisted to recover as much of her prior function as possible, applying metacognitive and processing strategies within occupations. This individualised approach to therapy utilises clinical reasoning and reflective practice essential for dealing with cognitive–perceptual problems (Bergquist *et al.*, 1994; Katz and Hartman-Maeir, 1997; Hochstenbach and Mulder, 1999; Cicerone *et al.*, 2000; Toglia, 2003). Case studies are reported in the literature as this is not an approach that lends itself easily to randomised controlled trials to prove its efficacy (Blair and Robertson, 2005); it is, however, based on sound theoretical principles.

Implementation of therapy

The facilitation techniques within the Bobath concept (BC) and strategies in the multicontext approach (MA) are used in all sessions. Sally is assisted to participate in a range of meaningful and purposeful occupations reflecting her goals, guided by HSIO. To illustrate the application of therapy, an example session has been selected. Sally was able to complete this occupation prior to her stroke.

Collect juice from the fridge and pour into a beaker for drinking

Sally has previously been in the kitchen for other therapy sessions and the occupational therapist asks, 'Bearing in mind what happened yesterday when you got some juice, what do you think might be difficult today?' (anticipation, MA).

Sally recalls that she kept catching the fridge door against her left foot so she must remember to alter how she stands near to the fridge so this does not happen today. Before Sally goes to the kitchen, the occupational therapist asks Sally to imagine the sequence she will perform to complete the occupation, using visual imagery (MA), including visualising herself opening the fridge door smoothly, without catching her foot.

She is assisted to walk to the kitchen. The occupational therapist facilitates external rotation at Sally's left shoulder to assist extension patterns for walking (BC) whilst Sally uses a stick in her right hand to aid stability. At the entrance to the kitchen, Sally is directed to look all over (MA), locate the fridge and the floor cupboard where the beakers are stored. She is instructed to scan the whole environment, turning her head, to compensate for her hemianopia. The occupational therapist reminds Sally that she has used these strategies in other occupations in the kitchen and bathroom. Sally walks to the work surface over the cupboard and places her walking stick against the row of cupboards. The occupational therapist prompts Sally about her checking questions. Sally uses one of her self-questions (MA), 'Is my walking stick safe?' checks it and then places both hands on to the work surface. Sally is able weakly but actively to flex her left elbow and shoulder joint to do this unassisted. Sally uses another self question, 'Am I in the right place?' (MA) whilst looking at the cupboard. She then moves to the right slightly so she can open the cupboard. The occupational therapist uses her left hand over Sally's left hand to assist her to open the cupboard (Fig. 9.4), helping Sally to slide her fingers into the D handle. Using her right hand, the occupational therapist supports and facilitates movements (BC) at Sally's left shoulder joint, to help her open the door. Sally does as much as she can unaided.

Whilst Sally holds the door open, maintaining her grip, she selects a plastic beaker with her right hand from the top shelf. This requires flexing forward in her hips and trunk and then realigning body segments to stand up straight to place the beaker on the counter. Sally then moves around the work surface to the fridge, using her self-questions. This pattern is repeated with the fridge, which she opens smoothly, as she imagined (MC). 'I've put myself into a better position today.'

Sally places the juice carton on to the work surface close to the beaker. She stabilises the carton in her left hand; the grip is facilitated by the occupational therapist, reflecting normal patterns for a cylinder grip (Fig. 9.5). Sally opens the carton

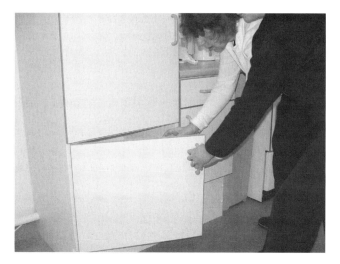

Figure 9.4 Opening the cupboard door.

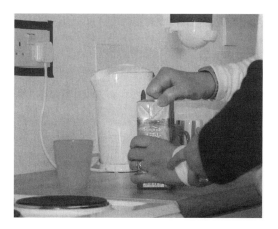

Figure 9.5 Opening juice carton.

with her right hand, then is assisted to release the carton from her left hand, using normal release patterns (BC), not just withdrawing her fingers. The occupational therapist then helps Sally to hold the beaker in her left hand, encouraging her to consciously think about maintaining her grip. Sally instructs herself (MA), 'Grip the beaker.' The beaker is light but has a firm surface, facilitating isometric muscle activity and an increase in tone. Sally has hypotonia in many left arm muscles at this stage, with resultant feelings of weakness. As Sally maintains her grip on the beaker, facilitated by the occupational therapist (Fig. 9.6), Sally pours juice with

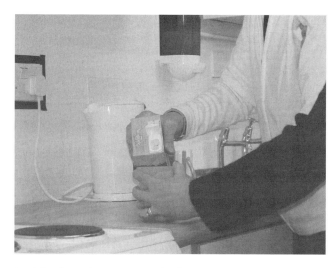

Figure 9.6 Pouring juice from the carton to a beaker.

her right hand. After putting the carton down, the occupational therapist then facilitates movements and grip in Sally's left arm and hand to enable her to drink the juice, using opportunities to put down and pick up the beaker numerous times (BC). This gives Sally practice in grasp and release patterns that she needs for many tasks. The occupational therapist asks Sally to think about the objects she gripped in the bathroom earlier that morning and when she was helped to tidy her locker the previous day (MA). Facilitation helps to overcome Sally's motor control difficulties and the structuring of the occupations makes relevant demands on her cognitive–perceptual processing.

Evaluation of therapy

Evaluation is used to appraise and monitor progress throughout intervention, and particularly at the end of the programme to plan for discharge. The outcomes of the intervention should be measured whilst acknowledging any constraints. Sally and her occupational therapist are interested in the therapy's effectiveness as recipient and professional respectively. Service managers and commissioners of services also concern themselves with outcomes to ensure appropriate use of resources (Pickering and Thompson, 2003).

Evaluation will be completed using a mix of formal and informal methods. Formally, all the assessments used with Sally will be scored again to measure outcome. Changes in scores will be noted to ascertain progress. In addition, during week 4, before Sally's discharge home, the Stroke Impact Scale (SIS) version 3.0 (Duncan *et al.*, 2002) will be used as an outcome measure to reflect activity and participation (World Health Organization, 2001). This is a comprehensive outcome measure investigating the multiple consequences of stroke, reflecting the perspectives of the individual, carers and health professionals (Finch *et al.*, 2002). It is a 59-item scale assessing eight domains:

- Strength.
- Hand function.
- Mobility.
- Activities of daily living.
- Emotion.
- Memory.
- Communication.
- Social participation.

Sally will be asked a series of questions for each of these domains and to rate her response to each question on a five-point scale. She will also be asked to rate her perception of her recovery on a visual analogue scale from 0 (no recovery) to 100 (full recovery). It is estimated to take 20 minutes. Validity and reliability studies continue to be completed, with some domains more sensitive than others; useful reviews may be found in Finch *et al.* (2002) and Salter *et al.* (2005). Sally has been referred to a community stroke service to continue her rehabilitation for 6 months where the SIS will be used to monitor change.

In addition to evaluating change in Sally's outcomes, the occupational therapist will evaluate her application of the therapy approaches, utilising reflective practice (Blair and Robertson, 2005). Evaluation will help the occupational therapist's future use of these interventions and how the experience she gained with Sally has informed her knowledge and expertise.

Reflections on the intervention

Numerous factors are apparent:

- The occupational therapist's skill and knowledge with the assessments and therapy approaches.
- The occupational therapist's clinical reasoning, knowledge of the evidence base and ability to use reflective practice to provide an individually tailored programme.
- The stroke unit environment. Hospitals are quite impoverished, unfamiliar settings that do not provide the most advantageous context for driving behaviour. An attempt to overcome this was completing some therapy sessions in Sally's home.

Challenges for the reader

- What alternative assessments could have been used to collect baseline data? What are their strengths and weaknesses?
- Which alternative restorative therapy approaches may have been selected? If Sally had stated her wish to adapt to her difficulties, which therapy approaches could be applied?
- How might the occupational therapist prioritise her work with individuals with stroke? Best results are achieved with regular therapy sessions, not 1 hour a day. Given that there are constraints on money, resources, available occupational therapists with expertise in stroke and limited numbers employed, how might this influence outcomes and areas for further research?
- How might occupational therapists act as advocates on behalf of people with stroke?

References

American Occupational Therapy Association (2002) Occupational Therapy Practice Framework: Domain and Process. *American Journal of Occupational Therapy*, **56**(6), 609–639

Appelros, P., Nydevik, I., Karlsson, G.M., Thorwalls, A. and Seiger, A. (2004) Recovery from unilateral neglect after right hemisphere stroke. *Disability and Rehabilitation*, **26**(8), 471–477

Bach-y-Rita, P. (2001) Theoretical and practical considerations in the restoration of function after stroke. *Topics in Stroke Rehabilitation*, **8**(3), 1–15

Bartels, M.N. (2004) Pathophysiology and medical management of stroke. In: *Stroke Rehabilitation. A Function-Based Approach*, 2nd edn. Ed. Gillen, G. and Burkhardt, A., pp. 1–30. Mosby, St. Louis

Bergquist, T.F., Boll, T.J., Corrigan, J.D., Harley, J.P., Malec, J. F., Millis, S.R. and Scmidt, M.F. (1994) Neuropsychological rehabilitation. Proceedings of a consensus conference. *Journal of Head Trauma Rehabilitation*, **9**(4), 50–61

Blair, S.E.E. and Robertson, L.J. (2005) Hard complexities – soft complexities: an exploration of philosophical positions related to evidence in occupational therapy. *British Journal of Occupational Therapy*, **68**(6), 269–276

Bowling, A. (2001) *Measuring Disease,* 2nd edn. Open University Press, Buckingham

Brown, A. (2005) *Fysioterapeuten.* Available from, www.fysio.dk (Accessed 4 October 2005) (English Translation)

Buxbaum, L.J., Ferraro, M.K., Veramonti, T., Farne, A., Whyte, J., Ladavas, E., Frassinetti, F. and Coslett, H.B. (2004) Hemispatial neglect: subtypes, neuroanatomy and disability. *Neurology*, **62**(5), 749–756

Carr, J.H. and Shepherd, R.B. (1998) *Neurological Rehabilitation. Optimising motor performance.* Butterworth Heinemann, Oxford

Carr, J.H. and Shepherd, R.B. (2003) *Stroke Rehabilitation. Guidelines for exercising and training to optimise motor skill.* Butterworth Heinemann for Elsevier Science, London

Cicerone, K.D., Dahlberg, C., Kalmar, K., Langenbahn, D.M., Malec, J.F., Bergquist, T.F., Felicetti, T., Giacino, J.T., Harley, J.P., Harrington, D.E., Herzog, J., Kneipp, S., Laatsh, L. and Morse, P.A. (2000) Evidence-based cognitive rehabilitation: recommendations for clinical practice. *Archives Physical Medical Rehabilitation*, **81**, 1596–1615

Clark, F. and Larson, E.A. (1993) Developing an academic discipline: the science of occupation. In: *Willard and Spackman's Occupational Therapy*, 8th edn. Ed. Hopkins H.L. and Smith H.D., pp. 44–57. J.B. Lippincott Company, Philadelphia

Clark, F., Parham, D., Carlson, M.E., Frank, G., Jackson, J., Pierce, D., Wolfe, R.J. and Zemke, R. (1991) Occupational science: academic innovation in the service of occupational therapy's future. *American Journal of Occupational Therapy*, **45(4)**, 300–310

Cochrane Database for Systematic Reviews: Stroke Group (2004) www.nelh.nhs.uk/cochrane.asp (Accessed 7 October 2005)

Cohn, E.S., Boyt Schell, B.A. and Neistatdt, M.E. (2003) Introduction to evaluation and interviewing. In: *Willard and Spackman's Occupational Therapy*, 10th edn. Ed. Crepeau, E.B., Cohn E.S. and Boyt Schell B.A., pp. 279–285. Lippincott Williams and Wilkins, Philadelphia

College of Occupational Therapists (2004) *Guidance on the use of The International Classification of Functioning, Disability and Handicap (ICF) and the Ottawa Charter for Health Promotion.* College of Occupational Therapists, London

Coull, A., Lovett, J. and Rothwell, P. on behalf of the Oxford Vascular Society (2004) Population based study of early risk of stroke after transient ischaemic attack or minor stroke: implications for public education and organisation of services. *British Medical Journal*, **328**, 326–328

Creek, J. (2003) *Occupational Therapy Defined as a Complex Intervention.* College of Occupational Therapists, London

Department of Health (1996) *Burdens of Disease. A discussion document.* National Health Service Executive, London

Department of Health (2001a) *NHS Plan: a Plan for Investment. A plan for reform.* Department of Health, London

Department of Health (2001b) *National Service Framework for Older People.* Department of Health, London

Dreissen, M.J., Dekker, J. and Van der Zee, J. (1997) Occupational therapy for patients with chronic disease. *Disability and Rehabilitation*, **19**, 198–204

Dromerick, A.W., Edwards, D.F. and Diringer, M.N. (2003) Sensitivity to changes in disability after stroke: a comparison of four scales useful in clinical trials. *Journal of Rehabilitation Research and Development*, **40(1)**, 1–8

Duncan, P.W., Wallace, D., Studenski, S., Lai, S.M. and Johnson, D. (2002) *Stroke Impact Scale Version, 3.0.* Available from, www2.kumc.edu/coa and wwwl.va.gov/rorc/stroke_impact.cfm. (Accessed 24 August 2005)

Finch, E., Brooks, D., Statford, P.W. and Mayo, N.E. (2002) *Physical Rehabilitation Outcome Measures*, 2nd edn. Canadian Physiotherapy Association, Hamilton

Fisher, A. (2003) *Assessment of Motor and Process Skills (AMPS)*, 4th edn. Three Star Press, Fort Collins

Fisher, B.E. and Sullivan, K.J. (2001) Activity dependent factors affecting post stroke functional outcomes. *Topics in Stroke Rehabilitation*, **8(3)**, 31–44

Foley, N.C., Teasell, R.W., Bhogal, S.K., Doherty, T. and Speechley, M.R. (2003) The efficacy of stroke rehabilitation: a qualitative review. *Topics in Stroke Rehabilitation*, **10(2)**, 1–18

Foster, M. (2002) Skills for practice. In: *Occupational Therapy and Physical Dysfunction*, 5th edn. Ed. Turner, A., Foster M. and Johnson S.E., pp. 85–105. Churchill Livingstone, Edinburgh

Gillen, R., Tennen, H. and McKee, T. (2005) Unilateral spatial neglect: relation to rehabilitation outcomes with right hemisphere stroke. *Archives of Physical and Medical Rehabilitation*, **86**, 763–767

Golisz, K.M. and Toglia, J.P. (2003) Perception and cognition. In: *Willard and Spackman's Occupational Therapy*, 10th edn. Ed. Crepeau, E.B., Cohn E.S. and Boyt Schell B.A., pp. 395–416. Lippincott Williams and Wilkins, Philadelphia

Golledge, J. (2004) Therapeutic occupation following stroke. In: *Occupation for Occupational Therapists*. Ed. Molineux, M., pp. 155–168. Blackwell Science, Oxford

Golledge, J. (2005a) Occupational therapy for cognitive–perceptual problems after stroke. *Therapy Weekly*, January 6, 9–12

Golledge, J. (2005b) Models of practice and therapy approaches in occupational therapy. *Therapy Weekly*, October 6, 13–16

Golledge, J. (2005c) Occupational therapy intervention approaches. *Therapy Weekly*, October 13, 11–14

Guide for Uniform Data Set for Medical Rehabilitation (1997) *Adult Functional Independence Measure (Adult FIM) Version 4.0.* Centre for Functional Assessment Research and Uniform Data System for Medical Rehabilitation, Buffalo

Hamilton, B.B., Laughlin, J.A., Fiedler, R.C. and Granger, C.V. (1994) Interrater reliability of the 7-level functional independence measure. *Scandinavian Journal of Rehabilitation Medicine*, **26(3)**, 115–119

Heddings, A.A., Friel, K.M., Plautz, S.B. and Nudo, R.J. (2000) Factors contributing to motor impairment and recovery after stroke. *Neurorehabilitation and Neural Repair*, **14(4)**, 301–310

Henry, A.D. (2003) The interview process in occupational therapy. In: *Willard and Spackman's Occupational Therapy*, 10th edn. Ed. Crepeau, E.B., Cohn E.S. and Boyt Schell B.A., pp. 285–297. Lippincott Williams and Wilkins, Philadelphia

Hochstenbach, J. and Mulder, T. (1999) Neuropsychology and the relearning of motor skills following stroke. *International Journal of Rehabilitation Research*, **22**, 11–19

Hsueh, I.P., Lin, J.H., Jeng, J.S. and Hsieh, C.L. (2002) Comparison of the psychometric characteristics of the functional independence measure, 5 item Barthel index, and 10 item Barthel index in patients with stroke. *Journal of Neurology Neurosurgery and Psychiatry*, **73**, 188–190

Intercollegiate Stroke Working Party (2000 and 2004) *National Clinical Guidelines for Stroke.* Royal College of Physicians, London, www.rcplondon.ac.uk

International Bobath Instructors Training Association (IBITA) (2005) *Theoretical Assumptions – Bobath Concept.* Available from www.ibita,org (Accessed 4 October 2005)

Itzkovich, M., Averbuch, S., Elazar, B. and Katz, N. (1990) *LOTCA Battery,* 1st edn. Maddack Inc, Pequannock

Johannsson, B.B. (2000) Brain plasticity and stroke rehabilitation. *Stroke*, **31(1)**, 223–230

Jutai, J.W. and Teasell, R.W. (2003) The necessity and limitations of evidence-based practice in stroke rehabilitation. *Topics in Stroke Rehabilitation*, **10(1)**, 71–78

Katz, N. (1998) *Cognition and Occupation in Rehabilitation. Cognitive Models for Intervention in Occupational Therapy.* American Occupational Therapy Association, Bethesda

Katz, N. and Hartman-Maeir, A. (1997) Occupational performance and metacognition. *Canadian Journal of Occupational Therapy*, **64**, 53–62

Katz, N., Hartman-Maeir, A., Ring, H. and Soroker, N. (2000) Relationship of cognitive performance and daily function of clients following right hemisphere stroke: predictive and ecological validity of the LOTCA Battery. *Occupational Therapy Journal of Research*, **20**(1), 3–17

King, R.B., Shade-Zeldow, Y., Carlson, C.E., Feldman, J.L. and Philip, M. (2002) Adaptation to stroke: a longitudinal study of depressive symptoms, physical health and coping process. *Topics in Stroke Rehabilitation*, **9**(1), 46–66

Lance, J.W. (1980) Synposium synopsis. In: *Spasticity: Disordered Motor Control.* Ed. Feldman R.G. and Young R.R., pp. 485–494. Year Book Medical Publishers, Chicago

Luke, C., Dodd, K.J. and Brock, K. (2004) Outcomes of the Bobath concept on upper limb recovery following stroke. *Clinical Rehabilitation*, **18**(8), 888–898

Lundgren-Nilsson, A., Grimby, G., Ring, H., Tesio, L., Lawton, G., Slade, A., Penta, M., Tripolski, M., Biering-Sorensen, F., Carter, J., Marincek, C., Phillips, S., Simone, A. and Tennant, A. (2005) Cross-cultural validity of functional independence measure items in stroke: a study using ranch analysis. *Journal of Rehabilitation Medicine*, **37**(1), 23–31

Lutz, B.J. (2004) Determinants of discharge destination for stroke patients. *Rehabilitation Nursing*, **29**(5), 154–163

Mant, J., Wade, D. and Winner, S. (2004) Health care needs assessment: stroke. In: *Health Care Needs Assessment: Epidemiologically Based Needs Assessment Reviews.* Ed. Stevens, A., Rafferty, J., Mant, J. and Simpson, S., pp. 141–243. Radcliffe Medical Press, Oxford

Mattingly, C. and Fleming, M.H. (1994) *Clinical Reasoning. Forms of Enquiry in a Therapeutic Practice.* F.A. Davis Company, Philadelphia

Mayo, N.E., Wood-Dauphinee, S., Cote, R., Durcan, L. and Carlton, J. (2002) Activity, participation and quality of life 6 months post stroke. *Archives of Physical and Medical Rehabilitation*, **83**, 1035–1042

Neistadt, M.E. (1994) Perceptual retraining for adults with diffuse brain injury. *American Journal of Occupational Therapy*, **48**(3), 225–233

Nudo, R.J., Barbay, S. and Kleim, J.A. (2000) Role of neuroplasticity in functional recovery after stroke. In: *Neuroplasticity and Reorganisation of Function after Brain Injury.* Ed. Levin, H. and Grafman, H., pp. 168–196. Oxford University Press, New York

Nudo, R.J., Plautz, E.J. and Frost, S.B. (2001) Role of adaptive plasticity in recovery of function after damage to motor cortex. *Muscle and Nerve*, **24**, 1000–1019

O'Dwyer, N.J., Ada, L. and Neilson, P.D. (1996) Spasticity and muscle contracture following stroke. *Brain*, **119**, 1737–1749

Paolucci, S., Antonucci, G. and Gialloreti, L.E. (1996) Predicting stroke inpatient rehabilitation outcome: the prominent role of neuropsychological disorders. *European Neurology*, **36**, 385–390

Paolucci, S., Antonucci, G., Pratesi, L., Trabellesi, M., Grasso, A. and Lubich, S. (1999) Post stroke depression and its role in rehabilitation of stroke patients. *Archives of Physical and Medical Rehabilitation*, **80**(9), 985–990

Park, S. (2004) Enhancing engagement in instrumental activities of daily living. In: *Stroke Rehabilitation. A Function-Based Approach,* 2nd edn. Ed. Gillen, G. and Burkhardt, A., pp. 447–482. Mosby, St. Louis

Patel, M., Coshall, C., Rudd, A.G. and Wolfe, C.D.A. (2003) Natural history of cognitive impairment after stroke and factors associated with its recovery. *Clinical Rehabilitation,* **17**, 158–166

Pickering, S. and Thompson, J. (2003) *Clinical Governance and Best Value. Meeting the Modernisation Agenda.* Churchill Livingstone, Edinburgh

Randall, K.E. and McEwen, I.R. (2000) Writing patient centred functional goals. *Physical Therapy,* **80**(12), 1197–1203

Rigler, S.K. (1999) Management of poststroke depression in older people. *Stroke,* **15**(4), 765–783

Robinson, S.E. and Fisher, A.G. (1996) A study to examine the relationship of the Assessment of Motor and Process Skills (AMPS) to other tests of cognition and function. *British Journal of Occupational Therapy,* **59**(6), 260–263

Salter, K., Jutai, J.W., Teasell, R., Foley, N.C., Bitensky, J. and Bayley, M. (2005) Issues for selection of outcome measures in stroke rehabilitation: ICF participation. *Disability and Rehabilitation,* **27**(9), 507–528

Sangha, H., Lipson, D., Foley, N., Salter, K., Bhogal, S., Pohani, G. and Teasell, R.W. (2005) A comparison of the Barthel index and the Functional Independence Measure as outcome measures in stroke rehabilitation: patterns of disability scale usage in clinical trials. *International Journal of Rehabilitation Research,* **28**(2), 135–139

Selzer, M.E. (2000) Neural plasticity and repair in rehabilitation. *Neurorehabilitation and Neural Repair,* **14**(4), 245–249

Sheean, G. (1998) Clinical features of spasticity and the upper motor neurone syndrome. In: *Spasticity Rehabilitation.* Ed. Sheean, G., pp. 7–15. Churchill Communications Europe Ltd, London

Stephen, A. and Rafferty, J. (1994) *Health Care Needs Assessment,* Volume 1. Radcliffe Medical Press, Oxford

Stephens, S., Kenny, R.A., Rowan, E., Kalaria, R.N., Bradbury, M., Pearce, R., Wesnes, K. and Ballard, C.G. (2005) Association between mild vascular cognitive impairment and impaired activities of daily living in older stroke survivors without dementia. *Journal of the American Geriatrics Society,* **53**(1), 103–107

Steultjens, E.M.J., Dekker, J., Bouter, L.M., van de Ness, J.C.M., Cup, E.H.C. and van den Ende, C.H.M. (2003) Occupational therapy for stroke patients. a systematic review. *Stroke,* **34**, 676–686

Stroke Association (2004) www.stroke.org.uk/media_centre/facts_and figures/index.html (Accessed 18 August 2005)

Tatemichi, T.K., Desmond, D.W., Stern, Y., Paik, M., Sano, M. and Babiella, E. (1994) Cognitive impairment after stroke: frequency, patterns, relationship to functional abilities. *Journal of Neurology, Neurosurgery, and Psychiatry,* **57**, 202–207

Teasell, R.W., Foley, N.C., Bhogal, S.K. and Speechley, M.R. (2003) An evidence-based review of stroke rehabilitation. *Topics in Stroke Rehabilitation,* **10**(1), 29–58

Timbeck, R. J. and Spaulding, S.J. (2004) Ability of the Functional Independence Measure-super (TM) to predict rehabilitation outcomes after stroke: a review of the literature. *Physical and Occupational Therapy in Geriatrics,* **22**(1), 63–76

Toglia, J.P. (1998) A dynamic interaction model to cognitive rehabilitation. In: *Cognition and Occupation in Rehabilitation*. Ed. Katz, N., pp. 5–50. American Occupational Therapy Association, Bethesda

Toglia, J.P. (2001) Generalisation of treatment: a multicontext approach to cognitive perceptual impairments in adults with brain injury. *American Journal of Occupational Therapy*, **45**(6), 505–515

Toglia, J.P. (2003) Multicontext treatment approach. In: *Willard and Spackman's Occupational Therapy*, 10th edn. Ed. Crepeau, E.B., Cohn E.S. and Boyt Schell B.A., pp. 264–267. Lippincott Williams and Wilkins, Philadelphia

Turner-Stokes, L. and Hassan, N. (2002) Depression after stroke: a review of the evidence base to inform the development of an integrated care pathway. Part 1: diagnosis, frequency and impact. *Clinical Rehabilitation*, **16**, 248–260

Umphred, D.A., Byl, N., Lazaro, R.T. and Roller, M. (2001) Interventions for neurological disabilities. In: *Neurological Rehabilitation*, 4th edn. Ed. Umphred, D.A., pp. 56–133. Mosby, St. Louis

Unsworth, C.A. and Cunningham, D.T. (2002) Examining the evidence base for occupational therapy with clients following stroke. *British Journal of Occupational Therapy*, **65**(1), 21–29

Wilson, B.A., Cockburn, J. and Halligan, P. (1987) *Behavioural Inattention Test (BIT)*. Thames Valley Test Company, Bury St. Edmunds

Winward, C.E., Halligan, P.W. and Wade, D.T. (2000) *Rivermead Assessment of Somatosensory Performance (RASP)*. Thames Valley Test Company, Bury St. Edmunds

Wolfe, C., Rudd, A. and Beech, R. (eds) (1996) *Stroke Services and Research. An Overview with Recommendations for Future Research.* Stroke Association, London

Wolfe, C.D.A., Rudd, A.G., Howard, R., Cashall, C., Stewart, J., Lawrence, E., Hajat, C. and Hillen, T. (2002) Incidence and case fatality of stroke subtypes in a multi ethnic population: the South London Stroke Register. *Journal of Neurology, Neurosurgery and Psychiatry*, **72**, 211–216

World Health Organization (2001) *International Classification of Functioning, Disability and Handicap (ICF)*. World Health Organization, Geneva

Zinn, S., Dudley, T.K., Bosworth, H.B., Hoenig, H.M., Duncan, P.W. and Horner, R.D. (2004) The effects of poststroke cognitive impairment on rehabilitation process and functional outcome. *Archives of Physical and Medical Rehabilitation*, **85**, 1084–1090

Zwecker, M., Levenkrohn, S., Fleisig, Y., Zeilig, G. and Ohry, A. (2002) Mini-mental State Examination, Cognitive FIM Instrument and the Lowenstein Occupational Therapy Cognitive Assessment: relation to functional outcome of stroke. *Archives of Physical and Medical Rehabilitation*, **83**, 342–345

10: A reflective challenge

Alex Clark

Introduction

The chapters in this text have explored the principles and practices underpinning occupational therapy intervention in relation to a spectrum of clinical conditions. The importance of evidence-based practice has been highlighted throughout, as have the philosophical paradigms, government policy agenda and professional practices (reflective practice) which shape intervention. Ideal principles have been argued to be fundamental to everyday practice so that all clients are offered the most appropriate and effective intervention. This final chapter will aim to contextualise and develop some of the generic themes and issues which were present in previous chapters. Philosophical, ethical and professional issues which arise when therapists aim to embody best practice in their everyday working lives will be explored. Intrinsic to such discussions is the belief that the tensions, conflicts and ambiguities inherent in translating abstract conceptual ideas into practice are not barriers or excuses for failing to aim for the best, but rather provide opportunities to reflect on and enhance personal practice. Such an approach is based upon the belief that the role of a modern day health and social care professional is not merely one of technical confidence, but also one of ability to engage in reflection and work with a degree of tension and uncertainty.

The concept of need

The relationship between the demand for health care and the ability to meet it, relates to the concept of need. Previous chapters have intrinsically defined need in relation to a variety of assessment tools. Such tools reflect the authors' ideas and perceptions as to how need is defined and measured. Assessment tools typically define need in relation to a variety of proxy indicators which reflect the extent to which an individual is in need; for example, aspects of daily living or the ability and ease with which functional tasks can be undertaken. Need within this context is therefore the gap between an individual's ability (to perform a task), compared with an average person's ability to undertake a functional task. Need is therefore a comparative deficient.

Historically, need has been defined as being clearly definable and measurable, or objective, universally applicable (based upon features of everyday life shared by everyone) and reflected in scientific technical procedures. This reflects the traditional medical model approach to need which occupational therapists have been striving to move away from; the idea that need is clinically based, rooted in biological structures, and is measurable and responsive to predefined clinical intervention. The NHS was, and to some extent still is, based upon the above assumptions. Such an approach also reflects the assumption that there are 'objective' and 'subjective' needs (Blakemore, 1998); objective needs are assumed to be historically and culturally universal and comprise of the meeting of basic needs that ensure one stays alive (food, basic health care and shelter). Subjective needs are above such basic needs and comprise those individual, cultural and economic needs relative to a particular point in time (Langan, 1999). It could be argued, however, that the division between objective and subjective needs is purely arbitrary and artificial (Hugman, 1999).

Recently the concept of need has become a more contested and debated entity (Endacott, 1997; Whitehead, 2000). This in part reflects issues related to the ability of the NHS to deploy resources to meet needs; it also reflects the transition to a post-modern society, in which human needs are perceived as being less fixed, certain and universal, as ideas relating to universal truth and certainty give way to a more fluid, diverse and questioning culture (Annandale, 1998). In the last 20 years, human need within welfare has been explored and discussed with less certainty and clarity than in previous decades (Doyal and Gough, 1991). The question as to who defines need is implicit within this change in emphasis; certainty placed in doctors previously determined as the 'experts' has been questioned and challenged (Scambler, 2003). The ability to define need reflects the status, authority and power of the individual(s) who are in the position to put forward collectively shared notions as to what need is, how it can be measured or assessed and how it can be met.

Bradshaw's (1972) typology of human need, although dated, provides a useful framework for exploring the different ways needs can be constructed. He argues that there are four ways need can be defined:

- **Felt need** is located within the individual requiring intervention, such as that of the young man who had suffered a series of fractures in Chapter 3.
- **Expressed need** reflects the individual's ability and willingness to articulate a need, such as that described by the woman with the diagnosis of multiple sclerosis in Chapter 4.
- **Normative need** is where an individual's need is judged is relation to professional/expert judgement or standard, such as the gentleman who underwent a total hip replacement in Chapter 7.
- **Comparative need** is where the needs of an individual are judged relative to the needs of other individuals, such as the child referred to in Chapter 2.

Whilst many assessment tools used by occupational therapists are based upon a normative approach (defined by tools which reflect expert classification), expressed needs are, to some extent, reflected in tools which include clients' views and those such as the Canadian Occupational Performance Measure (COPM) (Law *et al.*, 1990), which reflects a person-centred approach to practice. In reality, practice frequently adopts a comparative approach, with the needs and demands of a particular client being either formally or informally classified in relation to other clients. During the 1990s the classification of need within health and social care became more closely linked to the availability of resources (Langan, 1999). This reflected a judgment made in the High Court in 1995 that social services were only legally obliged to meet the needs of clients 'where resources permitted'. In essence, the availability or lack of financial resources became fundamental to the decision as to whether needs were defined as being 'appropriate' or 'legitimate'. Need is also a reflection of the organisational culture which a professional works for; the NHS, for example, tends to work to a much more rigid biomedical model of assessment and meeting of need, compared with social services, which adopts a more socially orientated focus to intervention.

When the NHS came into existence on 5 July 1948 there was an assumption that it could meet all clinical need. There was an assumption that there was a *'fixed quantity of illness'* (Timmins, 1995). Therefore, it was rather naively assumed that expenditure or need would decline as the impact of the newly created NHS became readily available. In fact the volume of clinical need and therefore expenditure grew and continues to grow in both absolute and relative terms. The NHS is *'a victim of its own success'* (Klein, 2001) because of the following factors:

- Life expectancy has grown because of the impact of the health service (and other factors), and so the proportion of older people has grown. Approximately 50% of the NHS budget is spent on the over 65s. Therefore in clinical terms the more people who are kept alive for longer, the more clinical need (particularly associated with old age) there will be.
- People's expectations in relation to health intervention continually rise, as what the NHS developed yesterday is commonly assumed to be readily available today. In other words there is a continual expectation that the health service can do more and more in relation to clinical need.
- The development of new medical procedures, treatments and prescriptions is relatively expensive; tremendous financial resources are spent on testing and refining such potential interventions, many of which are never fully developed and licensed. Therefore while the boundaries of clinical need are continually expanding, the relative costs of those procedures and interventions are extremely high.
- There is a range of social changes, such as the number of single parents, the stresses associated with modern living and individuals' greater awareness of health issues, which have all meant that many people turn to doctors and other health care professionals more readily (Scambler, 2003).

The notion of 'need' is, therefore, highly relative and expansive. In fact it has been argued that, in relation to health care, need is potentially infinite, with the resources (financial, time, infrastructural) available to meet need being finite.

Decisions regarding who would benefit from services were historically carried out by individual clinicians in a rather ad hoc and covert way, which lacked both accountability and consistency (Malin *et al.*, 2002). In many cases waiting lists were used to cope with the difference between the volume of clinical need and the ability of the NHS to meet it at any one time (Dunford and Richards, 2003). In theory a philosophy was adopted of 'Yes, you can have intervention for clinical need to be met, but you will have to wait for it'. In reality, waiting lists are crude in relation to the depth or urgency of an individual's clinical need, there are geographically large variations in terms of how long individuals have to wait, and a significant proportion of people died before they reached the top of a waiting list (Baggott, 2004).

With the development of the internal market in the 1980s, the issue of prioritising became more openly discussed and even used in relation to the setting of clinical objectives, particularly at the local level (Malin *et al.*, 2002). The words 'prioritising' and 'rationing' are often used interchangeably, although being distinct in relation to emphasis; 'prioritising' is frequently perceived to be more positive and about focusing on those in most need, whilst 'rationing' is seen as being negative and about denial of access to clinical procedures and services. In reality, one could argue that in fact the words mean exactly the same thing. However, Malin *et al.* (2002) suggest that 'prioritising' is about macro (group) decisions, whereas 'rationing' is micro, or to do with individual decisions.

The assumption that it is ethically advantageous to be explicit and open about rationing decisions, with a possible input from the general public, must mean that there is attention to the principles and procedures which underpin such decisions. There is a diverse range of possibilities, according to New and Le Grand (1997), which is outlined as follows:

- The 'rescue' principle of giving priority to those in greatest clinical need, or those whose condition is potentially most life threatening. The question as to who decides or labels an individual as being in such a category is interesting, as is the ultimate risk that the NHS ceases to be a health service, and only intervenes when there is an imminent threat to life. This criterion is used in social care where social services departments assess those most 'at risk' and give them priority in terms of intervention.
- Prioritising those patients to whom intervention might prove to be most effective, or treatments which have been proved to be most clinically effective. This approach has been translated by health economists into a statistical model known as 'QALYs' (Quality Adjusted Life Years). Basically, priority is given in relation to health expenditure which is the most clinically effective and would potentially benefit the greatest number of people. There are of course several ethical questions as to whether individuals should be denied treatment on relatively underdeveloped evidence surrounding clinical effectiveness, or because evidence relating to clinical effectiveness is hard, if not impossible, to formulate. There would also be obvious implications for older people whose capability to

benefit from interventions is compromised because they have fewer years left to live. This approach is based upon 'utility' or the 'ability to benefit' from intervention.

■ Age, until relatively recently (Department of Health, 2001b), was used as a cut-off marker whereby individuals were denied access to a whole range of medical interventions. This was not only based upon the ability to benefit clinically, but also a rather crude philosophy of 'you've had your chance', with the assumption that the young should have 'first bite' at the resource cake of the NHS! It could be argued that using age as a criterion for prioritising/rationing clinical service is not only discriminatory, but is a whole subjective and ambiguous process; on what basis is a certain numerical age decided, by whom and on what evidence? Age discrimination has recently been made illegal and has also been placed as the first standard in the National Service Framework for Older People (Department of Health, 2001b).

■ Criteria relating to individual behaviour have been argued to be a moral, legitimate basis for refusing individuals access to treatment. Those who have smoked, drink too much or are overweight could be argued to have ethically compromised their right to health care. Additionally such behaviours frequently have a clinical impact on the effectiveness of treatment, making it potentially less valuable. A distinction has to be made, however, between refusing treatment because past behaviour has had a direct impact of the person's chances of a successful clinical outcome, and refusing treatment because one is morally penalising an individual for contributing to their clinical condition. The issue of who decides what behaviours should attract such penalties and how conscious an individual needs to have been that a certain behaviour or habit was potentially harmful are very much open to debate.

■ Finally one could ration the 'menu' of health care procedures available to everyone. New Zealand adopted this approach in the 1990s where the government defined a 'core' package of interventions which were available to all free at the point of need (Cumming, 1994). Outside this package one had to either go private or go without. The most obvious problem with this approach is the question of to whom and on what basis inclusion in a 'core' package would be defined.

It is interesting that all of the above approaches assume that all individuals with a similar clinical condition benefit exactly the same from the same intervention. Evidence would suggest that this is not always the case (Scambler, 2003). In other words, just as in the case of 'need', there is an assumption that 'benefit' from intervention is clear, objective and measurable.

The introduction of care pathways, such as those described in Chapters 3 and 7, involves this assumption that clients with similar needs will benefit from packages of care specific to a given procedure, providing given timeframes for recovery and discharge. These were established to support the implementation of clinical guidelines and protocols. However they were also established to support clinical management, clinical and non-clinical resource management, clinical audit and financial management, which seems at variance with the concept of need and person-centred practice.

There are obviously fundamental implications for professional practice given the imbalance between clinical need and the ability of the NHS to meet it; morally one could argue from a Kantian point of view that honesty and telling clients the truth should be one's primary ethical duty. Whilst the founding principles of a health service being available to all and free at the point of need are highly commendable, they could be argued to be simplistic in a modern world of growing demands and expectations. Being upfront, even engaging in some sort of public debate about how the meeting of health needs is prioritised could be argued to be ethically appropriate and even socially inclusive. A consequentialist philosophical approach would demand that one should look at the consequences of one's actions in determining if it is ethically defensible; in other words, will the outcome of a decision or act do more good than harm? Therefore, in relation to making decisions about prioritising/rationing resources, a Kantian approach would examine the motives which were behind a decision, while a consequentialist would focus on the impact or result of a decision.

Challenge to the reader

Within this text you have considered a range of clinical conditions, with a rationale and strategy to support occupational therapy intervention. Each chapter has applied this material in relation to a specific individual. Suppose you are an occupational therapy service manager who is responsible for a team which accepts generic referrals from a range of acute hospital and community specialities. You have a gifted, able and highly motivated team. However, most of them are off work with a debilitating virus. You and a Senior II are left to run the department for the rest of the week and receive eight referrals reflected in the case studies outlined in previous chapters. Allocate a priority to each; rank them in order of urgency. Reflect on the issues, values and practical considerations which guide your decision-making. To what extent does policy, particularly the notion of evidence-based practice, inform the decisions and choices which you make?

Professional practice and the service user

The notion of intervention by human services based upon the objective of meeting need is located within a unique relationship: that between a professional and a service user. The fact that the service user typically has a need which the professional meets, makes the relationship complex and yet potentially very revealing, as will be explored later. The concept of power will be discussed in relation to professional–user relations, which will allow some of the issues which have been previously highlighted with reference to the concept of need to be developed. This conceptual discussion will then be used to evaluate the current policy agenda which aims to promote an inclusive and active role for the service user in relation to the processes which underpin service delivery. The notion of the professional, however, needs to be understood before the relationship with individuals who use human services can really be understood.

The notion of a selected range of employees or workers being categorised as a 'profession' has a long established and historical background (Hugman, 1991). A professional emerged out of the idea that selected workers have most if not all of the following characteristics:

- Their prime motivation was to serve others (the client) not self-interest.
- They behaved in ways which corresponded to an ethical code of conduct which was collectively maintained.
- The work they carried out was based upon specialised knowledge and skills.
- A professional group would be organised into a professional body which would control admission to the profession and ensure members maintained technical standards and behaved ethically once they gained entry into the group.

This approach to the notion of professionalisation reflects a consensus perspective of social relations; or, to put it another way, that 'experts' are a specialised group who hold selective abilities, behaving in ways which are morally commendable and virtuous. In contrast, social theorists such as Zola (1972) and Illich (1977) suggest that professional groupings merely reflect a process of social closure, whereby a group of workers organise themselves collectively into a monopoly which is based on covert self-interest; privilege in relation to skills, practices, freedoms and financial rewards are therefore defined and pro-tected. The relationship between the state and professional groups reflects both mutuality and conflict historically, sometimes with both being present at the same time! When the NHS was set up in the 1940s the medical profession were able to gain compromises in relation to professional autonomy and involvement in man-aging the service, which the government originally had refused to allow. In fact the Minster of Health at the time, when asked how much he had compromised with the British Medical Association (BMA) stated that he had 'stuffed their mouths full of gold' (Ham, 1999). The state has also been active in developing the remit of the medical profession, which is now crucial in many aspects of how individuals deal with the state of their daily lives: access to social security, time off work and life insurance. However, Conrad (2005) argues that the powerful role of the medical professional is subordinate to the commanding influence of biotechnol-ogy (especially the pharmaceutical industry), service user and managed care, these being driven more by commercial and market interests than the state itself.

Professional power is frequently talked and written about, but not always ana-lysed or understood. Power might seemly appear to be a relatively simple concept, if one accepts that the definition of power as the:

possibility of being able to carry out one's will in the pursuit of a goal of action, regardless of resistance (Hugman, 1991).

In other words, power is reflected in the ability to get one's own way or, as Westwood (2002) suggests, the capability of an agent (or individual) to influence a particular outcome. This, however, is a relatively simple perception of what power is: that it is visible, tangible and that one individual has power and others do not (Lukes, 1976). Tew (2002) argues that in reality power is very much more ambiguous, complex and abstract. In essence, power is covert and intrinsic to social interactions (Westwood, 2002). This reflects the writings of Foucault (1972), who argues that power is not a thing or a commodity but rather an imbedded aspect of everyday life located in discourse (language, shared meaning and values). Gramsci (1977) argues that power is the ability of one group in society to impose a *'world view'* in which ideas and perceptions are presented as natural, universal and historically constant.

Lukes (1976) places power within the context of health and social care. He suggests that there are three kinds or levels of power exercised by professionals:

▨ Power as in the ability to impose one's will so as to achieve a particular goal or intended outcome.
▨ Power to control the agenda.
▨ Power to control the behaviours, expectations and perceptions of individuals in a particular social situation.

The above three levels might be illustrated within the context of professional–client interactions. The first level would be reflected in the ability of the professional directly to control the client's behaviour. In the second level the professional would control the agenda: what issues/questions were addressed, what objectives were set, etc. At the third level the client would comply not merely with what the professional wanted, but also do so in ways which reflected the belief that the professional's expertise meant that they had to comply with and respect the authority of the professional. This is latent power. Thompson (2002) claims that professionals tend to be more powerful than service users because they typically:

▨ Control or influence the allocation of resources.
▨ Have knowledge, expertise and a monopoly of skills.
▨ Engage in a professional discourse which helps to legitimise what they do.
▨ Frequently can exercise statutory powers.
▨ Hold a high rank in relation to hierarchical power.

Professional discourse relates not merely to the language which professionals use when they are communicating with service users, but the values, attitudes and norms which underpin it. Although the technical nature of language used by professionals can be and is disempowering to service users, it is not the technical nature of wording per se which produces a power imbalance, but the context in which language is used. Language reflects values, stereotypes and stigmatises individuals; the way clients are diagnosed or labelled, for example, frequently constructs a sense of vulnerability, lack of social worth and powerlessness associated with particular clinical conditions (Addy and Dixon, 1996; Tew, 2002).

Language is part of the processes whereby individual difference is 'essentialised' or constructed as fixed, innate and beyond the control of the person.

Such a discussion risks highlighting individual professionals within human services as being completely dominant and socially marginalising clients. Simplistically, such an approach understands human behaviour solely in terms of 'agency' or the behaviour of individuals (the professional and service user). However, if one were to accept the concept of power as conceptual rather than the property of selected individuals, the processes and structures which underpin professional working are actually understood to be the causes of what might be termed the categorisation of some individuals as being socially different, inferior and vulnerable, rather than individual intent on the part of professionals. In other words, the organisational cultures, working practices, education and professional practices, which individual health care professionals work within, produce a discourse in which service users are marginalised and singled out as being different.

Professionals' obligation to work to a code of ethics reflects an ethos of service to others, motivated and guided by moral principles (Seedhouse, 1998). Collective self-policing ensures that all members of a professional group uphold ethical principles. However, one needs to reflect on the very notion of morals and ethics; Hugman (1991) comments that professional codes of ethics tend to be based on a Kantian approach to ethical behaviour (the belief that the underlying motives of an action are what is intrinsically important). In contrast, a consequentialist approach would suggest that the ethical worth of an action can be judged in terms of its outcome, not its underlying motives. Consequentialists would also argue that the moral worth of an action needs to be judged in terms of its impact on the majority of people affected by the act, as it is impossible to isolate the impact of an act simply in terms of one individual. One could also be critical of the ideal nature of codes of ethics; certainly, until relatively recently, little attention was paid to practical considerations, such as availability of resources, time or the diverse nature of human existence. Codes of ethics therefore could be argued to reflect a modernistic scientific–technical approach to life, where all human behaviour was 'rational' and predictable. In contrast, post-modern theory would suggest that human existence is highly fluid and relative. Therefore a simple code of ethics to guide professional behaviour at best misses the point, at worst compounds the imbalance of power between clients and professionals.

What is needed, therefore, is not merely to develop and update new codes of ethics, but to cultivate the ability of professionals to engage in constant ethical reflection. Thompson (2002) argues that a modern-day professional needs to be able to reflect on what is ethical in each and every situation, not merely follow a prescribed written code. Therefore, acting ethically is a way of thinking and reflecting in every situation on the part of each professional. Hugman (1999) argues that this should be considered to be the defining characteristic of a professional in contemporary society, with it separating them from social organisations, which are becoming more and more technically driven, and bureaucratic and legalistic in character.

The service user

Historically the relationship of the NHS to the medical model and a strongly centralised and bureaucratic organisational culture rendered little, if any, scope for active service user involvement (Ham, 1999). The 'patient' was encouraged to be grateful for and compliant with the intervention offered. This rather paternalistic model of health care contrasted with the historically relatively small private health care sector in the UK, which was perceived to be much more responsive to the wishes, needs and circumstances of the individual service user (North and Bradshaw, 1997). The first attempt to include service users in decision making was in 1976 with the introduction of community health councils (CHCs); these were independent bodies which gave a user input into the NHS at a local level. However, the role of CHCs was relatively tokenistic and their inclusion in decision making was merely advisory, as they had no statutory powers. When the Labour Party was elected to government in 1997 they introduced legislation which gave users of the NHS a real input into decision making at both a local and national level, with new statutory procedures which ensured multilayered redress procedures when 'patients' were not happy with the service they received. The document *Shifting the Balance of Power: The Next Steps* (Department of Health, 2002) claims that there will be a revolutionary change to ensure service users are not only placed at the centre of decision making, but that their views, aspirations and expectations will ensure a more responsive, effective and efficient service. A document published a year later stated that the objective of creating *'a culture of involvement, listening and feedback, was not merely radical in concept, but radical in reality'* (Department of Health, 2003, p. 2).

Service users' involvement will now be reflected in the inclusion of a 'patient representative' on the boards of primary care trusts (PCTs) and acute trusts; and in the review processes which underpin NICE and the Health Service Commission. Trusts will also have to undertake annual user evaluation in relation to the clinical areas they provide and service users' opinions of service will form part of the criteria for measuring quality. 'Patient advocate and liaison service' in PCTs and acute trusts will provide users with advice and ultimately support service users through complaint procedures; these are now formally organised both within each trust and externally through a Health Service Commissioner, who will act as the service users' national guardian. Together these changes are designed to make the NHS more responsive to the needs, wishes and preferences of the service user.

Further attempts have been made to shift the focus of power in favour of the service user by the introduction to the 'expert patient programme' referred to in Chapter 4. This programme was developed for those living with a long-term condition to *'take control'* of their illness. The premise was clear; that *'people who have the confidence, skills, information and knowledge would be able to play a central role in the management of life with chronic disease'* (Department of Health, 2001a). Interestingly only 21% of doctors were in favour of this programme (Association of the

British Pharmaceutical Industry, 1999), as there were fears of service users emerging from the programme with a *'sheaf of printouts from the internet, demanding a particular treatment that is unproved, manifestly unsuitable, astronomically expensive, or all three'* (Shaw, 2004).

The fact that this programme refers to the *expert patient* rather than service user is also interesting, as once again this infers a power position placing those who need help subject to those who are in a position to offer it. The grammatical term 'patient' refers to an entity upon whom an action is carried out. For example, in the sentence 'Jack kicked the ball', 'the ball' is the patient. Applied in a health context, *'the patient is the participant of a situation upon whom an action is carried out'* (Wickipedia on-line, 2006). In literal terms the word patient comes from the Latin verb 'patior' meaning to 'suffer', both in the sense of pain and forbearance (Medicinenet.com, accessed 2006); both of these definitions hardly denote a term which promotes a shift in power from service user to provider.

The notion of user involvement is more complex than merely providing individuals with the opportunity to express their views or concerns. Braye and Preston-Shoot (1995) point out the distinction between giving users the right to 'exist' (to choose one service instead of another) and 'voice', whereby they can express their view after receiving a service, in comparison to users having a sense of participation in the planning and delivery of services. There is an argument that 'voice' and 'exist' are merely a form of window-dressing, as users typically lack the time, motivation and knowledge to impact on service providers. Giving service users a participatory role actually ensures that they contribute to the processes and systems which shape service provision. One has to also bear in mind the distinction between the service user (individually) and service users (collectively). One has also got to give careful consideration to service users who do not have the experience, confidence or intellectual capability to participate in such processes.

There is sometimes an assumption that simply giving service users the forum and opportunity to contribute their views, experiences and opinions is sufficient to realise meaningful participation. However this is somewhat naïve; service users frequently lack the confidence, skills, knowledge and motivation that are intrinsic to enable meaningful involvement (Bray and Preston-Shoot, 1995). Giarchi (1998) terms the phrase 'information deprivation' to reflect the lack of knowledge many individuals hold in relation to public service provision. The concept of 'cultural capital' reflects the lack of skills and confidence which many social groups experience in relation to articulating aspirations and expectations. Being in need of human services means that individuals are also vulnerable, concerned and physically or psychologically weak. This could be argued to make it even more difficult for active participation to take place. Therefore empowering service users is not merely presenting them with an opportunity, but rather a process which provides them with the insights, experiences and skills over a period of time which enables individuals to realise and use such opportunities.

Modern professional–user relations

The notion of being a 'professional' and a 'service user' has been significantly challenged over the last two decades as alluded to above. The professional's role has been challenged, critiqued and opposed by the development of a post-modern era, in which absolute truth and authority have been rejected and public confidence in professionals somewhat displaced. The incorporation of market principles into welfare provision has, to some extent, allowed (some) service users to exercise a degree of choice and to articulate concerns and complaints. The question as to the long-term impact of such changes has already been debated; suggestions include the notion that professionals are a dying entity, with service users gradually acquiring the role of active consumer, to the idea that the role of the professional will be transformed to that of a source of technical expertise who will advise and empower the service user (Jones *et al.*, 1998). Professional practice, power relations and ethics will, however, certainly become more fluid, less certain and more open to scrutiny.

Challenge to the reader

Select any of the case studies from one of the previous chapters. Thinking about your potential role as a health and social care professional take some time to think through the Government's recently stated objective of promoting a greater sense of user involvement, with individual clients being given the opportunity to not merely give feedback, but to exercise choice and some degree of control. Reflect upon the following questions:

▪ How might your sense of authority and expertise as a professional help to shape the relationship you develop with the client?
▪ To what extent do you think the client might be willing and able to make demands and exercise choice?
▪ What ethical and practical issues might potentially impact on the choices and opportunities you might be able to allow the client to realise?

Disability and the caring professionals

Disability is frequently linked to the notions of normality and difference (Saraga, 1998). There is also a belief that the category 'disabled' is somehow fixed, universal and innate. Because such difference is linked to the biological, a process of essentialism takes place whereby it could and will be argued that social–cultural aspects of difference assume powerful positions because they are constructed around the biological (Corker and Shakespeare, 2002). Therefore intervention by professionals would not only be seen to be appropriate, but inevitable and legitimate (Drake, 1999). The disabled person is constructed as being needy, vulnerable and helpless rather than being socially marginalised and excluded. Such arguments provide a useful and highly appropriate focus when exploring the intervention of occupational therapists seeking to meet human need. This focus is particularly interesting as the professional has come under criticism by a number of disabled writers who have accused it of being disempowering and disabling (Apperby, 1995; Finklestein, 1999). There is a need to understand the nature of the argument posed by members of the disability movement, even if one does not fully accept them, so as to reflect critically on our clinical practice.

Disability is not a natural category of difference but a product of modernity, or modern industrial society (Barnes *et al.*, 1999). Industrialisation, with the development of formalised, standardised and bureaucratic working practices, marginalised people with certain impairments. It is important to recognise that impairment, or biological faults and limitations are common to all humanity and not confined to a small proportion of the population (Priestley, 2001). With industrialisation came the development of a scientific, 'rational' approach to life, and, more particularly, the development of medical science. The body and the person became separated as medical intervention developed an ethos of objectivity and authority in relation to involvement; health intervention became equated with biological repair and restoration. Such an approach constructed normality around the myth of biological purity and perfection, with intervention being capable of assessing and treating any deviation from this norm, in theory at least. Together, the dependency created by economic capitalism and classification and intervention by modern medicine created the illocution of a clearly definable group (the 'disabled') with needs that could only be met by scientific and 'objective' intervention. The categories of 'impairment' and 'disability' became interlinked, seemingly fixed, universal and clearly definable.

Intervention within the context of scientific and objective modernity was all about making the disabled individual 'fit' as well as possible into mainstream society; the rehabilitation model of intervention was based upon the need to restore a degree of normality, to the greatest extent possible (Priestley, 2001). The notion of 'special' became equated with difference, inferiority and need. The role of the professional within scientific medicine took on the authority, power and social status experienced by priests in pre-industrial, pre-modern society (Drake, 1999). The relationship between special provision and difference has been debated; whilst the theory of special or additional help is to empower or enable, it has been argued that, in reality, such provision actually highlights and compounds hierarchical difference (Drake, 1999).

The social model of disability developed from groups of disabled people who formed in the US and Britain in the 1970s and 1980s who challenged the traditional ethos and philosophy of health and social care intervention. Alongside this movement, a number of disabled academics developed a theoretical model which underpinned the approach adopted by disabled activists. Central to the social model of disability was the argument that disability was socially/culturally contracted rather than being the product of biological impairment. Oliver (quoted in Barnes *et al.*, 1999) suggests that disability is a product of:

The disadvantage or restriction caused by contemporary social organisation which takes little or no account of the needs of people with impairments and this excludes them from mainstream social activities.

Disability is, therefore, the product of the social processes which ignore, reject, marginalise and exclude people with impairments. Marks (1999) remarks that *'impairment only becomes disabling because of social structures and organisations'*. The social model of disability adopts a position shared by the women's and race equality movements, by arguing that society's unwillingness to incorporate needs and aspirations into everyday life results in second class citizenship.

The social model and the activists in the disability movement were particularly articulate and critical about the relationship between disability and medicine. In essence it was argued that the link of biological impairment with disability rendered disabled people powerless, vulnerable and requiring expert help. Not only were disabled people to be treated, modified and equipped to be as 'normal' as possible, but they were to be paternally 'looked after' and even controlled! Disability was constructed as a personal tragedy which was reflected in individual helplessness and dependency (Marks, 1999). Albrecht (1992) articulates a thesis based on the notion of 'The Disability Business', whereby it is argued a range of health and social care professionals have a vested interest in disabled peoples' dependency and need; basically it creates jobs for them. It is also provides meaning, status and authority to those who join the ranks of the professions. Intrinsic to this argument is the inherent power imbalance within the professional–disabled person relationship; the power to control disabled peoples' bodies, their access to a whole range of social opportunities (work, housing, social security) and, of course, to engage in processes whereby certain individuals are labelled as being different, needy and helpless (Marks, 1999). It has been argued that the notion of 'independence' and 'dependency' is a myth (Barnes *et al.*, 1999). In reality we are all *inter-dependent* in modern society, reliant on complex food chains, highly developed transportation systems and technology-based communication. Therefore, one has to answer the question as to why a selected and arbitrary collection of human abilities are used to define the notion of 'independence'? The labelling of disabled people as 'being in need' is about selected cultural values and norms, not about innate ability.

The notion of care

The notion of providing 'care' is similarly located within cultural norms and customs. 'Care' is inherently about being needy or being looked after. Care in relation to disability (and old age) could be argued to be not only about being in need, but having needs which are directly located within the body of the individual within which the person/identity/status is located in western culture (Marks, 1999). Such caring is, therefore, highly personal or intimate, being reflected in notions of social worth, identity and powerlessness. Such cultural norms and values also mean that the person providing the care is particularly well placed to assume power, authority and expertise – particularly when it is linked to techno-logical procedures or knowledge bases. With the emergence of risk as a criterion for eligibility to social care, there is again an equation of human need meaning that one is vulnerable and powerless, unable to look after oneself (Kemshall, 2002). The distinction between 'caring for' and 'caring about' is crucial in this context: 'caring for' is about doing (physical tasks), whereas 'caring about' is about ensur-ing individuals have the opportunities, support systems and resources to realise their ambitions and aspirations. Morris (1993) suggests that professionals confuse the concepts of 'independence' and 'autonomy'; whilst the former equates to per-forming physical tasks, the later is about having a sense of control and exercising choice. In other words, Morris is arguing that it should be possible to have control over how one's care needs are met, without actually carrying out the tasks oneself.

Exercising autonomy in relation to receiving care has been discussed both within the disability field and the wider context of health and social care for several decades. The typical consumerist model is based on empowerment through direct payment. The availability of direct payments to clients of social services under the Community Care (Direct Payments) Act 1995 modified this model, where clients were awarded a care budget by their local social service department from which they could put together their own package of care. Evidence to date, however, suggests the managers and professionals are highly selective in terms of which clients and what situations are deemed to be 'appropriate' to offer a particular client access to direct payments (Priestley, 2001). The disability move-ment was instrumental in setting up collective organisations run by and for dis-abled people, who planned and ran their own care infrastructure. The independent living movement has developed across Britain and in many instances has secured public funding. Members are educated, supported and empowered in both access-ing their own need and in putting together a care package. Whilst one could argue that such organisations are limited in membership to the relatively vocal, articu-late and educated minority, the principles behind them should provide some interesting ideas; Jones *et al.* (1998) suggest that occupational therapists could act as a resource, or facilitate clients to develop a sense of control and autonomy over their lives. Perhaps disabled clients could be equipped with knowledge, gradually encouraged to gain insight and experience and provided with the opportunities which enable them to gain a sense of control of the ways in which their needs are met (Priestley, 2001). One could even argue that such a process should develop so that clients can define their own needs more fully, as well as how they are met.

Challenge to the reader

Reflecting on the distinction between 'doing' and 'facilitating', select two or three case studies used in the previous chapters. To what extent is it important to enable the client through assessment and the provision of equipment and services, com-pared with the argument that what is really important is to develop a sense of autonomy and participation in clients' lives? To what extent are clients' needs a product of biological impairment or a disabling society?

Need, difference and client-centred professional practice

This chapter has explored a number of themes and issues which could be argued to be fundamental to being client-centred: to think critically about what we mean by 'need', thinking about the notion of user involvement or participation and by viewing the client as having a potential sense of autonomy and control and not merely being in need and dependent. And yet there are practical constraints (time, resources etc), potential ethical issues relating to acceptable risk and informed consent and professional issues relating to accountability and working on the basis of available evidence and organisational culture. Issues relating to the empowerment of clients in terms of defining, assessing and meeting need, with them exercising a sense of control and choice and of realising personal autonomy despite physical dependency and vulnerability place great demands on professionals working within contexts already characterised by tensions, conflicts and pressures (Malin *et al.*, 2002). How can the reality of an approach which incorporates diversity in relation to human need, is grounded in the expectations and aspirations of individual clients and enables individuals to realise a sense of control and autonomy, be developed?

Neil Thompson's (2002) highly readable text on anti-oppressive practice in health and social care explores the tensions produced by trying to promote change whilst faced by practical, ethical and personal constraints. He argues with a considerable degree of conviction that there is a process of professional change, rather than simply a predefined set of guidelines or ingredients. Intrinsic to such a process is the ability of professionals to engage in a process of constant curiosity or reflection; not to accept every clinical situation at face value, but continually to question the values, beliefs and motivations which underpin professional intervention. There is also a sensitivity to the historical forces which have typically disempowered clients; not merely in relation to knowledge, terminology and time factors, but also the relative powerlessness and dependency which is constructed around being a client in health and social care. Language (Tew, 2002) is perceived to be an important element in professional–user relations, not merely in terms of each party's ability to communicate, but in terms of how norms, values and stereotypes are constructed. Inherent to such an approach would be the ability not only to engage with clients, but also to work with a sense of uncertainty and with a 'blank piece of paper' rather than with clearly defined strategies and goals.

In relation to the themes and issues developed in this chapter, therefore, professionals would not simply accept needs in relation to predefined technical assessment tools, but would also engage with clients so as to facilitate an appreciation as to how the perceptions, aspirations and values of each and every individual relate to the concept of need. One can also reflect on the values which underpin how the health and social care system and individual professionals tend to prioritise one particular need in relation to other needs; the issues of the availability of resources, assessment of risk and the impact of statutory regulation need to be appreciated and reflected upon. The section of this chapter devoted to disability invited readers to explore the nature of the independent/dependency dualism, the impact of professional intervention and the potential for individuals to realise a sense of autonomy. Again, such issues could potentially provide the basis of a new approach to practice based upon reflection and analysis, in which practitioners constantly question what they are doing and seeking to achieve.

In many respects this chapter is distinct from previous chapters; it does not provide clearly defined and articulated suggested models to intervention, or give prescriptive steps which underpin clinical processes. Some of my fellow authors may feel a sense of unease about this. However, the aim of the chapter is to encourage reflection and thought – not instead of evidence-based formulated intervention, but as complementary to it. Remember that science itself is a product of individual curiosity and questioning – the idea that the world was flat, or was the centre of the universe, had to be challenged. Ideas in relation to disability were also displaced by science in modernity – disability was once believed to be the result of a mother's intercourse with the devil. Therefore to critique, challenge and question scientific ideas is intrinsically not 'unscientific', one could even argue that it is a part of scientific reasoning. Questioning, reflection and analysis may not be allied to personal security and comfort, but they will ultimately allow a professional to develop practice which is pitched to ensuring that clients' individual needs are met in ways which realise a sense of autonomy and worth. Perhaps it is a case of evidence to all (including clients) and not the few!

References

Addy, L.M. and Dixon, G. (1996) To label or not to label that is the question. *British Journal of Therapy and Rehabilitation*, **6(8)**, 394–397

Abberby, P. (1995) Disabling ideology in health and social care: the case of occupational therapy. *Disability and Society*, **10**, 221–231

Albrecht, G. (1992) *The Disability Business: Rehabilitation in America*. Sage, London

Annandale, E. (1998) *The Sociology of Health and Illness: A Critical Introduction*. Polity, Cambridge

Archeson, D. (1998) *Report of Independent Inquiry into Inequalities in Health*. Department of Health, London

Association of the British Pharmaceutical Industry (1999) *The Expert Patient – Survey*. ABPI, London. www.abpi.org.uk/publications/publication_details/expert_patient/survey.asp

Baggott, R. (2004) *Health and Health Care in Britain*. Palgrave Macmillan, London

Barnes, C., Mercer, G. and Shakespeare, T. (1999) *Exploring Disability; a Sociological Introduction*. Polity, Cambridge

Blakemore, K. (1998) *Social Policy: an Introduction*. Open University Press, Buckingham

Bradshaw, J. (1972) The concept of human need. *New Society*, **30**, 640–643

Braye, S. and Preston-Shoot, M. (1995) *Empowering Practice in Social Care*. Open University Press, Buckingham

Conrad, P. (2005) The shifting engines of medicalization. *Journal of Health and Social Behavior*, **46(1)**, 3–14

Corker, M. and Shakespeare, T. (2002) *Disability/Postmodernity: Embodying Disability Theory*. Continuum, London

Cumming, J. (1994) Core services and priority-setting: the New Zealand experience. *Health Policy*, **29**, 41–60

Department of Health (2001a) *The Expert Patient: a New Approach to Chronic Disease Management in the 21st Century*. Stationery Office, London

Department of Health (2001b) *National Service Framework for Older People*. Stationery Office, London

Department of Health (2002) *Shifting the Balance of Power: The Next Steps*. Stationery Office, London

Department of Health (2003) *The NHS Improvement Plan: Putting People at the Heart of Public Services*. Stationery Office, London. Cm 626.8

Doyal, L. and Gough, I. (1991) *A Theory of Human Need*. Macmillan, Basingstoke

Drake, R. (1999) *Understanding Disability Politics*. Macmillan, Basingstoke

Dunford, C. and Richards, S. (2003) *'Doubly Disadvantaged' Report of a Survey on Waiting Lists and Waiting Times for Occupational Therapy Services for Children with Developmental Coordination Disorder*. COT, London

Endacott, R. (1997) Clarifying the concept of need: a comparison of two approaches to concept analysis. *Journal of Advanced Nursing*, **25(3)**, 471–476

Finklestein, V. (1999) *Professions Allied to Medicine*. Unpublished paper

Foucault, M. (1972) *The Archaeology of Knowledge*. Tavistock, London

Giarchi, G. (1998) *Information Deprivation*. Citizens Advice Bureau, Devon

Glennester, H. (1995) *British Social Policy since 1945*. Blackwell, Oxford

Gramsci, A. (1977) *Selected Writings From the Prison Notebook*. Lawrence and Wishcart, London

Ham, C. (1999) *Health Policy in Britain: the Politics and Organisation of the National Health Service*. Palgrave, Basingstoke

Hartley, M. (1998) *The Social Context of Health*. Open University Press, Buckingham

Hugman, R. (1991) *Power in the Caring Professions*. Macmillan, London

Hugman, R. (1999) *Social Welfare and Social Values*. Macmillan, Basingstoke

Illich, I. (1977) *Limits to Medicine. Medical Nemesis: the Exploration of Health*. Penguin, Harmondsworth

Jones, D., Blair, S.E.E., Hartery, T. and Jones, R.K. (1998) *Sociology and Occupational Therapy: an integrated approach*. Churchill Livingstone, Edinburgh

Kemshall, H. (2002) *Risk, Social Policy and Welfare*. Open University Press, Buckingham

Klein, R. (2001) *The Politics of the New NHS*. Prentice Hall, London

Langan, M. (1999) *Welfare: Needs, Rights and Risks*. Routledge, London

Law, M., Baptiste, S., McColl, M., Opzoomer, A., Polatajko, H. and Pollock, N. (1990) The Canadian occupational performance measure: an outcome measure for occupational therapy. *Canadian Journal of Occupational Therapy*, **57(2)**, 82–87

Lukes, S. (1976) *Power*. Basil Blackwell, Oxford

Malin, N., Wilmot, S. and Manthorpe, J. (2002) *Key Concepts and Debates in Health and Social Policy*. Open University Press, Buckingham

Marks, D. (1999) *Disability: Contoversial Debates and Psychosocial Perspectives*. Routledge, London

Medicinenet.com definition of term 'patient' (accessed 11 January 2006)

Morris, J. (1993) *Independent Lives: Community Care and Disabled People*. Macmillan, Basingstoke

New, B. and Le Grand, J. (1997) *Rationing in the N.H.S.* King's Fund, London

North, N. and Bradshaw, Y. (1997) *Perspectives in Health Care*. Macmillan, Basingstoke

Oakley, A. (1981) *Subject Women*. Martin Robertson, Oxford

Priestley, M. (2001) *Disability and the Life Course: Global Perspectives*. Cambridge University Press, Cambridge

Randall, W. (1998) *Market and Health Care: A Comparative Analysis*. Longman, London

Saraga, E. (1998) *Embodying the Social: Construction of Difference*. Routledge, London

Scambler, G. (2003) *Sociology as Applied to Medicine*. Saunders, London

Shaw, J. (2004) Expert Patient – dream or nightmare. *British Medical Journal*, **328**, 723–724

Seedhouse, D. (1998) *Ethics: the Heart of Healthcare*. Wiley, London

Tew, J. (2002) *Social Theory, Power and Practice*. Palgrave Macmillan, Basingstoke

Thompson, N. (2002) *Theory and Practice in Human Services*. Open University Press, Maidenhead

Timmins, N. (1995) *The Five Giants: A Biography of the Welfare State*. Harper-Collins, London

Tudor-Hart, J. (1971) The Inverse Care Law. *The Lancet*, **27**, 405–412

Westwood, S. (2002) *Power and the Social*. Routledge, London

Whitehead, M. (2000) *The Concepts and Principles of Equity in Health*. World Health Organization, Copenhagen

en.wikipedia.org/wiki/Patient (grammar) definition of term 'patient' (accessed 11 January 2006)

Zola, I.K. (1972) Medicine as an institution of social control. *Sociological Review*, **20**, 487–504

Index